Gay, Lesbian, Bisexual & Transgender Aging

Gay, Lesbian, Bisexual & Transgender Aging

Challenges in Research, Practice, and Policy

Edited by

TARYNN M. WITTEN, PH.D., L.C.S.W., F.G.S.A.

Associate Professor
Center for the Study of Biological Complexity
Virginia Commonwealth University
Richmond, Virginia

and

A. EVAN EYLER, M.D., M.P.H.

Associate Professor of Family Medicine and Psychiatry
University of Vermont College of Medicine / Fletcher Allen Health Care
Burlington, Vermont

The Johns Hopkins University Press
Baltimore

© 2012 The Johns Hopkins University Press
All rights reserved. Published 2012
Printed in the United States of America on acid-free paper
2 4 6 8 9 7 5 3 1

The Johns Hopkins University Press
2715 North Charles Street
Baltimore, Maryland 21218-4363
www.press.jhu.edu

Library of Congress Cataloging-in-Publication Data

Gay, lesbian, bisexual, and transgender aging : challenges in research,
practice, and policy / edited by Tarynn M. Witten and A. Evan Eyler.
    p. ; cm.
Includes bibliographical references and index.
ISBN-13: 978-1-4214-0319-9 (hardcover : alk. paper)
ISBN-10: 1-4214-0319-6 (hardcover : alk. paper)
ISBN-13: 978-1-4214-0320-5 (pbk. : alk. paper)
ISBN-10: 1-4214-0320-X (pbk. : alk. paper)
1. Older gays—Care.   2. Older sexual minorities—Care.   3. Older
people—Abuse of—Prevention.   4. Preventive health services for older
people.   I. Witten, Tarynn.   II. Eyler, A. Evan.
[DNLM: 1. Aging.   2. Homosexuality.   3. Bisexuality.   4. Elder
Abuse—prevention & control.   5. Health Services for the Aged.
6. Social Stigma. WT 30]
RA564.9.H65G39 2011
362.1086'6—dc22   2011009997

A catalog record for this book is available from the British Library.

*Special discounts are available for bulk purchases of this book. For more
information, please contact Special Sales at 410-516-6936 or
specialsales@press.jhu.edu.*

The Johns Hopkins University Press uses environmentally friendly book
materials, including recycled text paper that is composed of at least
30 percent post-consumer waste, whenever possible.

To my children, Willow, Misty, and Amber, who are the best of my works;
and to my mother and father, who gave me so many gifts; and to Lynda.

TARYNN MADYSYN WITTEN

To my grandparents, three of whom were teachers; my mother, who
was my first teacher; my father, a wonderful teacher from whom I have
learned a great many things about medicine and about life; and to John.

A. EVAN EYLER

And to all of those individuals who have provided so much of
the information for the research cited in this book,
without whom we would have nothing about which to speak.

ALL THE FACES OF AGING

Aging claims its place.
Make room.
It does not ask
What is the gender of my pain?
What is the sex of my sadness?
What is the sexuality of my loneliness?
See me for what I am.
For I am all the faces of aging.
—TARYNN M. WITTEN

Contents

Preface

The idea for this book arose quite a number of years ago, when we realized that no integrative text addressed the unique problems of lesbian, gay, bisexual, and transgender aging, and that the concerns of intersex-identified older adults had not been addressed. To be sure, there were books that contained a chapter on some small subset of problems of LGBT aging. In the interim, a few books have appeared (Clunis, Fredricksen-Goldsen, Freeman, & Nystrom, 2005; Herdt & DeVries, 2004; Hunter, 2005; Kimmel, Rose, & David, 2006). However, this important area of study deserves ongoing, integrated, and comprehensive coverage, with attention to the details of what is known and what remains to be learned.

This book is written for students and professionals in gerontology, medicine, social work, psychology, nursing, public health, health care administration, and related fields who wish to learn more about the life experiences and concerns of sexuality and gender-minority-identified elderly persons, in order to effectively serve their patients, clients, and service consumers. Material is drawn from a wide cross section of available research literature, which is unfortunately scant in many important content areas. Questions are sometimes proposed and ideas extrapolated from the general gerontologic and geriatric literatures, from professional practice, from discussions with our colleagues, and from survey response data.

Chapter 1 offers basic demographic information regarding sexual and gender minority persons in the United States and worldwide. Specific data are lacking in many respects, so Tarynn M. Witten has extrapolated from existing census data and population estimates regarding LGBT persons. Information regarding gender identity and gender variance in a variety of indigenous cultural groups is also provided.

Many people might ask why LGBT aging should be any different from aging in any other population. In chapter 2, Karen I. Fredriksen-Goldsen discusses caregiving from the perspective of sexual minority persons. Using that as a single topic area, she examines the commonalities and differences associated with caregiving in the LGBT population versus other populations. Most older persons who are either married or partnered will attempt to maintain an independent residence as the health and capabilities of one or both partners decline. However, this can prove costly, and people who cannot legally marry are legally and financially disadvantaged, relative to their married peers. Elderly persons who are single, without strong connections with children or other relatives, face additional challenges. Fredriksen-Goldsen summarizes these realities from a legal, social, and practical perspective.

Gay men are the most visible group within LGBT communities. The current cohort of older gay men has had the unique experience of surviving the AIDS crisis, during which many friends and partners died and the future of the community appeared foreshortened. Now these individuals are at the life stage during which surviving loved ones die of other chronic illnesses. In chapter 3, Brian de Vries and Gil Herdt discuss the physical, emotional, and social health needs of older gay men.

Older lesbians have been leaders in advocacy and community visibility. Old Lesbians Organizing for Change is an advocacy and educational organization that addresses the concerns of lesbian women in middle age and beyond. In chapter 4, Nancy M. Nystrom and Teresa C. Jones employ a case-based format to examine the concerns of older lesbians and contrast them with those of their heterosexually identified peers. Practical advice for older lesbians and their service professionals is also provided.

Bisexual elders are often presumed to be either heterosexually or homosexually identified and are therefore less visible than their gay or lesbian peers. In chapter 5, Paula C. Rodríguez Rust discusses the life course dynamics and forms of bisexuality identified in the "International Bisexual Identities, Communities, Ideologies, and Politics" study, drawing from first-person accounts of study participants. Social, legal, and health concerns are also discussed and a resource list is provided.

Most people who socially and medically transition gender do so during young adulthood or middle adult years. Some do not publicly identify as transgender after transition has been completed. However, the physical and social changes of transition influence subsequent experiences and the elder years. Legal protections for transgender individuals and their families also remain incomplete. In chapter 6, Tarynn M. Witten and A. Evan Eyler discuss the health, legal, and practical aspects of life for older transgender persons, including palliative care and end-of-life concerns. This discussion is followed by general conclusions about aging among sexual- and gender-minority-identified persons.

Despite the growing voice of intersex-identified advocates and educators, little is known about the lived experience and concerns of elderly persons born with variations in sex development. In chapter 7, Heather Laine Talley and Monica J. Casper offer a provisional research agenda with respect to this population. The professional terminology and political culture regarding intersex/disorders of sex development/variation in sex development is evolving and, in some respects, being contested. The term *intersex* is used to refer to an aspect of personal identity, rather than medical biology. Many adults who use it consider the intersex identity a crucial aspect of their personhood.

The perspective of this book is *resilience* (Connolly, 2005; Harris, 2008). Many LGBT-identified elders have survived to old age in an invalidating, threatening, and persecuting social environment (Green, 2004; Russell & Richards, 2003; Scourfield, Roen, & McDemott, 2008). Despite the often severe difficulties they have encountered, many have achieved the wisdom that accompanies trials successfully faced and challenges mastered, and are living their final years with dignity and grace. Their first-person accounts permeate this volume, providing real-life examples that illustrate practical points and that illuminate areas of lived experience that have not yet been made explicit through comprehensive research.

The authors of these chapters include professionals in medicine, social work, psychology, gerontology, health administration, and health research. We, the editors, are a gerontologist/social worker and a psychiatrist/family physician. We have attempted to offer a useful combination of (unfortunately frequently scant) biological and social science research, case examples and first-person accounts, and practical advice for health professionals, service planners, and individuals interested in the field of LGBT aging.

The completion of this book has suffered through much the same life course as those who have contributed to it. Authors have dealt with life issues concerning their respective partners, parents, careers, and personal health, as they have moved through midlife. This book has waited for multiple heart surgeries to be completed, stents to open clogged blood vessels, serious back injuries, eye surgery for cataracts, relocations, hand surgery, job changes, and other traditional midlife and later-life crises. It is an avatar of our own lives over the past five years.

Each chapter author is an expert in his or her field, and we are excited to have been able to work with them and to see the fruition of years of labor. We express sincere appreciation to the contributors to this book. In particular, we thank them for their extra efforts in multiple reviews of their chapters. We thank them for their patience as we carefully reviewed their work, asked questions, and requested re-edits during the process.

Many people contributed to completing this book. It is beyond our power to mention all of them.

Normally, at this point, authors take a moment to thank their editor for her or his patience and diligence. However, TMW would like to do a bit more than the norm: Wendy Harris not only was my editor but also has been a treasured friend for nearly 30 years. Wendy and I grew gray haired together in parallel with this book's voyage to completion. When I first approached her with the idea for this book, she was excited about the possibilities and was most encouraging at every step along the way. From simple chapter outline to the final product, Wendy was there with encouragement and friendship; would that all of my other books have gone as smoothly. If Evan and I are metaphorically the pages of this book, Wendy was and remains its spine. Without doubt, her inordinate patience has allowed the book to come to fruition. Wendy was succeeded by Suzanne Flinchbaugh, who saw our book through its final production. We owe her thanks as well.

Ultimately, this book is the result of the willingness of patients, clients, research participants, and colleagues to share their experiences and opinions regarding life as sexual- or gender-minority-identified older persons. To all of these people and their families, we owe our thanks.

As this book was going to press, the Institute of Medicine (2011) issued a "seminovarian" report on the health of LGBT people. We, the editors and the contributing authors, are proud to be able to say that this book addresses the IOM's stated need for more information in this area.

REFERENCES

Clunis, D. M., Fredricksen-Goldsen, K. I., Freeman, P. A., & Nystrom, N. (2005). *Lives of lesbian elders: Looking back, looking forward*. Binghamton, NY: Haworth Press.

Connolly, C. M. (2005). A qualitative exploration of resilience in long-term lesbian couples. *Family Journal, 13*, 266–280.

Green, R. J. (2004). Risk and resilience in lesbian and gay couples: Comment on Solomon, Rothblum, and Balsam (2004). *Journal of Family Psychology, 18*(2), 290–292.

Harris, P. B. (2008). Another wrinkle in the debate about successful aging: The undervalued concept of resilience and the lived experience of dementia. *International Journal of Human Development, 67*(1), 43–61.

Herdt, G., & DeVries, B. (2004). *Gay and lesbian aging: Research and future directions*. New York: Springer.

Hunter, S. (2005). *Midlife and older GLBT adults: Knowledge and affirmative practice services*. New York: Taylor & Francis.

Institute of Medicine. (2011). *The health of lesbian, gay, bisexual and transgender people: Building a foundation for better understanding*. Washington, DC: National Academies Press.

Kimmel, D., Rose, T., & David, S. (2006). *Lesbian, gay, bisexual, and transgender aging*. New York: Columbia University Press.

Russell, G. B., & Richards, J. A. (2003). Stressor and resilience factors for lesbians, gay men, and bisexuals confronting antigay politics. *American Journal of Community Psychology, 31*(3–4), 313–328.

Scourfield, J., Roen, K., & McDermott, L. (2008). Lesbian, gay, bisexual and transgender young people's experiences of distress: Resilience, ambivalence and self-destructive behavior. *Health and Social Care in the Community, 16*(3), 329–336.

Contributors

Monica J. Casper, Ph.D., Professor of Social and Behavioral Sciences and Women's Studies and Director, Division of Humanities, Arts, and Cultural Studies, New College of Interdisciplinary Arts and Sciences, Arizona State University, Phoenix, Arizona

Karen I. Fredriksen-Goldsen, Ph.D., M.S.W., Associate Professor and Director, Institute for Multigenerational Health, School of Social Work, University of Washington, Seattle, Washington

Gil Herdt, Ph.D., Professor and Director, National Sexuality Resource Center, Department of Human Sexuality Studies, San Francisco State University, San Francisco, California

Teresa C. Jones, Ph.D., M.S.W., Lecturer, School of Social Work, University of Washington, Seattle, Washington

Nancy M. Nystrom, Ph.D., M.S.W., L.I.C.S.W., Lecturer, School of Social Work, University of Washington, Seattle, Washington

Paula C. Rodríguez Rust, Ph.D., Independent Consultant, Spectrum Diversity LLC, East Brunswick, New Jersey

Heather Laine Talley, Ph.D., Assistant Professor, Department of Anthropology and Sociology, Western Carolina University, Cullowhee, North Carolina

Brian de Vries, Ph.D., Professor, Department of Gerontology, San Francisco State University, San Francisco, California

Gay, Lesbian, Bisexual & Transgender Aging

CHAPTER ONE

The Aging of Sexual and Gender Minority Persons

An Overview

TARYNN M. WITTEN, PH.D., L.C.S.W.

Aging—being old—is defined both biomedically and psychosocioeconomically: "The geriatric or elderly patient is defined as an individual whose *biological age* is advanced. By definition, such an individual has one or more diseases, one or more silent lesions in various organ systems" (Aronheim, 1992, p. ix). However, there are also links between the biological aspects of aging and the social components of aging (Adams & White, 2004). Social aspects of aging are also complex, and they include, but are not limited to, adapting to lessened physical capabilities, reduced income, and limited social network support. Social support networks can decay as members age and die. Many older persons find themselves living alone after decades of marriage, partnership, and child rearing.

The current cohort of elderly persons reflects the wide diversity of the U.S. population (Fried, 2000; George, 2005). Life experience as a member of a particular gender, racial, or ethnic group—often in defined economic circumstances and in the context of regional culture—shapes the experience of aging and the skills and expectations with which individuals enter later years (Pampel, Krueger, & Denney, 2010). Recent research has focused on the effects of these demographic variables on health and social outcomes among elderly persons and groups (Rogers, Hummer, & Nam, 2000).

Members of sexual and gender minorities—persons identified as gay, lesbian, bisexual, or transgender (LGBT)—are a newly visible population of elderly persons (Cahill, South, & Spade, 2000; Fruhoff & Mahoney, 2010; Institute of Medicine [IOM], 2011). As a result of vigorous educational and activist efforts by a small number of intersex-identified persons, intersex/disorders of sex development (also abbreviated DSD in some political contexts) has also emerged as an enduring minority group (Brinkmann, Schuetzmann, & Richter-Appelt, 2007; Preves, 2000), though less is known about their experience of aging than for older adults who identify as lesbian, gay, bisexual, or transgender. Although variation in partnered, romantic, sexual behaviors, gender identity, and sex development is an inherent aspect of human biological and social evolution, the freedom to be publicly identified as an LGBT, or intersex/DSD, adult was not available, in any meaningful way, during the youth through middle adulthood of the current cohort of elderly persons in the United States and in other Western nations.

Over the past four decades, the public perception of homosexuality has transformed from a criminal act or a manifestation of mental illness (Warner et al., 2004) to a normal variation in emotional and social life; however, religious proscriptions have been slower to erode than medical and legal prohibitions. Bisexually identified persons still experience stigmatization and invisibility (Hylton, 2006; Saewyc et al., 2006; Ulrich, 2011), though bisexuality is now generally regarded as an enduring sexual identity, rather than as a manifestation of erotic ambivalence or a transitional or immature sexuality. For transgender-identified individuals, gender transition often continues to be a difficult experience, although in some respects, it has become more ordinary and increasingly less sensationalized. Services are slowly becoming more available and gender-transitioning persons have become more visible. Yet the legal status of transgender individuals often remains unprotected.* Public understanding of intersex/DSD has improved substantially during the past decade although pejorative terms such as *hermaphrodite* continue to be used as descriptors of this population. The focus of intersex/DSD concerns remains the medical treatment of children born with variation

---

* A major legal change was implemented when President Obama signed federal hate crimes legislation into law. The Matthew Shepard and James Byrd, Jr. Hate Crimes Prevention Act of 2009 "will help protect people against violence based on sexual orientation, gender identity, race, religion, gender, national origin and disability by extending the federal hate crimes statute" (www .thetaskforce.org/node/3438/print).

in sex development and little is known about the experience of middle and older adulthood for intersex-identified persons and their respective concerns and needs.

The current cohort of LGBT older persons came of age in an environment that sought to "normalize" them, that is, to make them gender and developmentally usual and heterosexual, through psychological or medical treatment, and to suppress those who did not conform. Suppression often took on many forms, from physical abuse and violence, to mental abuse, to denial of health care access. Many current elders therefore have difficulty seeking or accepting assistance through the helping professions because of their own past negative experiences or the experiences of their peers (Brotman et al., 2007; Clover, 2006; McNair, 2003; Witten, 2009, 2011; Witten & Whittle, 2004). When asked about their worries around growing older, one of Witten's survey respondents stated (Witten, 2011):

> [I am worried about] being abused, as my wife was, in health care settings at the end of life while in a state of complete dependency on others. My wife died horribly in pain and terror from overt homophobic physical abuse and denial of treatment for infection in a nursing home while I was incapacitated by serious complications following my double mastectomy for breast cancer, and unable to monitor her care and well being. She had had several strokes and was completely dependent upon nursing home staff for care, unable to ambulate or talk, or defend herself in any fashion.

This is but one in numerous responses that document the negative experiences and profound fears of many members of the LGBT population members.

In addition, gay and lesbian communities have emphasized youth concerns (Cochran, Stewart, Ginzler, & Cauce, 2002; Cocker, Austin, & Shuster, 2010; Magee, Bigelow, DeHaan, & Mustanski, 2011; Mustanski, Garofalo, & Emerson, 2010;), such as coming out and family support (Ryan, Huebner, Diaz, & Sanchez, 2009; Weber, 2010), establishing relationships, homelessness, tobacco and other substance abuse (Remafedi & Carol, 2005), and, more recently, parenting, over an awareness of the needs and preferences of older persons. While there has been a recent spurt in addressing the needs of the LGBT elders (IOM, 2011), much still remains to be both understood and implemented. The effort and commitment to medically and socially transition gender emphasize the time of life in which transition is undertaken, usually early or middle adulthood, rather than in fostering a long-term perspective and plan. Both transgender and intersex/DSD adults frequently have felt the need to conceal important aspects of their early lives, or have been instructed to, in order to preserve their social acceptance or safety.

Anecdotal evidence supports that some LGBT individuals "return to the closet" as they age.* For some transgender-identified individuals, this could mean removing implants or potentially undoing earlier surgeries or hormonal modifications. These practices have sometimes subtly undermined the development of a complete life cycle perspective, including reasonable expectations for the elder years. Such behavior patterns are now termed *de-transitioning* (Witten, 2011). A participant in Witten (2011) clearly makes the point:

> I am a late transitioner. I was in denial most of the years of my life. I did not seriously try to even begin to be full time until I retired. I am kind of afraid of surgeries and seem to pass without any. At my age it might be hard to find a surgeon anyway, so I probably won't get any. Being able to de-transition upon need for serious medical care might be handy too. Who knows.

Most profoundly, AIDS has interfered with the evolution of a normal, multigenerational, and long-term perspective for communities most heavily affected, particularly among urban gay men.

The cumulative effect of these events and experiences has been the emergence of a population of older LGBT persons who have experienced a wide variety of negative interactions in many areas of life. Many of these individuals have the same need for health and social services as their majority-identified peers. However, they may have insufficient community support, and, in many cases, helping professionals may lack familiarity with their concerns or simply be unwilling to serve them (Anderson, Patterson, Temple, & Inglehart, 2009; Kelly & Robinson, 2011; Makadon, 2006).

The bulk of the research dialogue in the LGBTI aging field has concerned gay and lesbian aging (Adelman, 1987). In the past 10 to 15 years, interest in the field of LGBT aging has increased significantly, with health needs that are now only truly being investigated (Bakker, Sandfort, Vanwesenbeeck, van Lindert, & Westert, 2006; Concannon, 2009; Conron, Mimiaga, & Landers, 2010; Fredriksen-Goldsen & Muraco, 2010; Harcourt, 2006; Hatzenbuehler, Keyes, & Hasin, 2009; Hellman & Drescher, 2004; Kuyper & Vanwesenbeeck, 2011; Landers, Mimiaga, & Krinsky, 2010; Smith, McCaslin, Chang, Martinez, & McGrew, 2010; Makadon, Mayer, Potter, & Goldhammer, 2007; Masiongale, 2009; McNair & Hegarty, 2010; MetLife Mature Market Institute [MMMI], 2010; Riorden, 2004; Scout, Bradford, & Fields, 2001; Shankle, 2006; Sullivan, 2003). In parallel with that interest

---

* A significant new movie *GenSilent*, released in 2010, documents that many elders of the GLBT-identified community are going back into the closet (http://gensilent.com).

has been a growing volume of research in transgender aging. Little has been written about bisexual aging or intersex/DSD aging.

This chapter summarizes the literature on the aging of sexual and gender minority persons to provide a context for discussion within the overall field of aging research and a focus on the challenges and unique demands in aging across the life course as a member of a sexual or gender population.

THE AGING POPULATION

Any contemporary analysis of health care policy and health care delivery in the global economy (Kinsella & Phillips, 2005) must include discussion of the *worldwide aging population* (Crato, Haase, Welsh, & Wasow, 2006; National Institute on Aging [NIA], 2007a), *global health care disparity* (Mullins, Blatt, Gbarayor, Yang, & Baquet, 2005; Singh & Siahpush, 2006), *ethnic* (Griffith, Moy, Reischl, & Dayton, 2006; Haviland, Morales, Dial, & Pincus, 2005) and *minority inclusion* (Anderson, Bulato, & Cohen, 2004; Committee on Population [CPOP], 2004; Fiscella, Franks, Gold, & Clancy, 2000; Smedley, Stith, & Nelson, 2003; Williams, 2005), *socioeconomic status* (Kahn & Fazio, 2005; Robert et al., 2009), *gender differences* (Crimmins, 2004; Pinn, 2003; Read & Gorman, 2010), and *rurality* (Hartley, 2004). These significant topics will remain so into the future. In light of the research on successful and productive aging (Bowling, 2007; Rowe & Kahn, 1998; Depp & Jeste, 2006), maintaining an effective health care system, particularly as related to the global aging population, is critical.

Birren (2007, p. 49) defines aging as "interacting biological, psychological and social processes that start with birth and end with death. The term is widely used to refer to the biopsychosocial changes in the later phases of the life course." Birren recognizes that aging is an intricate spatial and temporal hierarchy of dynamic behaviors coupled in a complex dance across the life span. Thus, aging is a complex process (Pearce & Merletti, 2006; Witten, 2004) not easily dissected into disjoint subprocesses. This understanding requires examining aging across multiple domains of organization.

As aging is a universally experienced process, it is within the collective biomedical, psychosocial, economic, cultural, and political dynamics of aging that members of the LGBT minority populations and associated subgroups (such as members of racial, ethnic, and ability minorities) experience the driving forces of growing older (Brotman, Ryan, & Cormier, 2003), the associated ageisms (Angus & Reeve, 2006; Dobson, 2007; Giles & Reed, 2005; Kane, Priester, & Neumann, 2007; Walsh et al., 2007), health and economic disparities, barriers to access to needed resources and services (Lurie & Dubowitz, 2007; Yagoda, 2005), and lack of knowledge regarding important aspects of planning and self-care (Baker et al., 2007; Kimmel, Rose, & David, 2006), all of which affect how an individual proceeds through the life course (Kuh, 2007). Even factors such as feelings of usefulness to others can affect disability and mortality in older adults (Gruenewald, Karlamangla, Greendale, Singer, & Seeman, 2007).

CONTEMPORARY DEMOGRAPHICS

Individuals are "living longer and, in some parts of the world, healthier lives" (NIA, 2007a, p. 1). The base statistics on worldwide population aging are staggering. In 2006, "almost 500 million people worldwide were 65 and older. By 2030, that total is projected to increase to 1 billion—1 in every 8 of earth's inhabitants" (NIA, 2007a, p. 2). Estimates indicate that "one million people turn 60 every month and 80% of those are in the developing world. Although the proportion of older people—out of the total population—is higher in developed nations, the percentage of increase of the elderly population is greater in the developing world" (World Health Organization [WHO], 2002, p. 2). "Significantly, the most rapid increases in the 65-and-older population are occurring in developing countries, which will see a jump of 140 percent by 2030" (NIA, 2007a, p. 2). By 2050, the number of individuals older than age 60 is expected to be 2 billion individuals, with 80% of them living in developing countries such as China, India, Mexico, Indonesia, Brazil, Japan, Pakistan, Bangladesh, the Russian Federation, Nigeria, and in the United States (Peterson & Yamamoto, 2005). "Aged populations in Germany, France or Sweden are expected to undergo 30 to 60% increases from 1990 to 2020, while developing countries such as Thailand, Kenya and Colombia are predicted to experience more than a 300% rise and a higher than 400% rise in Indonesia" (Ruger & Kim, 2006; WHO, 2002, p. 2).

U.S. statistics are equally startling. "Since 1900, the US population has tripled, but the number of older adults has increased 11-fold . . . to 35 million in 2000. By 2030, when all of the baby boomers (individuals born between 1946 and 1964) have reached 65, the number of older Americans is expected to reach 71 million, or roughly 20% of the U.S. population" (Merck, 2004, p. 2). WHO points out that "by 2020, countries such as Cuba, Argentina, Thailand and Sri Lanka will have a higher proportion of older people than the US" (WHO, 2002, p. 3). Perhaps the most amazing projection is that, "for the first time in history, and probably for the rest of human history, people age 65 and over will outnumber children under age 5" (NIA, 2007a, p. 3).

PATTERNS OF ILLNESS

As the global number of elderly persons increases and as the average human life expectancy rises, diverse trends regarding the health of this population are developing (Cigolle, Langa, Kabeto, Tian, & Blaum, 2007; Polivka, 2007a, 2007b). Concurrent with this population trend (NIA, 2007a; WHO, 2007a) a host of formidable fiscal (Costa, 2007) and functional health care challenges have been identified.

Noncommunicable diseases (Wong, Shapiro, Boscardin, & Ettner, 2002) have taken a larger share of the overall health care burden (Zack, Moriarty, Stroup, Ford, & Mokdad, 2004), and chronic noncommunicable diseases (Wen, 2004) are now the major cause of death among older people in both developed and less developed countries. The National Council on Aging [NCOA] estimates that "approximately 80% of older adults have at least one chronic disease, and 50% have at least two" (NCOA, 2011a). In addition, "chronic non-communicable disease can decrease the overall quality of life" (Merck, 2004, pp. 2–3). For example, Clark (2006) points out that "by the year 2030, the number of people with Alzheimer's in the U.S. is expected to increase by 70%." The NCOA (2011a) projects that "nearly 15 million [elders] will experience some mental disorder including depression, anxiety disorders and dementia." Other, more acute health risks sometimes complicate the burden of chronic illness. For instance, Clark (2006) also points out that "the suicide rate for older men, already the highest in the nation, will likely rise even further." In addition, suicidality, particularly among members of the LGBT population is now being recognized as a growing problem (House, Van Horn, Coppeans, & Stepelman, 2011; Paul et al., 2002).

Many other illnesses are equally problematic. Cancer rates in elderly people are higher than in any other segment of the U.S. population. Moreover, in the United States, 60% of new cancers occur in individuals older than 65 years of age, with more than 50% of cancer deaths occurring in those older than 70 years of age. SEER (National Cancer Institute Surveillance Epidemiology and End Results) estimates project that by 2020 the U.S. population of 85 years of age or older will have increased by 12% over that of 1990. If no significant environmental changes occur in this period, cancer incidence for this age group will increase by 60%.

Diabetes affects 12.2 million U.S. elders 60 years and older. "This represents 23.1% of the older population. 90% of Americans aged fifty-five and over are at risk for hypertension (high blood pressure). Women are more likely than men to develop this chronic condition, with half of women aged 60+ and 77% of women aged 75+ having this condition. Hypertension affects 64% of men aged 75+" (NCOA, 2011a, 2011b).

HIV in elderly people is also growing (Brown & Sankar, 1998; Mack & Ory, 2003; Lee, 2006; Wallace, Cochran, Durazo, & Ford, 2011; Waysdorf, 2002). Knodel, Watkins, and VanLandingham (2002, p. 3) report that 10.7% of U.S. AIDS cases occur in people older than age 50 years. Worldwide, the over-50-year-old occurrence rates range from 4.5% to 16%, with male percentages routinely higher than female percentages. Given the ability of new treatment protocols to extend the life span in individuals living with HIV/AIDS, normal, even successful, aging in the face of this disease (Sanchez Rodriguez & Rodriguez Alvarez, 2003) is becoming ever more important (AIDS Alert, 2004; Kahana & Kahana, 2001), particularly in light of out-of-pocket expenses for prescriptions as a percentage of total available income (Copeland, 2007; Crystal, Johnson, Harman, Sambamoorthi, & Kumar, 2000; Soumerai et al., 2006; Xu, 2003), treatment disparities associated with traditional socioeconomic indicators (Byrd, Fletcher, & Menifield, 2007; Ghilarducci, 2007), potential for drug-drug interactions (Marzolini et al., 2011), and overall importance to the field of geriatric medicine (Kearney, Moore, Donegan, & Lambert, 2010).

Sambamoorthi, Shea, and Crystal (2003) find, that in 1997, nearly 8% of the U.S. population older than 65 years of age (2.3 million people) spent more than 10% of their income on prescription drugs. Moreover, "despite pharmacy coverage, [the] out-of-pocket burden fell most heavily on women and those with chronic health conditions. Burden was also higher among those with self-purchased supplemental coverage" (p. 345). Kennedy and Erb (2002) found similar results: "Severe disability, poor health, low income, lack of insurance and high number of prescriptions increased the odds of being noncompliant [with medical treatment] as a result of cost" (p. 1120). Similar results are occurring in other countries worldwide (Goldman, Joyce, & Zheng, 2007; Kildemoes, Christiansen, Gyrd-Hansen, Kristiansen, & Anderson, 2006). Pollicino and Saltman (2000) address the interplay of elder functional status and physician cost, pointing out that higher cost is correlated with lower functional status (i.e., persons who are the least physically vigorous incur the most extensive health care costs).

Nationwide and worldwide increases in elderly populations imply an increase in Alzheimer's disease, other dementias, and mild cognitive impairments (Parker & Thorslund, 2007). Haan and Wallace (2004, pp. 1–24) point out that, "by the year 2020, the WHO predicts that there will be nearly 29 million demented people in both developed and developing countries." This implies a significant economic and staffing burden on the health care system. Similar arguments can be made concerning disabilities affecting activities of daily living, including instrumental activities of daily living: "Projections indicate that the cost of care for older adults with functional limitations will almost triple over the next 40 years, from $123 billion to $346 billion" (Spillman, 2004). Falls merit special mention: "Nearly one third of the older US population currently reports some lower body limitations, with women, minorities and those with low socioeconomic standing at higher risk" (Ostir, Kuo, Berges, Markides, & Ottenbacher, 2007). Moreover, "among older adults, falls are the leading cause of fracture, hospital admissions for trauma and injury deaths" (National Council on Aging, 2011a).

Oral health problems will be similarly affected by an increase in the elderly population. Priorities will include access to care (Dolan, Atchison, & Huynh, 2005; WHO, 2007b) in order to ensure adequate nutrition, treatment of caries, periodontal disease, and edentulism (Cunha-Cruz, Hujoel, & Nadanovsky, 2007). The relationship between poor dentition and diabetes, cardiovascular, and cardiopulmonary disease must also be addressed (Ettinger, 2005; WHO, 2007b).

PSYCHOSOCIAL ASPECTS OF AGING

Psychosocial aspects of aging are complex and include adapting to lessened physical capabilities, reduced income (Copeland, 2007; Ghilarducci, 2007), and a potentially weakened social network support structure (Ajrouch, Blandon, & Antonucci, 2005; Everard et al., 2000; Green, Rebok, & Lyketsos, 2008). Many older persons live alone (Greenfield & Russell, 2011; Hawkley & Cacippo, 2007) after decades of marriage (Van Baarsen, 2002), partnership, or child rearing and have a growing number of functional limitations (Angel, Jimenez, & Angel, 2007; Nummela, Sppanen, & Uutela, 2011).

Increased life span can leave elders with diminished social support networks at a time when human interaction (Grossman, D'Augelli, & Hershberger, 2000; Pinquart & Sorenson, 2000; Umberson, Brosnoe, & Reczek, 2010) is crucial to quality of life and overall health (Kraaj, Arensman, & Spinhoven, 2002; Shippy & Karpiak, 2005). Having fewer options for care because of alterations in overall family and social structure (Angel & Angel, 2006; Avison & Davies, 2005) can leave elderly family members emotionally and socially isolated and unable to care for themselves (Silverstein, Gans, & Yang, 2006; Tomaka, Thompson, & Palacios, 2006). Moreover, social isolation—independent of emotional isolation—can increase the risk of other diseases. Rurality also plays a part in this as smaller regions often have fewer resources for elders, and for LGBT members, the risk of outing oneself using the few resources is too great. For example, results of a critical study (Wilson et al., 2007) demonstrate that "social isolation (loneliness) nearly doubles the risk of Alzheimer's disease as compared with those persons who were not lonely." The impact of intergenerational identity and well-being and grand-parent identity is discussed in Reitzes and Mutran (2004) and in chapter 6.

Elders find their resources increasingly strained (Kahn & Pearlin, 2006; O'Rand & Shuey, 2007) by the demands of existing inflexible health care (Wei, Akincigil, Crystal, & Sambamoorthi, 2006) and pension systems (Copeland, 2007, p. 20): "77% of adults aged 65+ depend on Social Security for all or some of their monthly income, and almost 20% live at less than 150% of federal poverty level (FPL), $16, 245 annually for a single person" (NCOA, 2011b). Income is tight for those who are retired, and retirement is not golden for a large number of older adults. "White women aged 65+ comprise 50% of those living below poverty. 50% of African-American women aged 65+ have incomes at or below 200% of FPL" (NCOA, 2011b). Savings and debt are also problematic. "One third of senior households has no money left over each month or is in debt after meeting essential expenses" (NCOA, 2011b). Later-life care is increasingly expensive and problematic. According to Merck (2004, p. 2), "Nearly 79% of people who need long-term care live at home or in community settings rather than in institutions." This increases the demand for caregiving facilities and personnel. U.S. businesses lose between $11 billion and $29 billion each year because employees take time off to care for elderly family members (National Family Caregivers Association, 2004). Other, more large-scale problems include long-term stability of social insurance (Hu, 2005; Lurie, Jung, & Lavizzo-Mourey, 2005), as well as other social entitlement programs (Polivka, 2007b; Svihula & Estes, 2007).

Violence and abuse against and among elderly people is an international (Krug et al., 2002; WHO, 2007c) and a growing public health problem (Cooper, Selwood, & Livingston, 2008; Rutherford et al., 2007a, 2007b). Kleinschmidt's (1997) excellent review of early literature regarding elder abuse (Buzgová & Ivanová, 2009; Luo & Waite, 2011) and related problems points out that older patients "use EMS at twice the rate of other age groups and represented 22% of EMS users in one urban study." The U.S. House Select Committee on Aging (1990) estimated that 1 million to 2 million older Americans are abused each year. More recent estimates are that as many as 2.5 million older people are abused each year in the United States, and "the number of cases will likely increase as this population grows." Sexual abuse of elders is also a growing problem (Acierno et al., 2010; Ramsey-Klawsnik et al., 2007; Teaster & Roberto, 2004). Elder abuse receives less attention than many other forms of domestic violence, and fewer than 10% of cases are reported to the authorities (Kleinschmidt, 1997, p. 471). Moreover, assessment of the reported cases is often problematic (Nadien, 2006; Rudolph & Hughes, 2001), and outcomes can be unsatisfactory.

Although abuse and neglect are probably more common in home and in informal settings than in retirement facilities (Johnson, 2005) and care facilities, treatment in nursing homes remains a concern as well (Conrad, Iris, Ridings, Langley, & Anetzberger, 2011; Post et al., 2010). WHO (2002) reports that despite a "vast literature on quality of care issues in institutions, no prevalence or incidence data is available." A survey of nursing home personnel in one U.S. state disclosed that 36% of the staff reported having seen at least one incident of physical abuse in the preceding year by another staff member. Further, 10% of the respondents admitted to having committed at least one act of elder abuse (physical) themselves. Eighty-one percent of the sample had observed an incident of psychological abuse against a nursing home resident, and 40% of the respondents admitted to committing an act of psychological abuse (Pillemer & Moore, 1989). Elders who live alone may also experience self-neglect, which is considered a form of abuse (Dyer et al., 2007). Neglect of the self can lead to failure to eat, failure to bathe, and failure to maintain one's health. Financial abuse against elders can also be a problem, as elders are often vulnerable to scams. Moreover, many seniors give access to their financial accounts to their children (Davies et al., 2011), leaving the senior vulnerable to the potential depletion of funds by family members. Sexual abuse can also be problematic, from denial of partner access in care facilities, to more abusive sexual interactions or violations of genital privacy as in the case of transgender nonoperative or intersex/DSD community members (Teaster & Roberto, 2006).

Substance abuse, particularly alcohol, tobacco, and illicit drugs, in the elderly is a well-documented phenomenon (Dowling, Weiss, & Condon, 2008; Gfroerer, Penne, Pemberton, & Folsom, 2003; Stevenson, 2005; Wu & Blazer, 2011). It is also a well-known phenomenon in the LGBT community (Cochran & Cauce, 2006; Corliss, Grella, Mays, & Cochran, 2006; Substance Abuse and Mental Health Services Administration [SAMHSA], 2003).

Many members of the LGBT community have suffered life course histories of perceived and actual abuse and violence. Ramifications of life course abuse on later life morbidity and mortality are also important in understanding LGBT health (Balsam et al., 2010)

Cultural variation can affect perceptions of abuse and violence (Smyer & Clark, 2011; WHO, 2002, 2007c). In one study, "all [surveyed] groups denied the existence of physical violence in their communities. This created an issue of getting definitions of 'abuse,' because for them, 'abuse' does not exist in India. What they would talk about was 'emotional problems,' 'lack of emotional support,' 'neglect by the family members,' 'feeling of insecurity,' 'loss of dignity,' 'maltreatment,' 'disrespect by the family.' However, not a single person was willing to label it as 'abuse'" (WHO, 2002, p. 9).

Gender-based hate crimes and other forms of violence against women are a widespread global problem (McPhail, 2002; McPhail & DiNitto, 2005), and violence against elder women remains a growing concern (Fisher & Regan, 2006; WHO, 2007c).

The complexity of abuse and violence is illustrated in figure 1 of Rutherford et al. (2007a). They demonstrate that across the four major categories of the "nature of violence"—physical, sexual, psychological, and deprivation/neglect—are three major categories of violence (self-directed, interpersonal, and collective), under which fall 12 subcategories. Other types of abuse, including spiritual and financial, are described in Kleinschmidt (1997, p. 464). Risk factors associated with violence, and an ecological model demonstrating the hierarchy of complexity in dealing with violence and abuse, are conceptually detailed in Rutherford et al. (2007b). For example, Argentinian respondents, in the WHO (2002) research project, "defined societal abuse as age discrimination manifested particularly in inadequate pensions" (WHO, 2002, p. 10). Numerous respondents in the WHO report also discussed disrespect and ageist attitudes. As one Lebanese respondent stated, "One rude word said to an old man is stronger than stabbing him with a knife" (WHO, 2002, p. 13).

Several major themes emerged in the WHO (2007c) report:

- Neglect: isolation, abandonment and social exclusion
- Violation: of human, legal and medical rights
- Deprivation: of choices, decisions, status, finances and respect

Later-life violence in general (Lacks et al., 1998, 2002; National Center on Elder Abuse, 2005), intimate partner violence (Bonomi et al., 2007), caretaker abuse and violence (Nadien, 2006), and violence and abuse in the nursing home (from health service providers [Pillemer & Moore, 1989], family, or other residents [Shinoda-Tagawa et al., 2004]) are all growing problems magnified by increasing numbers of elderly persons worldwide (Johnson, 2000; Krug et al., 2002).

SOCIAL AND ECONOMIC INFLUENCES
ON AGING AND HEALTH

Numerous factors (Irwin et al., 2006) such as *birth (natal) sex* (Crimmins, Kim, & Solé-Auró, 2011; Hinton, Zweifach, Oishi, Tang, & Unützer, 2006), *increased life stress* (Kraaij, Arensman, & Spinoven, 2002), *family structure and social or socio-economic status* (Coppin et al., 2006; Ross et al., 2011; Turra & Goldman, 2007), *minority status (by race or ethnicity)* (Alvarado et al., 2007; Gaines, 2007; Shuey & Willson, 2008), *childhood disadvantage* (Bengtsson & Lindstrom, 2000; Braveman & Barclay, 2009; Luo & Waite, 2005), and even *negative life events* (Kraaij, Arensman, & Spinoven, 2002; Rosnick, Small, McEvoy, Borenstein, & Mortimer, 2007) have been shown to mediate the existence of health inequities across the life span (Feinglass et al., 2007; George, 2005). Moreover, the same factors have been shown to mediate life expectancy and quality of life (Singh & Siahpush, 2006). Some recent life span theoretic constructs (Alwin & Wray, 2005) demonstrate that life course experience (e.g., financial strain, economic status, material disadvantage, social status, education, degree of illness, gender, race) strongly mediates many variables related to health (e.g., self-reported health, depression status, cognitive status), quality of life, morbidity (e.g., functional disability status), and mortality (Kahn & Pearlin, 2006; Melchior et al., 2006). Strong social networks and a strong sense of faith, religiosity, or spirituality are positive mediators of quality of life, morbidity, and mortality mediators often denied to members of the LGBT population (Daaleman, Perera, & Studenski, 2004; Krause, 2006; Vance, Brennan, Enah, Smith, & Kaur, 2011; Wilcox, 2002; Witten & Whittle, 2004). An excellent discussion of the social determinants of health can be found in the work of Marmot and Wilkinson (2006) and Pampel et al. (2010).

To remain vigorous, productive, and independent, older adults often require a variety of health care and social services (Heathcote, 2000). It is therefore essential that professionals who work with elderly persons understand the needs of members of this demographic group (Abendstern, Hughes, Clarkson, Sutcliffe, & Challis, 2011; Atdjian & Vega, 2005; Byrd et al., 2007). This will be particularly true during the first three decades of this century, as the cohort born in the years 1945–1964—the largest demographic group in the history of the United States—moves from middle adulthood into the elder years. If demographic projections are accurate, the needs of elderly persons will significantly affect the organization and economic structure of Western nations into the foreseeable future (NIA, 2007a).

AGING AND HEALTH OF POPULATION SUBGROUPS

In the face of the growing acknowledgment of the importance of life span theories of aging, the increasing human life expectancy and population of older individuals, it is important that life experience as a member of a particular social group be considered. Salient characteristics include gender (Crimmins et al.,

2011; Moen & Chermack, 2005; Read & Gorman, 2006), race (Liao, McGee, Cao, & Cooper, 1999) and ethnic group (Ahmad & Bradby, 2008; Becker et al., 2006; Brister, Hamdulay, Verma, Maganti, & Buchanan, 2007), economic circumstances (Guralnick, Butterworth, Wadsworth, & Kuh, 2006; Ross et al., 2011), and regional culture (Becker, Gates, & Newson, 2004; Danzon, 2009). These factors influence the experience of aging in a variety of respects (Russell, 2007; Thompson, 2006), including the competencies and expectations (Sarkisian, Hays, & Mangione, 2002; Sarkisian, Shunkwiler, Aguilar, & Moore, 2006) with which individuals enter older adulthood (Kubzansky, Berkman, & Seeman, 2000) and can also affect quality of life (Angel & Angel, 2006), health span (Cutler & Mattson, 2006; Fontana & Klein, 2007), and the morbidity (Costa, 2007; Mangin, Sweeney, & Heath, 2007) and mortality rates (Feinglass et al., 2007; Lubin, Lusky, Chetrit, & Dankner, 2003) of a population.

The literature regarding the relationship between traditional demographic and socioeconomic factors and health care delivery, and the international disparity regarding lack of minority inclusion in health care–related research and practice, is robust and expanding. The ways in which membership in a specific subpopulation can affect aging are seen in the study of these subcultures, referred to as *groups* in the sociology literature. Examples include the homeless group (Crane et al., 2005; Wright, Tompkins, Oldham, & Kay, 2004), the incarcerated group (Alexander & Meshelemia, 2010; Jenness, 2011; Loeb & Abudagga, 2006; London & Myers, 2006; Rikard & Rosenberg, 2007), the less-abled group (Reuben, 2006), the Native American and Hawaiian group (Holkup, Salois, Tripp-Reimer, & Weinart, 2007; Morrow & Messinger, 2006), ethnic groups (i.e., Latino/Latina; Kuhns, Vazquez, & Ramirez-Valles, 2008), and the military group (Setterson, 2006; Setterson & Patterson, 2006). The LGBT population can be considered its own minority group (or groups). When coupled with disparities associated with membership in other groups (intersectionality) (Allen, 2003; Cronin & King, 2010; Dang & Vianney, 2007), significant problems across the later-life path are amplified and compounded. The following section briefly discusses disparity literature as a foundation for the chapters in this book.

DISPARITIES IN HEALTH CARE

In recent years, disparities in health care have become a central focus of research in gerontology, public health, health care administration, and other fields (Moy, Dayton, & Clancy, 2005; Victoria, 2006). Reports from federal agencies (Agency for Healthcare Research and Quality [AHRQ], 2006; CDC, 2003; Cigolle et al.,

2007; NIA, 2007b, 2007c) and private think tanks (Curry & Jackson, 2003; National Gay and Lesbian Task Force [NGLTF], 2005) document disparities in health care delivery, health status, and treatment outcome for various "US racial and ethnic minority groups" (Sheikh, 2006) as well as other subgroups, including persons who are LGBT identified. LGBT health status has historically not been a focus of governmental public health research in the United States, though this has been changing in recent years.

The term *disparity* implies the existence of a difference between one group and another that is "markedly distinct in quality or character" (*Merriam-Webster Online Dictionary*, 2006). Table H.1 of AHRQ (2006, p. 8) lists numerous "opportunities for reducing disparities" that remain in health status and care. Unfortunately, in many cases, adequate measures do not yet exist for evaluating the extent of the particular disparity. An excellent discussion of some of the limitations of these reports can be found in Moy et al. (2005) and through the Gay and Lesbian Medical Association (GLMA, 2000).

In the *National Healthcare Disparities Report* (AHRQ, 2005), the Agency for Healthcare Research and Quality defines disparities as "any differences among populations." They note that all disparities discussed in the National Healthcare Disparities Report must "meet criteria based on statistical significance and size of difference" and state that disparities "related to race, ethnicity and socio-economic status still pervade the American healthcare system" (AHRQ, 2006, p. 2).

The term *minority* recognizes the existence of a socially sanctioned "outgroup" or "group/subpopulation differing from others in some characteristics and often subjected to differential treatment" (*Merriam-Webster Online Dictionary*, 2006). Some minority groups are studied with regard to health disparities and others are not. In the AHRQ National Healthcare Disparities Reports, minority groups are defined by race, ethnicity, income, and education (AHRQ, 2006, pp. 3–4; Health Development Agency, 2006). Consequently, more newly recognized minority groups, such as the LGBT population (GLMA, 2000; Witten, 2008), men who have sex with men (MSM), women who have sex with women (WSW) (Young & Meyer, 2005), Arab Americans, Middle Eastern migrants, and Muslims (Salari, 2002) are not included in these analyses. Minority groups remain invisible in policy reports on health care disparity and aging until additional research efforts are focused on their behalf. The *2010 Healthcare Disparities Report* (www.ahrq.gov/qual/nhdr10/nhdr10.pdf) was similarly organized and did not emphasize disparities related to LGBT status.

The *Healthy People 2010* (2011) report stated, "all differences among populations in measures of health and healthcare are considered evidence of disparities" and emphasized that "within many subpopulations including: women, children, elderly, residents of rural areas, and individuals with disabilities and other special health care needs" (AHRQ, 2006, p. 2) are still prevalent health disparities. They failed to include any discussion concerning members of the LGBT community as a whole or in part. However, the *Healthy People 2020* report noted that "research suggests that LGBT individuals face health disparities linked to societal stigma, discrimination, and denial of their civil and human rights" and provided a list of efforts to improve LGBT health, demonstrating the improving awareness of LGBT health concerns that had taken place in the United States in less than a decade (http://healthypeople.gov/2020/topicsobjectives2020/overview.aspx?topicid=25). The publication of the Institute of Medicine report *The Health of Lesbian, Gay, Bisexual, and Transgender People: Building a Foundation for Better Understanding* (IOM, 2011) was a landmark event, signaling the inclusion of the LGBT community in the focus of the Board on the Health of Select Populations of that important research and policy organization.

Many health disparities can be regarded as a function of numerous demographic and socioeconomic status factors (Agabiti et al., 2007; Moy et al., 2005). However, health disparities are often most apparent in particular health care areas, such as the diagnosis and treatment of cancer (Crew et al., 2007; Harper et al., 2009; Newman et al., 2006); treatment of cardiovascular disease (Calvin et al., 2006; Eiras & Richardson, 2007); treatment of drug, alcohol abuse, and other substance abuse (Gruskin, Greenwood, Matevia, Pollack, & Bye, 2007; Knudsen, Ducharme, & Roman, 2007); severity of depression (Huang, Chung, Kroenke, & Spitzer, 2006; Mezuk et al., 2010); disability status (Iezzoni, Davis, Soukup, & O'Day, 2002); early childhood health and health care (Flores, Olsen, & Tomany-Korman, 2005); health financial status (Wasson & Benjamin, 2006); use of health services (Sherkat et al., 2007; Sudore et al., 2006); insurance coverage and treatment (Calvin et al., 2006); Medicare treatment (Schneider, Zaslavsky, & Epstein, 2002); access to and use of prescription drugs (Wang et al., 2006; Wei et al., 2006); psychiatric treatment and mental health care (Neighbors et al., 2007; Willging, Salvadore, & Kano, 2006); sexual health (Heaphy, 2007; Marshall & Katz, 2002); access to end-of-life facilities, treatment (Phillips et al., 2011), and other palliative care facilities (Haber, 1999; Kuschner, 2011; Witten, 2009); and self-care (Becker et al., 2004; Chin, 2007).

Disparities in information capture and data quality (Aspinall & Jacobson, 2007; Fikree & Pasha, 2004; Velkoff & Kinsella, 1998) are also problematic. Research on health disparities is based on available data, and many minority groups do not receive much research attention. In addition, data are often stratified by socioeconomic status, race or ethnicity, and gender. However, *gender*, often called *gender identity* (internal self-perception), and *gender role* are often conflated with natal *sex* (physical anatomy as identified at birth) (Pryzgoda & Chrisler, 2000). For example, a simple literature search with "gender AND disparity AND aging" as the key search terms can be used to find information regarding possible differences between women and men with regard to the treatment of behavior problems in people who have Alzheimer's disease (Ott, Lapane, & Gambassi 2000), disparities between men and women in the treatment of late-life depression (Herek & Garnets, 2007; Hinton et al., 2006), and many similar concerns in a variety of health conditions (Heaphy, 2007; Wei et al., 2006). However, this extensive literature has little to say about the experiences of transgender older adults.

Health disparity is a well-documented and continuing international problem (Das & Gertler, 2007; Loewy, 2004; Pan American Health Organization, 1998; United Nations [UN], 2001;) as well: Africa (Aikins & Marks, 2007), Argentina (Paganini, 1999), Asia and the Pacific Islands (Goh, 2005; UN, 2001), Brazil (Carvalho de Noronha & Rosa, 1999), Canada (Prus, 2000), India (Pandey et al., 2002; Prabhakar & Manoharan, 2005), Israel (Horev, Berg-Warman, & Zussman, 2004), Italy (Agabiti et al., 2007), Japan (Matsuda, 2002), Latin America and the Caribbean (Alvarado et al., 2007), the Netherlands (Mackenbach, 2003), South Africa (Myburgh, Solanki, Smith, & Lallo, 2005), South America (Pan American Health Organization, 1998), South Asia (Fikree & Pasha, 2004), Spain (Borrell et al., 2001; Carrasco-Garrido, De Miguel, Hernández Barreram, & Jiménez-Garcia, 2007), Sweden (Wamala, Merlo, Boström, & Hogstedt, 2007a; Wamala, Merlo, Bostrom, Hogstedt, & Agren, 2007b), Taiwan (Hsu, 2005), Turkey (Ciceklioglu, Soyer, & Öcek, 2005), and the United Kingdom (Mohammed, Man, Bentham, Stevens, & Hussain, 2006). Further, the aspirations (Sykes, 2006) of older people, worldwide and the cultural and regional realities interact in complex ways and significantly affect how disparities are managed in the health care system.

Within the global population of older adults who are LGBT identified, health disparities exist between groups, within each group because of other factors such as race, ethnicity, and socioeconomic status (intersectionality; Cronin & King, 2010), and relative to the majority population. In light of the international breadth of these health care disparities, and the visibility of the emerging LGBT population—with all its diversity—the concerns of the LGBT communities should no longer be ignored in health and in aging research and practice. Understanding the dynamic interplay of "normative" aging processes and their associated disparities, coupled with LGBT-related struggles in a multicultural environment, demands that these concerns be carefully addressed when dealing with members of the global LGBT populations.

The confluence of aging status and health care disparity level synergistically creates an elevated overall disparity for individuals who are, simultaneously, elders of a minority community and in need of health care support. This can be regarded as an expansion of the classic "double jeopardy"—aging and minority identified (Dowd & Bengston, 1978) to a "triple jeopardy"—aging, minority, and LGBT identified. Byrd et al. (2007) note that "minority elders are at great risk for missed diagnoses, greater disabilities, and higher death rates." This can have a profound influence on how these minority elder populations view the health care system (Moreno-John et al., 2004), access or interact with that same system (Dunlop, Manheim, Song, & Chang, 2002; Szczepura, 2005), receive competent help from that system (Brach & Fraser, 2000; Bruce, Fries, & Murtagh, 2007), and experience that system (Cook, Kosoko-Lasaki, & O'Brien, 2005; Gary, Narayan, Gregg, Beckles, & Saaddine, 2003). It also has a strong influence on how the system views the minority group and its needs.

Studies of aging processes in disparate populations have revealed much about patterns of behavior that foster successful aging and those that exacerbate morbidity and mortality risks. Lee (1987) and Witten (2008) expand on theories of aging, as derived from and applied to gay and transgender populations. Members of sexual and gender minorities—LGBT persons—represent a newly visible minority population of elderly persons. Quam (2005) estimates that there are "between 1 and 3 million LGBT adults over the age of 65 [in the United States]. This group will continue to increase in size as the overall population of elders increases and as aging adults become more comfortable with their sexual orientation" (Quam, 2005, p. 287). The same will likely be the case with respect to elders who become more comfortably open about having been born with variations in sex development and being intersex identified. Estimation of the sizes of these communities is nontrivial (Boemer, 2002; Corliss, Shankle, & Moyer, 2007; Meyer, 2001) and will be discussed in detail in chapter 7. Nevertheless, sexuality, health, and human rights remain an uneasy area of discussion (Miller, 2001).

Sell and Becker (2001, p. 876) state that "one of the greatest threats to the health of lesbian, gay and bisexual (LGB) Americans is the lack of scientific information about their health." However, this work and the work of others in this area, including Quam (2005), do not focus on the presence of transgender and intersex-identified persons within LGBT communities, and both groups remain greatly underrepresented in health research. Gay men have received the most research attention of any group within the LGBT population. Lesbians and bisexual women are significantly less likely to be included in scientific research literature than are gay or bisexual men (Lee & Crawford, 2007; Makadon, 2006), and both lesbians and bisexual women continue to face significant health disparities relative to their heterosexual peers (Crawford, 2006; McNair, 2003). Health research regarding bisexual men and women is still limited, and few studies have included many participants older than age 60 years (e.g., Hidaka & Operario, 2007; M. Crawford, personal communication, August 2007).

Public health concerns related to LGBT communities have only recently been accepted as important (IOM, 2011; Sanders & Reinisch, 1999; Silvestre, 2001) and, consequently, are being increasingly researched (McMahon, 2003; Meyer & Northridge, 2007). These include HIV/AIDS (Emlet, 2006; Orel, Spence, & Steele, 2005; Ramirez-Valles, Kuhns, Campbell, & Diaz, 2010), lesbian health (Bradford, Ryan, Honnold, & Rothblum, 2001a; Bradford, White, Honnold, Ryan, & Rothblum, 2001b; Cochran & Mays, 2007), smoking (Gruskin et al., 2007; Stevens, Carlson, & Hinman, 2004), sexually transmitted infections (Heintz & Melendez, 2006; Staley, Hussey, Roe, Harcourt, & Roe, 2001), and substance abuse (Cochran, Peavy, & Robohm, 2007; Finnegan & McNally, 2002; SAMHSA, 2003;).

The health care needs of Canadian elder lesbians and gay men have received some research attention (Brotman et al., 2003; Daley, 2006), and elder transgender persons are beginning to be recognized in the United States and other nations (Cook-Daniels, 2006; Witten & Whittle, 2004). However, many areas have yet to be addressed by federal (Craft & Mulvey, 2001; Epstein, 2003; IOM, 2011) and state governments (Clark, Landers, Linde, & Sperber, 2001; Nemoto, Operario, Keatley, Nguyen, & Sugano, 2005). Despite the recent increased interest in LGBT health, elders of the LGBT community (IOM, 2011; Kimmel et al., 2006; Price, 2007) remain very much an invisible population (Shankle, Maxwell, Katzman, & Landers, 2003; Staley et al., 2001). Moreover, their health care, social, and economic needs continue to remain little researched and poorly understood.

EMERGENCE: COMING OUT AS LGBT AND ELDERLY

Throughout the Western world, the possibility of identifying oneself as an LGBT person ("being out") was unavailable to elderly persons when they were young. Globally, depending on the cultural rules of the country, public identification as LGBT or its cultural equivalent varies, as do the consequences of such identification. This is particularly true within the global transgender community. Nonetheless, faced with mid- to late-life struggles, many closeted or "under the radar" individuals are coming out and coming to terms with their true gender identity or sexual orientation (Hidaka & Operario, 2006; Hunter, 2005; Roback & Lothstein, 1986), even in the face of the cultural stigma associated with those identifications.

During the lifetimes of people who are now elderly in Western nations, most legal sanctions against homosexuality have been abolished, and same-sex sexual behavior has been depathologized by the mental health and health care professions (Fetner, 2005; Kidd & Witten, 2007a), although many religious judgments remain (Herek, 2002; Tozer & Hayes, 2004). This is crucially important, given the significance of spirituality in the aging process (Daaleman et al., 2004; Smith & Horne, 2007), often particularly for elderly transgender persons (Kidd & Witten, 2007b).

Bisexually identified elderly persons still experience substantial stigma and, as a group, are less visible than are either gay men or lesbian women (Chung, 2003; de Gruchy, 2007). Although some progress has been made during recent decades, the current cohort of bisexual elders came of age when bisexuality was regarded as an immature sexuality, rather than a legitimate, and often permanent, personal identity. This has likely influenced both the willingness of elderly persons who are bisexual to be out regarding sexual orientation and their attitudes toward health services and health research.

Most transgender elders did not have the opportunity to be publicly identified or to transition gender during adolescence or young adulthood, and some older persons are now coming out and seeking health services to facilitate gender transition. Gender transition has become somewhat more publicly acceptable. (MSNBC, Discovery Health Channel, and *The Oprah Winfrey Show* have all presented relatively honest treatments of challenges of transsexualism. A number of made-for-TV movies have addressed the same subject matter.) However, transition in later life is still relatively uncommon. The legal rights* of transgender-identified individuals also remain unprotected, save for a relatively small number of American states and a few countries worldwide (HRC 2011a; NGLTF, 2007; TranScience Longitudinal Aging Research Study, 2007). For example, discrimination in employment on the basis of gender identity is unlawful in 16 states and the District of Columbia at the time of this writing.

Persons born with variations in sex development (Consortium on Disorders of Sex Development, 2007), previously referred to as hermaphrodites, have traditionally been treated as having abnormalities needing correction regardless of

---

* One exception is the Matthew Shepard and James Byrd, Jr. Hate Crimes Prevention Act of 2009.

the consequences to sexual functioning and appropriateness to future gender identity (Creighton, 2001; Greenberg, 1998; Intersex Society of North America [ISNA], 2007), though these policies have been reassessed in recent years (Consortium on Disorders of Sex Development, 2007). Public understanding and acceptance of variations in sex development, and of intersex personal identification, improved dramatically during the 1990s, primarily because of the efforts of a few dedicated activists and educators (ISNA, 2007). However, persons who are now elderly grew up during an era when sex development was surrounded in shame and secrecy; very few elders are publicly intersex identified.

Transsexual, transgender, and cross-dressing persons, as well as those who are intersex identified, may be experiencing some lessening of stigma (Tucker & Potocky-Tripodi, 2006) with improved understanding of gender identity and sex development (Arber, Andersson, & Hoff, 2007) as human characteristics that can be conceptualized on a spectrum (Worthington, Savoy, Dillon, & Vernaglia, 2002), rather than in a strictly binary system. Some people self-identify as fully female or fully male, while others view their gender in some alternate or in-between way.* Similarly, prenatal sex development can produce infants with a fully female or fully male genital appearance or can produce variations not congruent with either "majority" sexual anatomy. However, misunderstandings (Kon, 2006) still occur, and legal recognition and protections remain incomplete (Lombardi, Wilchins, Priestling, & Malouf, 2001; Witten & Eyler, 1999).

PALLIATIVE CARE AND END-OF-LIFE CHALLENGES

Some form of end-of-life/palliative care will be needed for nearly every individual (Hermann & Cooney, 2011; Kolsky, 2008; Lunney et al., 2003; Norton, Hobson, & Hulm, 2010; Richie & Wieland, 2007). Very little has been written about palliative care and end-of-life challenges for the LGBT population. Almack, Seymour, and Bellamy (2010) explore the role of sexual orientation of end-of-life concerns and bereavement for GLB elders. Transgender elders (Redman, 2011; Witten, 2011) express great concern about how they will be treated, whether they will be respected or abused.

---

* The fifth edition of the *Diagnostic and Statistical Manual of Mental Disorders* (DSM-5) is in preparation at this writing. Revisions regarding "gender dysphoria" in children and adults will likely occur (DSM5.org).

I would hate to be in a nursing home where people know my past (and I can't imagine they won't because I worked in a nursing home as a student and know how medical info was not totally confidential) and being treated like I was trans, rather than just a regular woman as I am now. It would be like the final insult after a life of blending. I have joked (not seriously) about ending my life before such a thing happens but it really does depress me to think of such a situation if I allow myself to think about it. (Witten, 2011)

Many, when asked about their later life care plans, responded with very disturbing statements (Witten, 2011):

I plan on committing suicide at 60 or earlier.

If I become incapacitated, I plan to end my life.

Other transgender concerns are discussed in Witten (2008, 2009) and Witten and Whittle (2004). Members of the LGBTI/DSD population also express concerns about how they will be viewed and subsequently treated (Corbett, 2007; Fish, 2010; Friend, 1987; Grant, 2001; Hatzenbuehler et al., 2010; Knochel, Quam, & Crogham, 2011; Rondahl, 2007; Ward, Vass, Aggarwal, Garfield, & Cybyk, 2005). Very little is written about family needs after the death of a LGBTI/DSD-identified loved one. Issues around bereavement and support remain unstudied (Green & Grant, 2008; Witten, 2009). Rurality also plays a factor in LGBT fears for elder treatment (Jackson, Johnson, & Roberts, 2008; Willging, Salvador, & Kano, 2006). Research on late-life, hospice, and end-of-life care for prisoners who are LGBTI/DSD identified is marginal (Linder, Enders, Craig, Richardson, & Meyers, 2002; MacKinlay, 2006). Similarly, needs around dementia care for the LGBTI/DSD-identified population is lacking (Murray & Boyd, 2009). Respondents to the Witten (2011) survey routinely express fears around developing dementia and of not being treated with respect. "[I am afraid of] developing dementia and referring to myself in the wrong terms." More profound is the following respondent comment from the same survey:

[I am afraid of] being trapped in a nursing home and forced to live on an institutional schedule with bigoted attendants who try to treat me like a woman or harass me about my gender, out me to other residents. Especially if that takes place in a conservative state where fellow residents in the nursing home would also jump on the bigotry bandwagon. Terror, degradation and imprisonment. I do not want to be institutionalized. I don't want to die in a hospital either. I hate hospitals. I have been treated so badly in them because of my gender and had so many medical mistakes than in any medical institution. I feel as if I am taking my life in my hands. It's so easy to make a fatal mistake with someone's treatment. I've had to deflect wrong prescriptions for medications I'm allergic to in EVERY hospitalization in my life. I'm just lucky I never wound up unconscious in a hospital. They get so scared and freaked out by the trans that they can't handle the conditions I'm there for, and they don't listen to my list of disabilities so often cause me serious harm expecting me to be physically normal. I do not trust institutions as far as I can throw them.

THE RESULTS OF STIGMA: VIOLENCE AND ABUSE

Violence and victimization within the LGBT communities, and against persons who are LGBT identified, are problems that have only recently come to public health attention. Statistics on hate crime can be found in Los Angeles County Commission on Human Relations (2005); National Coalition of Anti-Violence Programs (2005, 2011); Herek (2009); Herek, Gillis, Cogan, and Glunt (1997); Herek, Cogan, and Gillis (2002); and other sources. The Matthew Shepard and James Byrd, Jr. Hate Crimes Prevention Act (HCPA), signed into law by President Barack Obama on October 28, 2009, gave the U.S. Department of Justice the authority to investigate and prosecute violent crimes involving bias based on gender, gender identity, and sexual orientation and required the FBI to keep statistics regarding these crimes (Human Rights Campaign, 2011b),

Violence directed toward gay men remains widespread (Bartlett, 2007; Parrott & Zeichner, 2006); hate crimes based on sexual orientation also occur against lesbians and bisexual women and men, although data collection has been less thorough (Blackwell, 2008). Fernandez (1998), Lombardi et al. (2001), and Kidd and Witten (2007a) provide information regarding hate crimes, violence, and abuse against the transgender community, while Herek (2002) and Herek et al. (1997) discuss hate crimes and violence against the lesbian, gay, and bisexual communities. Additional resources are available through the Human Rights Campaign (2011c). Violence and abuse can take on complex forms likely to be overlooked or to go unreported because of the multiple layers of stigma associated with them (Brown, 2007). Domestic violence also occurs within same-sex relationships; Burke, Jordan, and Owen (2002) provide a multinational comparison in that regard.

Estimating actual rates of violence against elderly persons who are members of sexual and gender minorities is often hampered by both traditional gerontological reasons for nonreport (e.g., dependence on the perpetrator, family loyalty)

and LGBT-related stigma and feared or actual consequences to the victim if a report is made (Cook-Daniels, 2006; Otis, 2007). In addition, many members of LGBT communities experience abuse early on and across the life span (D'Augelli, 2002; Paul et al., 2002), leading to a decreased desire to discuss experiences of abuse or violence, particularly if earlier responses to victimization have been inadequate or demeaning.

The study of abuse and violence against LGBT communities, from an international perspective, is just beginning, although anecdotal reports indicate that, in some countries, prevalence of these crimes is very high. Throughout much of the world, members of LGBT communities are aware that they are vulnerable to "hate crime" attacks (Poteat & Espelage, 2007; Rooke, 2007) and often restrict their lives accordingly. In a Dutch population study, Bakker et al. (2006) report on the physical and mental health consequences of the cultural stress and potential hate-crime victimization associated with sexual orientation.

Perception of violence and abuse is culturally influenced, with regard to both perpetration (whether it is acceptable to commit hate crimes against members of certain groups) and victimization (the personal meaning of having been harmed). Seelau and Setlaw (2005) address gender role stereotypes and perceptions of gay and lesbian domestic violence, while Heinz and Melendez (2006) address HIV/STD risk and partner violence. Witten (2008) examines perceptions of transgender violence and hate crimes and how they mediate use of the health care system, such as whether the victim seeks assistance. Witten and Whittle (2004) provide some examples regarding abuse of sexual and gender minority persons by the health care system, from an international perspective. Kidd and Witten (2007b) examine the effects of faith, religiosity, and spirituality on perceptions of victimization by members of the LGBT communities. The literature barely mentions the cohort effects within the LGBT populations. Steinberg, Brooks, and Remtulla (2003) discuss youth hate crimes; however, little systematically collected or robust information about the effects on the biological and psychosocial development on younger persons (Huebner, Rebchook, & Kegeles, 2004; Witten, 2003) suffering from such crimes is currently available.

MAJORITY PERCEPTION OF LGBT PERSONS, STIGMA, AND RESILIENCY

Non-Western nations and cultures treat persons who are members of sexual and gender minorities in various ways. Some cultures have particular recognition or roles for persons who have certain intersex conditions, such as the huevodoce ("eggs at twelve") of the Dominican Republic. However, many areas of the world still seek to suppress (Kidd & Witten, 2007a; NGLTF, 2007) or "normalize" (Kon, 2006) persons whose sex development, gender identity, or sexual orientation is outside majority norms, and these efforts were much more pervasive and virulent during the years when people who are now elderly were in their youth. Therefore, the status of LGBT elders is often difficult to research effectively. Additional information is needed regarding persons who are intersex, transgender, or bisexually identified and are now aged.

Many LGBT elders have difficulty seeking or accepting assistance through the helping professions because of their own, or their peers', past negative experiences (D'Augelli & Grossman, 2001; Witten, 2008). The combination of health services providers' normative ageism, membership in a sexual or gender minority group, and often other minority status (based on economic level, racial identification, etc.) can elevate the potential for health disparity to a higher level of complexity and difficulty (Mays et al., 2002). Additional outcomes health research is needed, as are efforts to reduce these negative societal dynamics and their effects on vulnerable elders.

"Multiple jeopardy" (Miksad et al., 2006; Thompson, 2006) for persons who are members of sexual and gender minority groups refers to the potential for misperception and perhaps multiple discrimination due to nontraditional self-identifications or lack of identification with more widely recognized societal groups. For example, a transgender person who has male genital anatomy and who has sex with men but does not self-identify as a gay man may be more marginalized and, in some ways, at higher risk for poor health outcomes, than a gay man who is not transgender. The complexity of transgender medical care for transgender persons, and lack of research in this area, may amplify these challenges (Ettner, Mostrey, & Eyler, 2007; Moffatt, 2006). More complex scenarios can also occur. A case was recently reported (Miksad et al., 2006) in which an elderly male-to-female transsexual person developed prostate cancer 41 years after beginning the feminization process with supplemental hormones.

Multiple jeopardy can take other forms, as well. For example, older LGBT persons who are developmentally disabled or mentally challenged because of some other cause, and persons who are members of disadvantaged racial or ethnic minorities, often face a constellation of related difficulties (Allen, 2003). Bisexual Latino men who are older and HIV positive may face greater risks of neglect and victimization than their younger peers (Muñoz-Laboy & Dodge, 2007). Homeless elder members of the LGBT community are clearly at risk for a variety of poor outcomes (O'Connell, 2004; Wright et al., 2004).

Similar results are found in other countries. For example, Pirner (2005) discusses the multifaceted marginalization of being older, a woman, and a visible minority in Canada, while Kabir et al. (1998) address the "invisible elderly" in Bangladesh. The increasing income inequality (Prus, 2000) for older persons in many countries compounds the depth of suffering elders facing multiple stigmatization experience.

CHALLENGES FOR THE HEALTH AND SERVICE PROFESSIONS

Despite the stereotypes regarding old age, the need for intimacy and sexual expression for elderly persons is recognized in numerous environments, from private life to nursing homes and care facilities to palliative care settings, jails and prisons (Rikard & Rosenberg, 2007), and homes for developmentally disabled and brain-injured persons (Marshall & Katz, 2002). Discussing sexuality in the context of sexual or gender minority status can be more complex than in heteronormative culture (Corbett, 2007). Variation in sex development and the possibility of intersex identity, gender identity and its congruence (or lack or congruence) with genital anatomy, sexual orientation, and partner choice can all be significant to the individual, and usual terminology may be insufficient, such as on clinical intake forms. For example, an older person who is male-to-female transgender, and who has not had any gender confirmation surgery, may self-identify as female and heterosexual, although her male genital anatomy and long-term relationship with a male partner may cause her to be regarded as an unusual gay man by the service providers involved in her care. Although a thorough discussion of some of these concerns appears later in this book, a general principle to follow is that the personal identity and individual needs of the elderly person should receive primary consideration (Kertzner, 2001; Witten, 2004).

Outreach to LGBT persons who are multiply marginalized, for purposes of health and community service or health research, is difficult, because of past experiences of judgment or victimization and the need for protection from the possibility of further abuse. However, although obstacles clearly exist (States, Susman, Riquelme, Godwin, & Greer, 2007; Steen et al., 2006), it is nevertheless important that efforts be made (Franks, 2004; Kehoe, 1989; Slusher, Mayer, & Dunkle, 1996). Older adults should not have to suffer because of the legacy of discrimination and persecution that characterized their earlier lives.

Socioeconomic status and educational attainment also influence the ability of older LGBT-identified persons to find and access appropriate services, and technological availability can be crucial for service organizations. Many elders are not "out" with regard to their self-identification and personal life and would be open to victimization if personal information were publicized. Service organizations need secure population-based, culturally relevant methods to electronically communicate material that, in the wrong hands, could result in problems for the client or patient. Furthermore, lack of internet access and digital capability can impede provision of treatment to distant locations where limited treatment resources are available, such as by telemedicine or electronic consultation, and can inhibit gathering important information about population needs. The research literature regarding telemedicine and tele–mental health care for LGBT elders is currently limited. Low literacy among certain LGBT subpopulations can further obstruct quality health care delivery (Baker et al., 2007; Sudore et al., 2006).

In addition to the difficulties in health service provision or access faced by many older members of LGBT communities, persons in some subgroups who are even more marginalized—sometimes referred to as "invisible" or "erased" (Young & Meyer, 2005)—face even greater obstacles. Health service research is also compromised by these barriers, because of inadequate definitions in study protocols, definitional inaccuracy, and misdirected focus (Bradford et al., 2001b). Concerns have been raised regarding the most invisible minorities within the LGBT elderly population, such as persons who are intersex identified and older or, concurrently, members of other disadvantaged groups (Adams, Horn, & Bader, 2006). Atdjian and Vega (2005) discuss health disparities by race and ethnicity in mental health treatment, while Ayala and Coleman (2000) discuss predictors of depression among lesbian women. It is likely that age, race, and membership in the LGBT community may make the development of clinical depression more likely, and treatment outcomes may be less favorable. Similar concerns can be raised regarding treatments for conditions such as coronary bypass surgery (Brister et al., 2007), arthritis treatment (Bruce et al., 2007), HIV/AIDS treatment (Clements-Nolle, Marx, Guzman, & Katz, 2001), and substance abuse treatment (Cochran & Cauce, 2006; Cochran et al., 2002, 2007; Corliss et al., 2006).

Generational differences within the LGBT community generally have not benefited elder members of this population. Gay and lesbian community centers have traditionally focused on concerns of younger members, such as coming out, forming relationships, learning HIV prevention and negotiation skills, and, during the last decade, parenting. Elder groups and multigenerational activities are few. The AIDS crisis has also given many communities of urban gay men both a sense of foreshortened future and a lack of usual, long-term, and multigenerational perspective. Transgender organizations often emphasize the gender transition process, which is most commonly undertaken in early or middle adulthood, more recently in adolescence, rather than the concerns of older persons, many of whom transitioned decades ago (Witten, 2004). The secrecy that elderly persons who are transgender or intersex identified maintain has often not fostered development of a long-term perspective, which would be beneficial in later years (Witten 2003, 2008).

Knowledge gained from clinical and social science research highlights current informational deficits and avenues for further exploration. As some data have become available regarding older sexual and gender minorities in Western nations, the need for cultural and health research in other parts of the world has become more apparent.

RESEARCH ON LGBT AGING

Understanding the complex, multifaceted dynamics of LGBT communities requires both qualitative (e.g., Butler & Hope, 1999; McBride & Lewis, 2004) and quantitative (Johnson, 2003) data. In particular, if we are to understand the aging process, its perceptions (Rooke, 2007; Seelau & Seelau, 2005) and expectations (Sarkisian et al., 2002), and the needs of the elders of this population, we must make an effort to reach out to elderly persons and to engage them in the research process so that their life experience can benefit others in the LGBT population. Such data are not sufficiently available, particularly for transgender, bisexual, and intersex-identified elders, so that reasonable planning and policy can be undertaken and developed on behalf of those communities. While a more general discussion of LGBT medicine and public health concerns has taken place for years, little research literature focuses on the needs of older persons in the LGBT communities, though there has been some recent improvement in that regard (Healthy People 2020; Institute of Medicine, 2011; Landers, Mimiaga, & Krinsky, 2010; MMMI, 2010; Smith et al., 2010). Moreover, the conflation of sex and gender (Boyle, Smith, & Liao, 2005; Heaphy, 2007) and the definitions of these concepts within a binary system (Greenberg, 1998; Witten, 2005) perpetuate the invisibility of many individuals who identify as members of the LGBT population (Belongia & Witten, 2006) and reduces appropriate health service access for members of these populations.

Despite these difficulties, in recent years, larger numbers of older LGBT persons have come out. It has become clear that most have the same need for health and social services as their majority-identified peers. Unfortunately, they experience this need in the context of insufficient support from within the LGBT community and lack of familiarity with their life experience and health concerns from health and social service professionals.

CONCLUSION

One of the first major attempts to address the public policy concerns affecting LGBT elders was the National Gay and Lesbian Task Force report *Outing Age* (Cahill et al., 2000). More recently, challenges of aging in the LGBT population have been discussed in the IOM report (2011). In both reports, the authors have defined a number of critical concerns regarding aging for LGBT elders. (Intersex/DSD-identified persons were not yet included in discussion of sexual and gender minority concerns.) At the time of this writing, many of the challenges in both reports remain unaddressed (Corliss et al., 2007). However, much new research and literature have appeared regarding aging and the experiences of the LGBT-identified persons and populations, although data are still lacking in many respects.

It is hoped that the current generation of health and social service clinicians and researchers will accept the limitations of the current literature and recognize that these omissions are an outgrowth of generations of discrimination—in many respects, active persecution—against members of sexual and gender minorities, yet respect the resilience with which many elders of these communities have lived their lives. It is also to hoped that each passing year will witness more successful efforts at redressing errors of the past and improving prospects for a future filled with respect and caring for elderly persons, regardless of life path or minority status.

REFERENCES

Abendstern, M., Hughes, J., Clarkson, P., Sutcliffe, C., & Challis, D. (2011). The pursuit of integration in the assessment of older people with health and social care needs. *British Journal of Social Work, 41*, 467–485.

Acierno, R., Hernandez, M. A., Amstadter, A. B., Resnick, H. S., Steve, K., Muzzy, W., & Kilpatrick, D. G. (2010). Prevalence and correlates of emotional, physical, sexual, and financial abuse and potential neglect in the United States: The National Elder Mistreatment Study. *American Journal of Public Health, 100*, 292–297.

Adams, C. E., Horn, K., & Bader, J. (2006). Hispanic access to hospice services in a predominantly Hispanic community. *American Journal of Hospice and Palliative Care, 23*, 9–16.

Adams, J. M., & White, M. (2004). Biological ageing: A fundamental, biological link between socio-economic status and health? *European Journal of Public Health, 14,* 331–334.

Adelman, M. (1987). *Long time passing: Lives of older lesbians.* Boston: Alyson.

Agabiti, N., Picciotto, S., Cesaroni, G., Bisanti, L., Forastiere, F., Onorati, R., . . . Perucci, C. A. (2007). The influence of socioeconomic status on utilization and outcomes of elective total hip replacement: A multicity population-based longitudinal study. *International Journal for Quality in Health Care, 19*(1), 37–44.

Agency for Healthcare Research and Quality. (2005). *2004 National healthcare disparities report* (AHRQ Publication No. 05-0014). Rockville, MD: Author.

Agency for Healthcare Research and Quality. (2006). *National healthcare disparities report.* (AHRQ Publication No. 06-0017). Rockville, MD: Author. Retrieved from ahrq.gov/qual/nhdr05/nhdr05.htm

Ahmad, W., & Bradby, H. (2008). Ethnicity and health: Key themes in a developing field. *Current Sociology, 56,* 47–56.

AIDS Alert. (2004). Special report: The aging AIDS epidemic. More normal lifespans present next hurdle: Experts discuss longevity with HIV infection. *AIDS Alert, 19*(9), 101–102.

Aikins, A. D., & Marks, D. F. (2007). Health, disease and healthcare in Africa. *Journal of Health Psychology, 12,* 387–402.

Ajrouch, K. J., Blandon, A. Y., & Antonucci, T. C. (2005). Social networks among men and women: The effects of age and socioeconomic status. *Journal of Gerontology, Series B, Psychological Sciences and Social Sciences, 60B*(6), 5311–5317.

Alexander, R., & Meshelemia, J. C. A. (2010). Gender identity disorders in prisons: What are the legal implications for prison mental health professionals and administrators. *Prison Journal, 90,* 269–287.

Allen, J. D. (2003). *Gay, lesbian, bisexual, and transgender people with developmental disabilities and mental retardation: Stories of the Rainbow Support Group.* Binghamton, NY: Haworth Press.

Almack, K., Seymour, J., & Bellamy, G. (2010). Exploring the impact of sexual orientation on experiences and concerns about end of life care and on bereavement for lesbian, gay and bisexual older people. *Sociology, 44,* 908–924.

Alvarado, B. E., Zunzunegui, M. V., Beland, F., Sicotte, M., & Tellechea, L. (2007). Social and gender inequalities in depressive symptoms among urban older adults of Latin America and the Caribbean. *Journal of Gerontology, Series B, Psychological Sciences and Social Sciences, 60B*(4), S226–S237.

Alwin, D. F., & Wray, L. A. (2005). Life-span developmental perspective on social status and health [Special issue 2]. *Journal of Gerontology, Series B, Psychological Sciences and Social Sciences, 60B,* 7–14.

Anderson, J. I., Patterson, A. N., Temple, H. J., & Inglehart, M. R. (2009). Lesbian, gay, bisexual and transgender (LGBT) issues in dental school environments: Dental student leaders' perceptions. *Journal of Dental Education, 73,* 105–118.

Anderson, N. B., Bulatao, R. A., & Cohen, B. (2004). *Critical perspectives on racial and ethnic differences in health in late life.* Washington, DC: National Academy Press.

Angel, J. L., & Angel, R. J. (2006). Minority group status and healthful aging: Social structure still matters. *American Journal of Public Health*, 96, 1152–1159.

Angel, J. L., Jimenez, M. A., & Angel, R. J. (2007). The economic consequences of widowhood for older minority women. *Gerontologist*, 47(2), 224–234.

Angus, J., & Reeve, P. (2006). Ageism: A threat to "aging well" in the 21st century. *Journal of Applied Gerontology*, 25, 137–152.

Arber, S., Abdersson, L., & Hoff, A. (2007). Changing approaches to gender and aging: Introduction. *Current Sociology*, 55, 147–153.

Aronheim, J. C. (1992). *Handbook of prescribing medications for geriatric patients*. New York: Little, Brown.

Aspinall, P. J., & Jacobson, B. (2007). Why poor quality of ethnicity data should not preclude its use for identifying disparities in health and healthcare. *Quality and Safety in Healthcare*, 16, 176–180.

Atdjian, S., & Vega, W. A. (2005). Disparities in mental health treatment in U.S. racial and ethnic minority groups: Implications for psychiatrists. *Psychiatric Services*, 56, 1600–1602.

Avison, W. R., & Davies, L. (2005). Family structure, gender, and health in the context of the life course. *Journal of Gerontology, Series B, Psychological Sciences and Social Sciences*, 60B, S113–S116.

Ayala, J., & Coleman, H. (2000). Predictors of depression among lesbian women. *Journal of Lesbian Studies*, 4(3), 71–86.

Baker, D. W., Wolf, M. S., Feinglass, J., Thompson, J. A., Gazmararian, J. A., & Huang, J. (2007). Health literacy and mortality among elderly persons. *Archives of Internal Medicine*, 167(14), 1503–1509.

Bakker, F. C., Sandfort, T. G., Vanwesenbeeck, I., van Lindert, H., & Westert, G. P. (2006). Do homosexual persons use healthcare services more frequently than heterosexual persons: Findings from a Dutch population study. *Social Science and Medicine*, 63(8), 2022–2030.

Balsam, K. F., Lehavot, K., Beadnell, B., & Circo, E. (2010). Childhood abuse and mental health indicators among ethnically diverse lesbian, gay and bisexual adults. *Journal of Consulting Clinical Psychology*, 78(4), 459–468.

Bartlett, P. (2007). Killing gay men, 1976–2001. *British Journal of Criminology*, 47, 573–595.

Becker, C., Crow, S., Toman, J., Lipton, C., McMahon, D. J., Macaulay, W., & Siris, E. (2006). Characteristics of elderly patients admitted to an urban tertiary care hospital with osteoporotic fractures: Correlations with risk factors, fracture type, gender and ethnicity. *Osteoporosis International*, 17(3), 410–416.

Becker, G., Gates, R. A., & Newson, E. (2004). Self-care among chronically ill African Americans: Culture, health disparities, and health insurance status. *American Journal of Public Health*, 94, 2066–2073.

Belongia, L., & Witten, T. M. (2006). We don't have that kind of client here: Institutionalized bias against and resistance to transgender and intersex aging research and training in elder care facilities. White paper download. Retrieved from www.transcience.org

Bengtsson, T., & Lindstrom, M. (2000). Childhood misery and disease in later life: The effects on mortality in old age of hazards experienced in early life, southern Sweden, 1760–1894. *Population Studies, 54*, 263–277.

Birren, J. (Ed.). (2007). *The encyclopedia of gerontology* (2nd ed.). Amsterdam, the Netherlands: Academic Press.

Blackwell, C. W. (2008). Registered nurses' attitudes toward the protection of gays and lesbians in the workplace. *Journal of Transcultural Nursing, 19*, 347–353.

Boehmer, U. (2002). Twenty years of public health research: Inclusion of lesbian, gay, bisexual and transgender populations. *American Journal of Public Health, 92*, 1125–1130.

Bonomi, A. E., Anderson, M. L., Reid, R. J., Carrell, D., Fishman, P. A., Rivara, F. P., & Thompson, R. S. (2007). Intimate partner violence in older women. *Gerontologist, 47*(1), 34–41.

Borrell, C., Fernandez, E., Schiaffino, A., Benach, J., Rajmil, L., Villalbí, J. R., & Segura, A. (2001). Social class inequalities in the use of and access to health services in Catalonia, Spain: What is the influence of supplemental private health insurance? *International Journal for Quality in Health Care, 13*, 117–125.

Bowling, A. (2007). Aspirations for older age in the 21st century: What is successful aging? *International Journal of Aging and Human Development, 64*(3), 263–297.

Boyle, M. E., Smith, S., & Liao, L.-M. (2005). Adult genital surgery for intersex: A solution to what problem? *Journal of Health Psychology, 10*, 573–584.

Brach, C., & Fraser, I. (2000). Can cultural competency reduce racial and ethnic health disparities? A review and conceptual model. *Medical Care Research and Review, 57*, 181–217.

Bradford, J., Ryan, C., Honnold, J., & Rothblum, E. (2001a). Expanding the research infrastructure for lesbian health. *American Journal of Public Health, 91*, 1029–1032.

Bradford, J., White, J., Honnold, J., Ryan, C., & Rothblum, E. (2001b). Improving the accuracy of identifying lesbians for telephone surveys about health. *Women's Health Issues, 11*(2), 126–137.

Braveman, P., & Barclay, C. (2009). Health disparities beginning in childhood: A life-course perspective. *Pediatrics, 124*, S163–S175.

Brinkmann, L., Schuetzmann, K., & Richter-Appelt, H. (2007). Gender assignment and medical history of individuals with different forms of intersexuality: Evaluation of medical records and the patients' perspective. *Journal of Sexual Medicine, 4*(4 Pt. 1), 964–980.

Brister, S. J., Hamdulay, Z., Verma, S., Maganti, M., & Buchanan, M. R. (2007). Ethnic diversity: South Asian ethnicity is associated with increased coronary artery bypass grafting mortality. *Journal of Thoracic and Cardiovascular Surgery, 133*, 150–154.

Brotman, S., Ryan, B., Collins, S., Chamberland, L., Cormier, R., Julien, D., . . . Richard, B. (2007). Coming out to care: Caregivers of gay and lesbian seniors in Canada. *Gerontologist, 47*, 490–503.

Brotman, S., Ryan, B., & Cormier, R. (2003). The health and social service needs of gay and lesbian elders and their families in Canada. *Gerontologist, 43*, 192.

Brown, D. R., & Sankar, A. (1998). HIV/AIDS and aging minority populations. *Research on Aging, 20*, 865–884.

Brown, N. (2007). Stories from outside the frame: Intimate partner abuse in sexual-minority women's relationships with transsexual men. *Feminism Psychology, 17*, 373–393.

Bruce, B., Fries, J. F., & Murtagh, K. N. (2007). Health status disparities in ethnic minority patients with rheumatoid arthritis: A cross-sectional study. *Journal of Rheumatology, 34*(7), 1475–1479.

Burke, T. W., Jordan, M. L., & Owen, S. S. (2002). Cross-national comparison of gay and lesbian domestic violence. *Journal of Contemporary Criminal Justice, 18*(3), 231–257.

Butler, S. S., & Hope, B. (1999). Health and well-being for late middle-aged and old lesbians in a rural area. *Journal of Gay and Lesbian Social Services, 9*(4), 27–46.

Buzgová, R., & Ivanová, K. (2009). Elder abuse and mistreatment in residential facilities. *Nursing Ethics, 16*, 110–125.

Byrd, L., Fletcher, A., & Menifield, C. (2007). Disparities in health care: Minority elders at risk. *ABNF Journal, 18*(2), 51–55.

Cahill, S., South, K., & Spade, J. (2000). *Outing aging: Report of the NGLTF Task Force on Aging.* Washington, DC: National Gay and Lesbian Task Force. Retrieved from www.ngltf.org

Calvin, J. E., Roe, M. T., Chen, A. Y., Mehta, R. H., Brogan, G. X., DeLong, E. R., . . . Peterson, E. D. (2006). Insurance coverage and care of patients with non-ST-segment elevation acute coronary syndromes. *Annals of Internal Medicine, 145*(10), 739–748.

Carmel, S., Morse, C. A., & Torres-Gill, F. M. (Eds.). (2007). *Lessons on aging from three nations: Vol. 1. The art of aging well.* Amityville, NY: Baywood Publishing.

Carrasco-Garrido, P., Gil De Miguel, A., Hernández Barreram, V., & Jiménez-Garcia, R. (2007). Health profiles, lifestyles and use of health resources by the immigrant population resident in Spain. *European Journal of Public Health.* doi:10.1093/eurpub/ckl279.

Carvalho de Naronha, J., & Rosa, M. L. G. (1999). Country report. Quality of health care: Growing awareness in Brazil. *International Journal for Quality in Health Care, 11*, 437–441.

Centers for Disease Control and Prevention. (2003). Public health and aging: Trends in aging, United States and worldwide. *JAMA, 289*, 1371.

Chin, M. H., Walters, A. E., Cook, S. C., & Huang, E. S. (2007). Interventions to reduce racial and ethnic disparities in health care. *Medical Care Research Review, 64*, 7S–28S.

Chung, Y. B. (2003). Ethical and professional issues in career assessment with lesbian, gay, and bisexual persons. *Journal of Career Assessment, 11*, 96–112.

Ciceklioglu, M., Soyer, M. T., & Öcek, Z. (2005). Factors associated with the utilization and content of prenatal care in a western urban district of Turkey. *International Journal for Quality in Health Care, 17*, 533–539.

Cigolle, C. T., Langa, K. M., Kabeto, M. U., Tian, Z., & Blaum, C. S. (2007). Geriatric conditions and disability: The Health and Retirement Study. *Annals of Internal Medicine, 147,* 156–164.

Clark, E. J. (2006). Preparing for the aging boom. *NASW News, 51*(3), 3.

Clark, M. E., Landers, S., Linde, R., & Sperber, J. (2001). The GLBT Health Access Project: A state-funded effort to improve access to care. *American Journal of Public Health, 91,* 895–896.

Clements-Nolle, K., Marx, R., Guzman, R., & Katz, M. (2001). HIV prevalence, risk, behaviors, health care use, and mental health status of transgender persons: Implications for public health intervention. *American Journal of Public Health, 91*(6), 915–921.

Clover, D. (2006). Overcoming barriers for older gay men in the use of health services: A qualitative study of growing older, sexuality and health. *Health Education Journal, 65,* 41–52.

Cochran, B. N., & Cauce, A. M. (2006). Characteristics of lesbian, gay, bisexual and transgender individuals entering substance abuse treatment. *Journal of Substance Abuse Treatment, 30*(2), 135–146.

Cochran, B. N., Peavy, K. M., & Robohm, J. S. (2007). Do specialized services exist for LGBT individuals seeking treatment for substance misuse? A study of available treatment programs. *Substance Use and Misuse, 42*(1), 161–176.

Cochran, B. N., Stewart, A. J., Ginzler, J. A., & Cauce, A. M. (2002). Challenges faced by homeless sexual minorities: Comparison of gay, lesbian, bisexual and transgender homeless adolescents with their heterosexual counterparts. *American Journal Public Health, 92,* 773–777.

Cochran, S. D., & Mays, V. M. (2007). Physical health complaints among lesbians, gay men, and bisexual and homosexually experienced heterosexual individuals: Results from the California Quality of Life Survey. *American Journal of Public Health, 97*(6). doi:10.2105/AJPH.2006.087254.

Cocker, T. R., Austin, S. B., & Schuster, M. A. (2010). The health and care of lesbian, gay, and bisexual adolescents. *Annual Reviews of Public Health, 31,* 457–477.

Committee on Population (CPOP). (2004). *Understanding racial and ethnic differences in health in late life: A research agenda.* Washington, DC: National Academies Press.

Concannon, L. (2009). Developing inclusive health and social care policies for older LGBT citizens. *British Journal of Social Work, 39,* 403–417.

Conrad, K. J., Iris, M., Ridings, J. W., Langley, K., & Anetzberger, G. J. Self-report measure of psychological abuse of older adults. *Gerontologist, 51,* 354–366.

Conron, K. J., Mimiaga, M. J., & Landers, S. J. (2010). A population-based study of sexual orientation identity and gender differences in adult health. *American Journal of Public Health, 100,* 1953–1960.

Consortium on Disorders of Sex Development. (2007). Retrieved from www.dsdguidelines.org

Cook, C. T., Kosoko-Lasaki, O., & O'Brien, R. (2005). Satisfaction with and perceived cultural competency of healthcare providers: The minority experience. *Journal of the National Medical Association, 97*(8), 1078–1087.

Cook-Daniels, L. (2006). Transaging. In D. Kimmel, T. Rose, & S. David (Eds.), *Lesbian, gay, bisexual and transgender aging: Research and clinical perspectives* (pp. 290–335). New York: Columbia University Press.

Cooper, C., Selwood, A., & Livingston, G. (2008). The prevalence of elder abuse and neglect: A systematic review. *Age Ageing, 37,* 151–160.

Copeland, C. (2007). Increasing debt risk of those aged 55 or old, 1992–2004. *Public Policy and Aging Report, 17*(2), 20–23.

Coppin, A. K., Ferrucci, L., Lauretani, F., Phillips, C., Chang, M., Bandinelli, S., & Guralnik, J. M. (2006). Low socioeconomic status and disability in old age: Evidence from the InChianti Study for the mediating role of physiological impairments. *Journal of Gerontology, Series A, Biological Sciences and Medical Sciences,* 61A(1), 86–91.

Corbett, K. (2007). Lesbian women and gay men found that nurses often assumed they were heterosexual, which led to feelings of discomfort and insecurity. *Evidenced Based Nursing, 10,* 94. doi:10.1136/ebn.10.3.94.

Corliss, H. L., Grella, C. E., Mays, V. M., & Cochran, S. D. (2006). Drug use, drug severity and help-seeking behaviors of lesbian and bisexual women. *Journal of Womens Health (Larchmt), 15*(5), 556–568.

Corliss, H. L., Shankle, M. D., & Moyer, M. B. (2007). Research, curricula, and resources related to lesbian, gay, bisexual and transgender health in US schools of public health. *American Journal of Public Health, 97,* 1023–1027.

Costa, D. L. (2007). The economics and demography of aging. *Proceedings of the National Academy of Sciences of the United States of America, 104*(33), 13217–13218.

Craft, E. M., & Mulvey, K. P. (2001). Addressing lesbian, gay, bisexual and transgender issues from the inside: One federal agency's approach. *American Journal of Public Health, 91,* 889–891.

Crane, M., Byrne, K., Fu, R., Lipmann, B., Mirabelli, F., Rota-Bartelin, A., . . . Warnes, A. N. (2005). The causes of homelessness in later life: Findings from a 3-nation study. *Journal of Gerontology, Series B, Psychological Sciences and Social Sciences, 60*B, S152–S159.

Crato, C., Haase, L. W., Welsh, M. P., & Wasow, B. (2006). *Public policy in an older America: A Century Foundation guide to the issues.* New York: Century Foundation.

Crawford, M. (2006). *Transformations: Women, gender, and psychology.* New York: McGraw-Hill.

Creighton, S. (2001). Surgery for intersex. *Journal of the Royal Society of Medicine,* 94, 218–220.

Crew, K. D., Neugut, A. I., Wang, X., Jacobson, J. S., Grann, V. R., Raptis, G., & Hershman, D. L. (2007). Racial disparities in treatment and survival of male breast cancer. *Journal of Clinical Oncology, 25,* 1089–1098.

Crimmins, E. M. (2004). Trends in the health of the elderly. *Annual Review of Public Health, 25,* 79–98.

Crimmins, E. M., Kim, J. K., & Solé-Auró, A. (2011). Gender differences in health: Results from SHARE, ELSA and HRS. *European Journal of Public Health, 21,* 81–91.

Cronin, A., & King, A. (2010). Power, inequality and identification: Exploring diversity and intersectionality amongst older LGB adults. *Sociology, 44*, 876–892.

Crystal, S., Johnson, R. W., Harman, J., Sambamoorthi, U., & Kumar, R. (2000). Out-of-pocket healthcare costs among older Americans. *Journal of Gerontology, Series B, Psychological Sciences and Social Sciences, 55B*(1), S51–S62.

Cunha-Cruz, J., Hujoel, P. P., & Nadanovsky, P. (2007). Secular trends in socioeconomic disparities in edentulism: USA, 1972–2001. *Journal of Dental Research, 86*, 131–136.

Curry, L., & Jackson, J. (Eds.). (2003). *The science of inclusions: Recruiting and retaining racial and ethnic elders in health research*. Washington, DC: Gerontological Society of America.

Cutler, R. G., & Mattson, M. P. (2006). The adversities of aging. *Ageing Research Reviews, 5*(3), 221–238.

Daaleman, T. P., Perera, S., & Studenski, S. A. (2004). Religion, spirituality, and health status in geriatric outpatients. *Annals Family Medicine, 2*(1), 49–53.

Daley, A. (2006). Lesbian and gay health issues: OUTside of Canada's health policy. *Critical Social Policy, 26*, 794–816.

Dang, A., & Vianney, C. (2007). *Living in the margins: A national survey of lesbian, gay, bisexual and transgender Asian and Pacific Islander Americans*. New York: National Gay and Lesbian Task Force Policy Institute.

Danzon, M. (2009). Crossing cultures: The European regional approach to addressing the social determinants and health equity. *Global Health Promotion, 16*, 28–29.

Das, J., & Gertler, P. J. (2007). Variations in practice quality in five low-income countries: A conceptual overview. *Health Affairs, 26*(3), w296–w309.

D'Augelli, A. R. (2002). Mental health problems among lesbian, gay and bisexual youths ages 14 to 21. *Clinical Child Psychology and Psychiatry, 7*, 433–456.

D'Augelli, A. R., & Grossman, A. H. (2001). Disclosure of sexual orientation, victimization, and mental health among lesbian, gay, and bisexual older adults. *Journal of Interpersonal Violence, 16*(10), 1008–1102.

Davies, M., Harries, P., Cairns, D., Stanley, D., Gilhooly, M., Hilhooly, K., . . . Hennessy, C. (2011). Factors used in the detection of elder financial abuse: A judgement and decision-making study of social workers and their managers. *International Journal of Social Work, 54*, 404–420.

de Gruchy, J. (2007). Straight talking? *BMJ, 334*, 1167.

Depp, C. A., & Jeste, D. V. (2006). Definitions and predictors of successful aging: A comprehensive review of large quantitative studies. *American Journal of Geriatric Psychiatry, 14*, 6–120.

Disparity. (n.d.). In *Merriam-Webster online dictionary*. Retrieved from www.m-w.com/dictionary

Dobson, R. (2007). Report calls for urgent action on ageism in treating stroke patients. *BMJ, 334*, 607.

Dolan, T. A., Atchison, K., & Huynh, T. N. (2005). Access to dental care among older adults in the United States. *Journal of Dental Education, 69*, 961–974.

Dowd, J. J., & Bengtson, V. L. (1978). Aging in minority populations: An examination of the double jeopardy hypothesis. *Journal of Gerontology, 33*(3), 427–436.

Dowling, G. J., Weiss, S. R., & Condon, T. P. (2008). Drugs of abuse and the aging brain. *Neuropsychopharmacology, 33*(2), 209–218.

Dunlop, D. D., Manheim, L. M., Song, J., & Chang, R. W. (2002). Gender and ethnic/racial disparities in health care utilization among older adults. *Journal of Gerontology, Series B, Psychological Sciences and Social Sciences, 57B*, 221.

Dyer, C. B., Goodwin, J. S., Pickens-Pace, S., Burnett, J., & Kelly, P. A. (2007). Self-neglect among the elderly: A model based on more than 500 patients seen by a geriatric medicine team. *American Journal of Public Health, 97*(9), 1–6.

Eiras, D., & Richardson, L. (2007). Disparities in the treatment of acute chest pain. *Academic Emergency Medicine, 14*, S105–S106.

Emlet, C. A. (2006). "You're awfully old to have *this* disease": Experiences of stigma and ageism in adults 50 years and older living with HIV/AIDS. *Gerontologist, 46*, 781–790.

Epstein, S. (2003). Sexualizing governance and medicalizing identities: The emergence of "state-centered" LGBT health politics in the United States. *Sexualities, 6*, 131–171.

Ettinger, R. (2005). Oral health in aging societies: A global view. *Special Care Dentist, 25*(5), 225–226.

Ettner, R., Mostrey, S., & Eyler, A. E. (Eds.). (2007). *Principles of transgender medicine and surgery.* New York: Haworth Press.

Everard, K. M., Lach, H. W., Fisher, E. B., & Baum, M. C. (2000). Relationship of activity and social support to the functional health of older adults. *Journal of Gerontology, Series B, Psychological Sciences and Social Sciences, 55B*(4), S208–S212.

Feinglass, J., Lin, S., Thompson, J., Sudano, J., Dunloop, D., Song, J., & Baker, D. W. (2007). Baseline health, socioeconomic status, and 10-year mortality among older middle-aged Americans: Findings from the Health and Retirement Study, 1992–2002. *Journal of Gerontology, Series B, Psychological Sciences and Social Sciences, 62B*(4), S209–S217.

Fernandez, M. E. (1998, December 12). Death suit costs city $2.9 million; mother of transgendered man wins case. *Washington Post*, p. C01.

Fetner, T. (2005). Ex-gay rhetoric and the politics of sexuality: The Christian antigay/pro-family movement's "Truth in Love" ad campaign. *Journal of Homosexuality, 50*(1), 71–75.

Fikree, F. F., & Pasha, O. (2004). Role of gender in health disparity: The South Asian context. *BMJ, 328*, 823–826.

Finnegan, D. A., & McNally, E. B. (2002). *Counseling GLBT substance abusers: Dual identities.* Binghamton, NY: Haworth Press.

Fiscella, K., Franks, P., Gold, M. R., & Clancy, C. M. (2000). Inequality in quality: Addressing socioeconomic, racial, and ethnic disparities in health care. *JAMA, 283*, 2579–2584.

Fish, J. (2010). Conceptualising social exclusion and lesbian, gay, bisexual and transgender people: The implications for promoting equity in nursing policy and practice. *Journal of Research in Nursing, 15*, 303–312.

Fisher, B. S., & Regan, S. L. (2006). The extent and frequency of abuse in the lives of older women and their relationship with health outcomes. *Gerontologist, 46*(2), 200–209.

Flores, G., Olsen, L., & Tomany-Korman, S. C. (2005). Racial and ethnic disparities in early childhood health and health care. *Pediatrics, 115*, e183–e193.

Fontana, L., & Klein, S. (2007). Aging, adiposity, and calorie restriction. *JAMA, 297*, 986–994.

Franks, J. (2004). Sunset Pink Villa: A home for gay and lesbian elders. *Gerontologist, 44*, 856–857.

Fredriksen-Goldsen, K. I., & Muraco, A. (2010). Aging and sexual orientation: A 25-year review of the literature. *Research on Aging, 32*, 372–413.

Fried, L. P. (2000). Epidemiology of aging. *Epidemiologic Reviews, 22*(1), 95–106.

Friend, R. A. (1987). The individual and social psychology of aging: Clinical implications for lesbians and gay men. *Journal of Homosexuality, 14*(1–2), 307–331.

Fruhoff, G. A., & Mahoney, D. (Eds.). (2010). *Older GLBT family and community life.* New York: Routledge Press.

Fulmer, E. M. (1995). Challenging biases against families of older gays and lesbians. In G. C. Smith, S. S. Tobin, E. A. Robertson-Tchabo, & P. W. Power. (Eds.), *Strengthening aging families: Diversity in practice and policy.* Thousand Oaks, CA: Sage.

Gaines, J. S. (2007). Social correlates of psychological distress among adult African American males. *Journal of Black Studies, 37*, 827–858.

Gary, T. L., Narayan, K. M., Gregg, E. W., Beckles, G. L., & Saaddine, J. B. (2003). Racial/ethnic differences in the healthcare experience (coverage, utilization and satisfaction) of US adults with diabetes. *Ethnicity and Disease, 13*(1), 47–54.

Gay and Lesbian Medical Association (GLMA). (2000). *Healthy People 2010: Companion document for lesbian, gay, bisexual, and transgender (LGBT) health.* San Francisco: Author. Retrieved from www.glma.org

George, L. K. (2005). Socioeconomic status and health across the life course: Progress and prospects [Special issue 2]. *Journal of Gerontology, Series B, Psychological Sciences and Social Sciences, 60B*, 135–139.

Gfroerer, J., Penne, M., Pemberton, M., & Folsom, R. (2003). Substance abuse treatment need among older adults in 2020: The impact of the aging baby-boom cohort. *Drug and Alcohol Dependence, 69*(2), 127–135.

Ghilarducci, T. (2007). Pressures on retirement income security. *Public Policy and Aging Report, 17*(2), 8–12.

Giles, H., & Reid, S. A. (2005). Ageism across the lifespan: Towards a self-categorization model of ageing. *Journal of Social Issues, 61*(2), 389–404.

Goh, V. H. (2005). Aging in Asia: A cultural, socio-economical and historical perspective. *Aging Male, 8*(2), 90–96.

Goldman, D. P., Joyce, G. F., & Zheng, Y. (2007). Prescription drug cost sharing: As- sociations with medication and medical utilization and spending and health. *JAMA*, 298(1), 61–69.

Grant, A. M. (2001). Health of socially excluded groups: Lessons must be applied. *BMJ*, 323, 1071.

Green, A. F., Rebok, G., & Lyketsos, C. G. (2008). Influence of social network char- acteristics on cognition and functional status with aging. *International Journal of Geriatric Psychiatry*, 23(9), 972–978.

Green, L., & Grant, V. (2008). "Gagged grief and beleaguered bereavements?" An analysis of multidisciplinary theory and research relating to same sex partnership bereavement. *Sexualities*, 11(3), 275–300.

Greenberg, J. A. (1998). Defining male and female: Intersexuality and the collision between law and biology. *Arizona Law Review*, 41(2), 265–328.

Greenfield, E. A., & Russell, D. (2011). Identifying living arrangements that heighten risk for loneliness in later life: Evidence from the US National Social Life, Health and Aging Project. *Journal of Applied Gerontology*, 30, 524–534.

Griffith, D. M., Moy, E., Reischl, T. M., & Dayton, E. (2006). National data for monitoring and evaluating racial and ethnic health inequalities: Where do we go from here? *Health Education and Behavior*, 33, 470–487.

Grossman, A. H., D'Augelli, A. R., & Hershberger, S. L. (2000). Social support net- works of lesbian, gay, and bisexual adults 60 years of age and older. *Journal of Ger- ontology, Series B, Psychological Sciences and Social Sciences*, 55B(3), P171–P179.

Gruenewald, T. L., Karlamangla, A. S., Greendale, G., Singer, B. H., & Seeman, T. E. (2007). Feelings of usefulness to others, disability and mortality in older adults: The MacArthur Study of Successful Aging. *Journal of Gerontology, Series B, Psy- chological Sciences and Social Sciences*, 62B(1), P28–P37.

Gruskin, E. O., Greenwood, G. L., Matevia, M., Pollack, L. M., & Bye, L. L. (2007). Disparities in smoking between the lesbian, gay, and bisexual population and the general population in California. *American Journal of Public Health*, 97, 1496–1502.

Guralnick, J. M., Butterworth, S., Wadsworth, E. J., & Kuh, D. (2006). Childhood socioeconomic status predicts physical functioning a half century later. *Journal of Gerontology, Series A, Biological Sciences and Medical Sciences*, 61B(7), 694–701.

Haan, M. N., & Wallace, R. (2004). Can dementia be prevented? Brain aging in a population-based context. *Annual Review of Public Health*, 25, 1–24.

Haber, D. (1999). Minority access to hospice. *American Journal of Hospice and Pallia- tive Care*, 16, 386–389.

Harcourt, J. (2006). *Current issues in GLBT health*. Binghamton, NY: Haworth Press.

Harper, S., Lynch, J., Meersman, S. C., Breen, N., Davis, W. W., & Reichman, M. C. (2009). Trends in area-socioeconomic and race-ethnic disparities in breast cancer incidence, stage at diagnosis, screening, mortality and survival among women ages 50 years and over (1987–2005). *Cancer Epidemiological Biomarkers Preven- tion*, 18, 121–131.

Hartley, D. (2004). Rural health disparities, population health and rural culture. *American Journal of Public Health, 94,* 1675–1678.

Hatzenbuehler, M. L., Keyes, K. M., & Hasin, D. S. (2009). State-level policies and psychiatric morbidity in lesbian, gay and bisexual populations. *American Journal of Public Health, 99,* 2275–2281.

Hatzenbuehler, M. L., McLaughlin, K. A., Keyes, K. M., & Hasin, D. S. (2010). The impact of institutional discrimination in psychiatric disorders in lesbian, gay and bisexual populations: A prospective study. *American Journal of Public Health, 100,* 452–459.

Haviland, M. G., Morales, L. S., Dial, T. H., & Pincus, H. A. (2005). Race/ethnicity, socioeconomic status, and satisfaction with health care. *American Journal of Medical Quality, 20,* 195–203.

Hawkley, L. C., & Cacioppo, J. T. (2007). Aging and loneliness: Downhill quickly? *Current Directions in Psychological Science, 16,* 187–191.

Health Development Agency. (2006). *Health inequalities: Concepts, frameworks and policies.* London: Author.

Healthy People 2010. (2011). Retrieved from www.healthpeople.gov

Heaphy, B. (2007). Sexualities, gender, and aging: Resources and social change. *Current Sociology, 55,* 193–210.

Heathcote, G. (2000). Autonomy, health, and ageing: Transnational perspectives. *Health Education Research, 15,* 13–24.

Heintz, A. J., & Melendez, R. M. (2006). Intimate partner violence and HIV/STD risk among lesbian, gay, bisexual, and transgender individuals. *Journal of Interpersonal Violence, 21,* 193–208.

Hellman, R. E., & Drescher, J. (2004). *Handbook of LGBT issues in community mental health.* Binghamton, NY: Haworth Press.

Herek, G. M. (2002). Gender gaps in public opinion about lesbians and gay men. *Public Opinion Quarterly, 66,* 40–66.

Herek, G. M. (2009). Hate crimes and stigma-related experiences among sexual minority adults in the United States: Prevalence estimates from a national probability sample. *Journal of Interpersonal Violence, 24,* 54–74.

Herek, G. M., Cogan, J. C., & Gillis, J. R. (2002). Victim experiences in hate crimes based on sexual orientation. *Journal of Social Issues, 58*(2), 319–339.

Herek, G. M., & Garnets, L. D. (2007). Sexual orientation and mental health. *Annual Review of Clinical Psychology, 3,* 353–375.

Herek, G. M., Gillis, J. R., Cogan, J. C., & Glunt, E. K. (1997). Hate crime victimization among lesbian, gay, and bisexual adults: Prevalence, psychological correlates, and methodological issues. *Journal of Interpersonal Violence, 12,* 195–215.

Hermann, C. P., & Looney, S. W. (2011). Determinants of quality of life in patients near the end of life. *Oncological Nursing Forum, 38*(1), 23–31.

Hidaka, Y., & Operario, D. (2006). Attempted suicide, psychological health, and exposure to harassment among Japanese homosexual, bisexual, or other men questioning their sexual orientation recruited via the internet. *Journal of Epidemiology and Community Health, 60,* 962–967.

Hinton, L., Zweifach, M., Oishi, S., Tang, L., & Unützer, J. (2006). Gender disparities in the treatment of late-life depression: Qualitative and quantitative findings
from the IMPACT trial. *American Journal of Geriatric Psychiatry, 14*, 884–892.

Holkup, P. A., Salois, E. M., Tripp-Reimer, T., & Weinart, C. (2007). Drawing on
wisdom from the past: An elder abuse intervention with tribal communities. *Gerontologist, 47*(2), 248–254.

Horev, T., Berg-Warman, A., & Zussman, S. P. (2004). Disparities in the Israeli oral
healthcare delivery system. *Refuat Hapeh Vehashinayim, 24*, 35–42.

House, A., Van Horn, E., Coppeans, C., & Stepelman, L. (2011). Interpersonal trauma
and discriminatory events as predictors of suicidal and nonsuicidal self-injury in gay,
lesbian, bisexual and transgender persons. *Traumatology.* doi:10.1177/1534765610395621.

Hsu, H. C. (2005). Gender disparity of successful aging in Taiwan. *Women's Health,
42*(1), 1–21.

Hu, M. (2005). *Selling us short: How the Social Security privatization will affect lesbian, gay, bisexual and transgender Americans.* New York: National Gay and Lesbian Task Force Policy Institute.

Huang, F. Y., Chung, H., Kroenke, K., & Spitzer, R. L. (2006). Racial and ethnic
differences in the relationship between depression severity and functional status.
Psychiatric Services, 57, 498–503.

Huebner, D. M., Rebchook, G. M., & Kegeles, S. M. (2004). Experiences of harassment, discrimination and physical violence among young gay and bisexual men.
American Journal of Public Health, 94, 1200–1203.

Human Rights Campaign. (2011a). Retrieved February 4, 2012, from www.hrc.org
/workplace

Human Rights Campaign. (2011b). Retrieved February 4, 2012, from http://www.hrc
.org/laws_and_elections/5660.htm

Human Rights Campaign. (2011c). Retrieved from www.hrc.org/issues/hate_crimes

Hunter, S. (2005). *Midlife and older LGBT adults.* New York: Haworth Press.

Hyde, J., Perez, R., & Forester, B. (2007). Dementia and assisted living. *Gerontologist,
47*, 51–67.

Hylton, M. E. (2006). Queer in southern MSW programs: Lesbian and bisexual
women discuss stigma management. *Journal of Social Psychology, 146*(5), 611–618.

Iezzoni, L. I., Davis, R. B., Soukup, J., & O'Day, B. (2002). Satisfaction with quality
and access to healthcare among people with disabling conditions. *International
Journal for Quality in Health Care, 14*, 369–381.

Institute of Medicine (2011). *The health of lesbian, gay, bisexual, and transgender
people: Building a foundation for better understanding.* Washington, DC: National Academies Press. Retrieved from www.nap.edu/catalog/13128.html, Washington, DC [Pre-publication online uncorrected proof copy downloaded April
25, 2011].

Intersex Society of North America (ISNA). (2007). Retrieved from www.isna.org

Irwin, A., Valentine, N., Brown, C., Loewenson, R., Solar, O., Brown, H., . . . Vega,
J. (2006). The commission on social determinants of health: Tackling the roots of
health inequities. *PLoS Medicine, 3*(6), 749–751.

Jackson, N. C., Johnson, M. J., & Roberts, R. (2008). The potential impact of discrimination fears of older gays, lesbians, bisexuals and transgender individuals living in small- to moderate-sized cities on long-term health care. *Journal of Homosexuality*, 54(3), 325–339.

Jenness, V. (2010). From policy to prisoners to people: A "soft mixed methods" approach to studying transgender prisoners. *Journal of Contemporary Ethnography*, 39, 517–553.

Johnson, C. W. (2003). How will we get the data and what will we do with it then? Issues in the reporting of adverse healthcare events. *Quality and Safety in Health Care*, 112, 64–67.

Johnson, M. J. (2005). Gay and lesbian perceptions of discrimination in retirement care facilities. *Journal of Homosexuality*, 49(2), 83–102.

Johnson, N. E. (2000). Aging and eldercare in lesser developed countries. *Journal of Family Issues*, 21, 683–691.

Kabir, Z. N., Szebehely, M., Tishelman, C., Chowdhury, A. H. R., Höjer, B., & Winblad, B. (1998). Aging trends—making an invisible population visible: The elderly in Bangladesh. *Journal of Cross-Cultural Gerontology*, 13, 361–378.

Kahana, E., & Kahana, B. (2001). Successful aging among people with HIV/AIDS. *Journal of Clinical Epidemiology*, 54(Suppl 1), S53–S56.

Kahn, J. R., & Fazio, E. M. (2005). Economic status over the life course and racial disparities in health. *Journal of Gerontology, Series B, Psychological Sciences and Social Sciences*, 60B, S76–S84.

Kahn, J. R., & Pearlin, L. I. (2006). Financial strain over the life course and health among older adults. *Journal of Health and Social Behavior*, 47(1), 17–31.

Kane, R. L., Priester, R., & Neumann, D. (2007). Does disparity in the way disabled older adults are treated imply ageism? *Gerontologist*, 47(3), 271–279.

Kearney, F., Moore, A. R., Donegan, C. F., & Lambert, J. (2010). The ageing of HIV: Implications for geriatric medicine. *Age Ageing*, 39, 536–541.

Kehoe, M. (1989). *Lesbians over sixty speak for themselves*. New York: Haworth Press.

Kelly, R. J., & Robinson, G. C. (2011). Disclosure of membership in the lesbian, gay, bisexual and transgender community by individuals with communication impairments: A preliminary web-based survey. *American Journal of Speech & Language Pathology*, 20, 86–94.

Kennedy, J., & Erb, C. (2002). Prescription noncompliance due to cost among adults with disabilities in the United States. *American Journal of Public Health*, 92, 1120–1124.

Kertzner, R. M. (2001). The adult life course and homosexual identity in midlife gay men. *Annual Review of Sex Research*, 12, 75–92.

Kidd, J., & Witten, T. M. (2007a). Transgender and transsexual identities. The next strange fruit: Hate crimes, violence, and genocide against trans-communities. *Journal of Hate Studies*, 6(1), 31–63.

Kidd, J., & Witten, T. M. (2007b). Assessing spirituality, religiosity, and faith in the transgender community: A case study in violence and abuse—implications for the aging transgender community and for gerontological research. *Journal of Religious Gerontology*, 20(1–2), 29–62.

Kildemoes, H. W., Christiansen, T., Gyrd-Hansen, D., Kristiansen, I. S., & Anderson, M. (2006). The impact of population ageing on future Danish drug expenditure. *Health Policy*, 75(3), 298–311.

Kimmel, D., Rose, T., & David, D. (2006). *Lesbian, gay, bisexual, and transgender aging: Research and clinical perspectives*. New York: Columbia University Press.

Kinsella, K., & Phillips, D. R. (2005). Global aging: The challenge of success. *Population Bulletin*, 60(1), 1–44.

Kleinschmidt, K. C. (1997). Elder abuse: A review. *Annals of Emergency Medicine*, 30, 463–472.

Knochel, K. A., Quam, J. K., & Croghan, C. F. (2011). Are old lesbian and gay people well served? Understanding the perceptions, preparation, and experiences of aging services providers. *Journal of Applied Gerontology*, 30, 270–389.

Knodel, J., Watkins, S., & VanLandingham, M. (2002). *AIDS and older persons: An international perspective* (PSC Research Report No. 02-495). Retrieved from Population Studies Center at the Institute for Social Research, University of Michigan. www.psc.isr.umich.edu/pubs/

Knudsen, H. K., Ducharme, L. J., & Roman, P. M. (2007). Racial and ethnic disparities in SSRI availability in substance abuse treatment. *Psychiatric Services*, 58, 55–62.

Kolsky, K. (2008). *End of life: Helping with comfort and care* (Publication No. 08-0636). Bethesda, MD: U.S. Department of Health and Human Services, National Institutes of Health, National Institute on Aging.

Kon, A. A. (2006). Normalization. *JAMA*, 296(21), 2621–2622.

Kraaij, V., Arensman, E., & Spinhoven, P. (2002). Negative life events and depression in elderly persons: A meta-analysis. *Journal of Gerontology, Series B, Psychological Sciences and Social Sciences*, 57B(1), P87–P94.

Krause, N. (2006). Gratitude toward God, stress, and health in late life. *Research on Aging*, 28, 163–183.

Krug, E., Dahlberg, L., Mercy, J. A., Zwi, A. B., & Lozano, R. (2002). *World report on violence and health*. Geneva: World Health Organization. Retrieved from www.searo.who.int/LinkFiles/Disability,_Injury_Prevention_&_Rehabilitation_injuries-3.pdf

Kubzansky, L. D., Berkman, L. F., & Seeman, T. E. (2000). Social conditions and distress in elderly persons: Findings from the MacArthur Studies of Successful Aging. *Journal of Gerontology, Series B, Psychological Sciences and Social Sciences*, 55B(4), P238–P246.

Kuh, D. (2007). A life course approach to healthy aging, frailty, and capability. *Journal of Gerontology, Series A, Biological Sciences and Medical Sciences*, 62, 717–721.

Kuhns, L. M., Vazquez, R., & Ramirez-Valles, J. (2008). Researching special populations: Retention of Latino gay and bisexual men and transgender persons in longitudinal health research. *Health Education Research*, 23, 814–825.

Kuschner, W. G. (2011). Racial disparities in end-of-life care. *Archives of Internal Medicine*, 171, 949–950.

Kuyper, L., & Vanwesenbeeck, I. (2011). Examining sexual health differences between lesbian, gay, bisexual and heterosexual adults; the role of sociodemographics, sexual behavior characteristics and minority health. *Journal of Sexuality Research*, 48(2–3), 263–274.

Lacks, M. S., Williams, C. S., O'Brien, S., Charlson, M. E., & Pillemer, K. A. (2002). Adult protective service use and nursing home placement. *Gerontologist*, 42(6), 734–739.

Lacks, M. S., Williams, C. S., O'Brien, S., Pillemer, K. A., & Charlson, M. E. (1998). The mortality of elder mistreatment. *JAMA*, 280(5), 428–432.

Landers, S., Mimiaga, M. J., & Krinsky, L. (2010). The Open Door Project Task Force: A qualitative study on LGBT aging. *Journal of Gay & Lesbian Social Services*, 22, 316–336.

Lee, I.-C., & Crawford, M. (2007). Lesbians and bisexual women in the eyes of scientific psychology. *Feminism Psychology*, 17, 109–127.

Lee, J. A. (1987). What can homosexual aging studies contribute to theories of aging? *Journal of Homosexuality*, 13(4), 43–71.

Lee, S. (2006). Women and HIV: Aging with HIV. *Beta*, 18(2), 33–35.

Liao, Y., McGee, D. L., Cao, G., & Cooper, R. S. (1999). Black-white differences in disability and morbidity in the last years of life. *American Journal of Epidemiology*, 149(12), 1097–1103.

Linder, J. F., Enders, S. R., Craig, E., Richardson, J., & Meyers, F. J. (2002). Hospice care for the incarcerated in the United States: An introduction. *Journal of Palliative Medicine*, 5, 4549–4552.

Loeb, S. J., & Abudagga, A. (2006). Health-related research on older inmates: An integrative review. *Research in Nursing and Health*, 29(6), 556–565.

Loewy, M. (2004). Aging in the Americas. *Perspectives in Health*, 9(1). Retrieved from www.paho.org/English/DD/PIN/Number19_article02.htm

Lombardi, E. L., Wilchins, R. A., Priestling, D., & Malouf, D. (2001). Gender violence: Transgender experiences with violence and discrimination. *Journal of Homosexuality*, 42(1), 89–101.

London, A. S., & Myers, N. A. (2006). Race, incarceration, and health: A life-course approach. *Research on Aging*, 28, 409–422.

Los Angeles County Commission on Human Relations. (2006). *2005 hate crime report*. Los Angeles, CA: Author.

Lubin, F., Lusky, A., Chetrit, A., & Dankner, R. (2003). Lifestyle and ethnicity play a role in all-cause mortality. *Journal of Nutrition*, 133, 1180–1185.

Lunney, J. R., Foley, K. M., Smith, T. J., & Gellband, H. (Eds.). (2003). *Institute of Medicine—describing death in America: What we need to know*. Washington, DC: National Academies Press.

Luo, Y., & Waite, L. J. (2005). The impact of childhood and adult SES on physical, mental, and cognitive well-being in later life. *Journal of Gerontology, Series B, Psychological Sciences and Social Sciences*, 60B, S93–S101.

Luo, Y., & Waite, L. J. (2010). Mistreatment and psychological well-being among older adults: Exploring the role of psychological resources and deficits. *Journal of Gerontology: Social Sciences, 66B*(2), 217–229.

Lurie, N., & Dubowitz, T. (2007). Health disparities and access to health. *JAMA, 297*, 1118–1121.

Lurie, N., Jung, M., & Lavizzo-Mourey, R. (2005). Disparities and quality improvement: Federal policy levers. *Health Affairs, 24*(2), 354–364.

Mack, K. A., & Ory, M. G. (2003). AIDS and older Americans at the end of the twentieth century. *Journal of Acquired Immune Deficiency Syndromes, 33*, S68–S75.

Mackenbach, J. P. (2003). An analysis of the role of health care in reducing socioeconomic inequalities in health: The case of the Netherlands. *International Journal of Health Services, 33*, 523–541.

MacKinlay, E. (Ed.). (2006). *Aging, spirituality & palliative care.* Binghamton, NY: Haworth Pastoral Press.

Magee, J. C., Bigelow, L., DeHaan, S., & Mustanski, B. S. (2011). Sexual health information seeking behavior online: A mixed-methods study among lesbian, gay, bisexual and transgender young people. *Health and Education Behavior.* doi:10.1177/1090198111401384.

Makadon, H., Mayer, K. H., Potter, J., & Goldhammer, H. (Eds.). (2007). *The Fenway guide to lesbian, gay, bisexual and transgender health.* Philadelphia, PA: American College of Physicians.

Makadon, H. J. (2006). Improving health care for the lesbian and gay communities. *New England Journal of Medicine, 354*, 895–897.

Mangin, D., Sweeney, K., & Heath, I. (2007). Preventative health care in elderly people needs rethinking. *BMJ, 335*(7614), 285–287.

Marmot, M., Wilkinson, R., & Wilkinson, R. G. (2006). *The social determinants of health.* Oxford: Oxford University Press.

Marshall, B. L., & Katz, S. (2002). Forever functional: Sexual fitness and the ageing male body. *Body and Society, 8*, 43–70.

Marzolini, C., Back, D., Weber, R., Furrer, H., Cavassini, M., Calmy, A., . . . Elzi, L.; on behalf of the Swiss HIV Cohort Study. (2011). Aging with HIV: Medication use and risk for potential drug-drug interactions. *Journal of Antimicrobial Chemotherapy.* doi:10.1093/jac/dkr248.

Masiongale, T. (2009). Ethical service delivery to culturally and linguistically diverse populations: A specific focus on gay, lesbian, bisexual and transgender populations. *Perspectives on Communication Disorders & Sciences in Culturally and Linguistically Diverse Populations.* doi:10.1044/cds16.1.20.

Matsuda, S. (2002). The health and social system for the aged in Japan. *Aging Clinical and Experimental Research, 14*(4), 265–270.

Mays, V. M., Yancey, A. K., Cochran, S. D., Weber, M., & Fielding, J. E. (2002). Heterogeneity of health disparities among African American, Hispanic, and Asian American women: Unrecognized influences of sexual orientation. *American Journal of Public Health, 92*, 632–639.

McBride, M. R., & Lewis, I. D. (2004). African American and Asian American elders: An ethnogeriatric perspective. *Annual Review of Nursing Research, 22,* 161–214.

McMahon, E. (2003). The older homosexual: Current concepts of lesbian, gay, bisexual, and transgender older Americans. *Clinics in Geriatric Medicine,* 19(3), 587–593.

McNair, R. P. (2003). Lesbian health inequalities: A cultural minority issue for health professionals. *Medical Journal of Australia,* 178(12), 643–645.

McNair, R. P., & Hegarty, K. (2010). Guidelines for the primary care of lesbian, gay and bisexual people: A systematic review. *Annals of Family Medicine, 8,* 533–541.

McPhail, B. A. (2002). Gender-bias hate crimes: A review. *Trauma, Violence and Abuse,* 3(2), 125–143.

McPhail, B. A., & DiNitto, D. M. (2005). Prosecutorial perspectives on gender-bias hate crimes. *Violence against Women,* 11(9), 1162–1185.

Meezan, W., & Martin, J. I. (2003). *Research methods with GLBT populations.* Binghamton, NY: Haworth Press.

Melchior, M., Berkman, L. F., Kawachi, I., Krieger, N., Zins, M., Bonenfant, S., & Goldberg, M. (2006). Lifelong socioeconomic trajectory and premature mortality (35–65 years) in France: Findings from the GAZEL Cohort Study. *Journal of Epidemiology and Community Health,* 60, 937–944.

Merck Institute of Aging and Health. (2004). *The state of aging and health in America, 2004.* Retrieved from www.miaonline.org

MetLife Mature Market Institute (MMMI). (2010). Out and aging: The MetLife Study of Lesbian and Gay Baby Boomers. *Journal of GLBT Family Studies, 6,* 40–57.

Meyer, I. H. (2001). Why gay, lesbian, bisexual, and transgender public health? *American Journal of Public Health,* 91(6), 856–859.

Meyer, I. H., & Northridge, M. E. (Eds.). (2007). *The health of sexual minorities: Public health perspectives on lesbian, gay, bisexual, and transgender populations.* New York: Springer.

Mezuk, B., Rafferty, J. A., Kershaw, K. N., Hudson, D., Abdou, C. M., Lee, H., . . . & Jackson, J. S. (2010). Reconsidering the role of social disadvantage in physical and mental health: Stressful life events, health behaviors, race and depression. *American Journal of Epidemiology,* 172, 1238–1249.

Miksad, R. A., Bubley, G., Church, P., Sanda, M., Rofsky, N., Kaplan, I., & Cooper, A. (2006). Prostate cancer in a transgender woman 41 years after initiation of feminization. *JAMA,* 296L, 2316–2317.

Miller, A. M. (2001). Uneasy promises: Sexuality, health, and human rights. *American Journal Public Health,* 91(6), 861–864.

Moen, P., & Chermack, K. (2005). Gender disparities in health: Strategic selection, careers, and cycles of control [Special issue 2]. *Journal of Gerontology, Series B, Psychological Sciences and Social Sciences,* 60B, 99–108.

Moffat, S. D. (2006). Does testosterone mediate cognitive decline in elderly men? *Journal of Gerontology, Series A, Biological Sciences and Medical Sciences,* 61A(5), 521.

Mohammed, M. A., Man, J., Bentham, L., Stevens, A., & Hussain, S. (2006). Process of care and mortality of stroke patients with and without a do not resuscitate order in the West Midlands, UK. *International Journal for Quality in Health Care, 19,* 102–106.

Moreno-John, G., Gachie, A., Fleming, C. M., Napoles-Springer, A., Mutran, E., Manson, S. M., & Perez-Stable, E. J. (2004). Ethnic minority older adults participating in clinical research: Developing trust. *Journal of Aging and Health,* 16(5), 93S–123S.

Morrow, D. F., & Messinger, L. (2006). *Sexual orientation and gender expression in social work practice: Working with GLBT people.* New York: Columbia University Press.

Moy, E., Arispe, I. E., Holmes, J. S., & Andrews, R. M. (2005). Preparing the national healthcare disparities report: Gaps in data for assessing racial, ethnic, and socioeconomic disparities in healthcare. *Medical Care,* 43(3 Suppl), 9–16.

Moy, E., Dayton, E., & Clancy, C. M. (2005). Compiling the evidence: The National Healthcare Disparities Reports. *Health Affairs,* 24, 376–387.

Mullins, C. D., Blatt, L., Gbarayor, C. M., Yang, H.-W. K., & Baquet, C. (2005). Health disparities: A barrier to high-quality care. *American Journal of Health-Systems Pharmacy,* 62, 1873–1882.

Muñoz-Laboy, M., & Dodge, B. (2007). Bisexual Latino men and HIV and sexually transmitted infections risk: An exploratory analysis. *American Journal of Public Health,* 97(6), 1102–1106.

Murray, L. M., & Boyd, S. (2009). Protecting personhood and achieving quality of life for older adults with dementia in the U.S. health care system. *Journal of Aging & Health,* 21, 350–373.

Mustanski, B. S., Garofalo, R., & Emerson, E. M. (2010). Mental health disorders, psychological distress, and suicidality in a diverse sample of lesbian, gay, bisexual and transgender youths. *American Journal of Public Health,* 100, 2426–2432.

Myburgh, N. G., Solanki, G. C., Smith, M. H., & Lallo, R. (2005). Patient satisfaction with healthcare providers in South Africa: The influences of race and socioeconomic status. *International Journal for Quality in Health Care,* 17, 473–477.

Nadien, M. B. (2006). Factors that influence abusive interactions between aging women and their caregivers. *Annals of the New York Academy of Sciences,* 1087, 158–169.

National Center on Elder Abuse. (2005). *Fact sheet on elder abuse prevalence and incidence.* Washington, DC: Author.

National Coalition of Anti-Violence Programs. (2005). *Anti-lesbian, gay, bisexual and transgender violence in 2004.* Retrieved from www.ncavp.org

National Coalition of Anti-Violence Programs. (2011). *Hate violence against lesbian, gay, bisexual, transgender, queer and HIV-affected communities: A report from the*

National Coalition of Anti-Violence Programs. Retrieved from www.avp.org
/documents/NCAVPHateViolenceReport2011Finaledjlfinaledits.pdf

National Council on Aging. (2011a). *Economic security: Fact sheet.* Retrieved from
www.ncoa.org/press-room/fact-sheets/economic-security-fact-sheet.html

National Council on Aging. (2011b). *Health aging: Fact sheet.* Retrieved from www
.ncoa.org/press-room/fact-sheets/healthy-aging-fact-sheet.html

National Family Caregivers Association. (2004). *Fact sheet: Family caregiving statistics.* Retrieved from www.nfcacares.org

National Gay and Lesbian Task Force (NGLTF). (2005). *Make room for all: Diversity,
cultural competency and discrimination in an aging America.* Retrieved from www
.thetaskforce.org/reslibrary/list.cfm?pubTypeID=2#pub304

National Gay and Lesbian Task Force (NGLTF). (2007). Retrieved from www
.ngltf.org

National Institute on Aging (NIA). (2007a). *Why population aging matters: A global
perspective.* (NIA/NIH Publication No. 07-6134). Bethesda, MD: Author.

National Institute on Aging (NIA). (2007b). *Review of minority aging research at the
NIA.* Retrieved from www.nia.nih.gov/AboutNIA/MinorityAgingResearch.htm

National Institute on Aging (NIA). (2007c). *Strategic plan to address health disparities, 2000–2005.* Retrieved from www.nia.nih.gov/AboutNIA/StrategicPlan

Neighbors, H. W., Caldwell, C., Williams, D. R., Nesse, R., Taylor, R. J., Bullard,
K. M., . . . Jackson, J. S. (2007). Race, ethnicity, and the use of services for mental
disorders: Results from the National Survey of American Life. *Archives of General
Psychiatry, 64*(4), 485–494.

Nemoto, T., Operario, D., Keatley, J., Nguyen, H., & Sugano, E. (2005). Promoting
health for transgender women: Transgender Resources and Neighborhood Space
(TRANS) Program in San Francisco. *American Journal of Public Health, 95*,
382–384.

Newman, L. A., Griffith, K. A., Jatoi, I., Simon, M. S., Crowe, J. P., & Colditz, G. A.
(2006). Meta-analysis of survival in African-American and White-American patients with breast cancer: Ethnicity compared with socioeconomic status. *Journal
of Clinical Oncology, 24*, 1342–1349.

Norton, C. K., Hobson, G., & Kulm, E. (2010). Palliative and end-of-life care in the
emergency department: Guidelines for nurses. *Journal of Emergency Nursing, 37*(3),
240–245.

Nummela, O., Seppanen, M., & Uutela, A. (2011). The effect of loneliness and
change in loneliness on self-rated health (SRH): A longitudinal study among aging
people. *Archives of Gerontology and Geriatrics, 53*(2), 163–167.

O'Connell, H., Chin, A.-V., Cunningham, C., & Lawlor, B. A. (2004). Recent developments: Suicide in older people. *BMJ, 329*, 895–899.

O'Connell, J. J. (2004). Dying in the shadows: The challenge of providing healthcare
for homeless people. *Canadian Medical Association Journal, 170*, 1251–1252.

O'Rand, A. M., & Shuey, K. M. (2007). Gender and the devolution of pension risks
in the US. *Current Sociology, 55*, 287–304.

Orel, N. A., Spence, M., & Steele, J. (2005). Getting the message out to older adults: Effective HIV health education risk reduction publications. *Journal of Applied Gerontology, 24*, 490–508.

Ostir, G. V., Kuo, Y.-F., Berges, I. M., Markides, K. S., & Ottenbacher, K. J. (2007). Measures of lower body function and risk of mortality over 7 years of follow-up. *American Journal of Epidemiology, 166*, 599–605.

Otis, M. D. (2007). Perceptions of victimization risk and fear of crime among lesbians and gay men. *Journal of Interpersonal Violence, 22*, 198–217.

Ott, B. R., Lapane, K. L., & Gambassi, G. (2000). Gender differences in the treatment of behavior problems in Alzheimer's disease. *Neurology, 54*, 427.

Paganini, J. M. (1999). Country report: Argentina. Current activities in the field of quality in health care. *International Journal for Quality in Health Care, 11*, 435–436.

Pampel, C. C., Krueger, P. M., & Denney, J. T. (2010). Socioeconomic disparities in health behaviors. *Annual Reviews of Sociology, 36*, 349–370.

Pan American Health Organization. (1998). *Health in the Americas*. Washington, DC: Author.

Pandey, A., Sengupta, P. G., Mondal, S. K., Gupta, D. N., Manna, B., Ghosh, S., . . . Bhattacharya, S. K. (2002). Gender differences in healthcare-seeking during common illnesses in a rural community of West Bengal, India. *Journal of Health, Population Nutrition, 20*(4), 206–311.

Parker, M. G., & Thorslund, M. (2007). Health trends in the elderly population: Getting better and getting worse. *Gerontologist, 47*, 150–158.

Parrott, D. J., & Zeichner, A. (2006). Effect of psychopathy on physical aggression toward gay and heterosexual men. *Journal of Interpersonal Violence, 21*(3), 390–410.

Paul, J. P., Catania, J., Pollack, L., Moskowitz, J., Canchola, J., Mills, T., . . . Stall, R. (2002). Suicide attempts among gay and bisexual men: Lifetime prevalence and antecedents. *American Journal of Public Health, 92*, 1338–1345.

Pearce, N., & Merletti, F. (2006). Complexity, simplicity, and epidemiology. *International Journal of Epidemiology, 35*(3), 515–519.

Peterson, P. E., & Yamamoto, T. (2005). Improving the oral health of older people: The approach of the WHO Global Oral Health Programme. *Community Dentistry and Oral Epidemiology, 33*, 81–92.

Phillips, L. L., Allen, R. S., Harris, G. M., Presnell, A. H., DeCoster, J., & Cavanaugh, R. (2011). Aging prisoners' treatment selection: Does prospect theory enhance understanding of end-of-life medical decisions? *Gerontologist.* doi:10.1093/geront/gnr039.

Pillemer, K. A., & Moore, D. W. (1989). Abuse of patients in nursing homes: Findings from a survey of staff. *Gerontologist, 29*(3), 314–320.

Pinn, V. W. (2003). Sex and gender factors in medical studies: Implications for health and clinical practice. *JAMA, 289*(4), 397–400.

Pinquart, M., & Sorenson, S. (2000). Influences of socio-economic status, social network, and competence on subjective well-being in later life: A meta-analysis. *Psychology and Aging, 14*(2), 187–224.

Pirner, D. (2005). "Multiple margins" (being older, a women, or a visible minority) constrained older women's access to Canadian health care. *Evidence-Based Nursing, 8,* 128.

Polivka, L. (2007a). Growing risk in an aging nation. *Gerontologist, 46,* 255–263.

Polivka, L. (2007b). Medicare and the future of retirement security. *Gerontologist, 47*(1), 123–130.

Pollicino, C. A., & Saltman, D. C. (2000). The relationship between physician cost and functional status in the elderly. *International Journal for Quality in Health Care, 12,* 425–431.

Post, L., Page, C., Conner, T., Prokhorov, A., Fang, Y., & Biroscak, B. J. (2010). Elder abuse in long-term care: Types, patterns and risk factors. *Research on Aging, 32,* 323–348.

Poteat, V. P., & Espelage, D. L. (2007). Predicting psychosocial consequences of homophobic victimization in middle school students. *Journal of Early Adolescence, 27,* 175–191.

Prabhakar, H., & Manoharan, R. (2005). The Tribal Health Initiative for Healthcare Delivery: A clinical and epidemiological approach. *National Medical Journal of India, 18*(4), 197–204.

Preves, S. E. (2000). Negotiating the constraints of gender binarism: Intersexuals' challenge to gender categorization. *Current Sociology, 48,* 27–50.

Price, E. (2007). Pride or prejudice? Gay men, lesbians, and dementia. *British Journal of Social Work.* doi:10.1093/bjsw/bcm027.

Prus, S. G. (2000). Income inequality as a Canadian cohort ages: An analysis of the later life course. *Research on Aging, 22,* 211–237.

Pryzgoda, J., & Chrisler, J. C. (2000). Definitions of gender and sex: The subtleties of meaning. *Sex Roles, 43*(7/8), 553–569.

Quam, J. K. (2005). Ruthie and Connie: Every room in the house. *Gerontologist, 45,* 286–287.

Ramirez-Valles, J., Kuhns, L. M., Campbell, R. T., & Diaz, R. M. (2010). Social integration and health: Community involvement, stigmatized identities, and sexual risk in Latino sexual minorities. *Journal of Health and Social Behavior, 51,* 30–47.

Ramsey-Klawsnik, H., Teaster, P. B., Mendiondo, M. S., Abner, E. L., Cecil, K. A., & Tooms, M. R. (2007). Sexual abuse of vulnerable adults in care facilities: Clinical findings and a research initiative. *Journal of the American Psychiatric Nurses Association, 12,* 332–339.

Read, J. G., & Gorman, B. K. (2006). Gender inequalities in US adult health: The interplay of race and ethnicity. *Social Science and Medicine, 62*(5), 1045–1065.

Read, J. G., & Gorman, B. K. (2010). Gender and health inequality. *Annual Reviews of Sociology, 36,* 371–386.

Redman, D. (2011). Fear, discrimination and abuse: Transgender elders and the perils of long-term care. *Aging Today, 32*(2), 1–2.

Reitzes, D. C., & Mutran, E. J. (2004). Grandparent identity, intergenerational identity, and well-being. *Journal of Gerontology, Series B, Psychological Sciences and Social Sciences, 59B,* S213–S219.

Remafedi, G., & Carol, H. (2005). Preventing tobacco use among lesbian, gay, bisexual and transgender youths. *Nicotine & Tobacco Research*, 7, 249–256.

Reuben, D. B. (2006). Meeting the needs of disabled older persons: Can the fragments be pieced together [Guest editorial]? *Journal of Gerontology, Series A, Biological Sciences and Medical Sciences*, 61A(4), 365–366.

Rikard, R. V., & Rosenberg, E. (2007). Aging inmates: A convergence of trends in the American criminal justice system. *Journal of Correctional Health Care*, 13, 150–162.

Riorden, D. C. (2004). Interaction strategies of lesbian, gay, and bisexual healthcare practitioners in the clinical examination of patients: Qualitative study. *BMJ*, 328. doi:10.1136/bmj.38071.774525.EB.

Ritchie, C. S., & Wieland, G. D. (2007). Improving end-of-life care for older adults: An international challenge [Editorial]. *Journal of Gerontology, Series A, Biological Sciences and Medical Sciences*, 62A(4), 393–394.

Roback, H. B., & Lothstein, L. M. (1986). The female mid-life sex change applicant: A comparison with younger female transsexuals and older male sex-change applicants. *Archives of Sexual Behavior*, 15(5), 401–415.

Robert, S. A., Cherepanov, D., Palta, M., Dunham, N. C., Feeny, D., & Fryback, D. G. (2009). Socioeconomic status and age variations in health-related quality of life: Results from the National Health Measurement Study. *Journal of Gerontology B, Psychological Science and Social Science*, 64B, 378–389.

Rogers, R. G., Hummer, P. A., & Nam, C. B. (2000). *Living and dying in the USA: Behavioral, health and social differentials of adult mortality*. San Diego, CA: Academic Press.

Rondahl, G., Innala, S., & Carlsson, M. (2006). Heterosexual assumptions in verbal and non-verbal communication in nursing. *Journal of Advanced Nursing*, 56(4), 373–381.

Rooke, A. (2007). Navigating embodied lesbian cultural space: Toward a lesbian habitus. *Space and Culture*, 10, 231–252.

Rosnick, C. B., Small, B. J., McEvoy, C. L., Borenstein, A. R., & Mortimer, J. A. (2007). Negative life events and cognitive performance in a population of older adults. *Journal of Aging & Health*, 19, 612–629.

Ross, N. A., Garner, R., Bernier, J., Feeny, D. H., Kaplan, M. S., McFarland, B., . . . Oderkir, J. (2011). Trajectories of health-related quality of life by socio-economic status in a nationally representative Canadian cohort. *Journal of Epidemiology and Community Health*. doi:10.1136/jech.2011.115378.

Rowe, J. R., & Kahn, R. L. (1998). *Successful aging*. New York: Pantheon Books.

Rudolph, M. N., & Hughes, D. H. (2001). Emergency assessments of domestic violence, sexual dangerousness and elder and child abuse. *Psychiatric Services*, 52(3), 281–282.

Ruger, J. P., & Kim, H.-J. (2006). Global health inequalities: An international comparison. *Journal of Epidemiology and Community Health*, 60, 928–936.

Russell, C. (2007). What do older women and men want? Gender differences in the "lived experience" of ageing. *Current Sociology*, 55, 173–192.

Rutherford, A., Zwi, A. B., Grove, N. J., & Butchart, A. (2007a). Violence: A glossary. *Journal of Epidemiology and Community Health*, 61, 676–680.

Rutherford, A., Zwi, A. B., Grove, N. J., & Butchart, A. (2007b). Violence: A priority for public health? Pt. 2. *Journal of Epidemiology and Community Health, 61,* 764–770.

Ryan, C., Huebner, D., Diaz, R. M., & Sanchez, J. (2009). Family rejection as a predictor of negative health outcomes in White and Latino lesbian, gay and bisexual young adults. *Pediatrics, 123,* 346–352.

Ryan, C., Russell, S. T., Huebner, D., Diaz, R., & Sanchez, J. (2010). Family acceptance in adolescence and the health of LGBT young adults. *Journal of Child and Adolescent Psychiatric Nursing, 23*(4), 205–213.

Saewyc, E. M., Skay, C. L., Pettingell, S. L., Reis, E. A., Bearinger, L., Resnick, M., . . . Combs, L. (2006). Hazards of stigma: The sexual and physical abuse of gay, lesbian and bisexual adolescents in the United States and Canada. *Child Welfare, 85*(2), 195–213.

Salari, S. (2002). Invisible in aging research: Arab Americans, Middle Eastern immigrants, and Muslims in the United States. *Gerontologist, 42,* 580.

Sambamoorthi, U., Shea, D., & Crystal, S. (2003). Total and out-of-pocket expenditure for prescription drugs among older persons. *Gerontologist, 43,* 345–359.

Sanchez Rodriguez, J. L., & Rodriguez Alvarez, M. (2003). Normal aging and AIDS. *Archives of Gerontology and Geriatrics, 36*(1), 57–65.

Sanders, S. A., & Reinisch, J. M. (1999). Would you say you "Had sex" if . . . ? *JAMA, 281,* 275–277.

Sarkisian, C. A., Hays, R. D., & Magione, C. M. (2002). Do older adults expect to age successfully? The association between expectations regarding aging and beliefs regarding healthcare seeking among older adults. *Journal of the American Geriatrics Society, 50*(11), 1837–1843.

Sarkisian, C. A., Shunkwiler, S. M., Aguilar, I., & Moore, A. A. (2006). Ethnic differences in expectations for aging among older adults. *Journal of the American Geriatrics Society, 54*(8), 1277–1282.

Schneider, E. C., Zaslavsky, A. M., & Epstein, A. M. (2002). Racial disparities in the quality of care for enrollees in Medicare managed care. *JAMA, 287*(10), 1288–1294.

Scout, Bradford, J., & Fields, C. 2001. Removing the barriers: Improving practitioners' skills in providing health care to lesbians and women who partner with women. *American Journal of Public Health, 91,* 892–894.

Seelau, S. M., & Seelaw, E. P. (2005). Gender-role stereotypes and perceptions of heterosexual, gay, and lesbian domestic violence. *Journal of Family Violence, 20*(6), 363–371.

Sell, R. L., & Becker, J. B. (2001). Sexual orientation data collection and progress toward Healthy People 2010. *American Journal of Public Health, 91,* 876–882.

Setterson, R. A. (2006). When nations call: How wartime military service matters for the life course and aging. *Research on Aging, 28,* 12–36.

Setterson, R. A., & Patterson, R. S. (2006). Military service, the life course, and aging: An introduction. *Research on Aging, 28,* 5–11.

Shankle, M. D. (Ed.). (2006). *The handbook of lesbian, gay, bisexual, and transgender public health: A practitioner's guide to service.* New York: Harrington Park Press.

Shankle, M. D., Maxwell, C. A., Katzman, E. S., & Landers, S. (2003). An invisible population: Older lesbian, gay, bisexual, and transgender individuals. *Clinical and Regulatory Affairs, 20*(2), 159–182.

Sheikh, A. (2006). Why are ethnic minorities under-represented in US research studies? *PLoS Medicine, 3*(2), 166–167.

Sherkat, D. E., Kilbourne, B. S., Cain, V. A., Hull, P. C., Levine, R. S., & Husaini, B. A. (2007). The impact of health service use on racial differences in mortality among the elderly. *Research on Aging, 29*(3), 207–224.

Shinoda-Tagawa, T., Leonard, R., Pontikas, J., McDonough, J. E., Allen, D., & Dreyer, P. I. (2004). Resident-to-resident violent incidents in nursing homes. *JAMA, 291*, 591–598.

Shippy, R. A., & Karpiak, S. E. (2005). The aging HIV/AIDS population: Fragile social networks. *Aging and Mental Health, 9*(3), 246–254.

Shuey, K. M., & Willson, A. E. (2008). Cumulative disadvantage and Black-White disparities in life-course health trajectories. *Research on Aging, 30*, 200–225.

Silverstein, M., Gans, D., & Yang, F. M. (2006). Intergenerational support to aging parents: The role of norms and needs. *Journal of Family Issues, 27*, 1068–1084.

Silvestre, A. (Ed.). (2001). *Lesbian, gay, bisexual and transgender health issues: Selections from the* American Journal of Public Health. Washington, DC: American Journal of Public Health.

Singh, G. K., & Siahpush, M. (2006). Widening socioeconomic inequalities in US life expectancy, 1980–2000. *International Journal of Epidemiology, 35*, 969–979.

Slusher, M. P., Mayer, C. J., & Dunkle, R. E. (1996). Gays and Lesbians Older and Wiser (GLOW): A support group for older gay people. *Gerontologist, 36*(1), 118–123.

Smedley, B. D., Stith, A. Y., & Nelson, A. R. (Eds.). (2003). *Unequal treatment: Confronting racial and ethnic disparities in healthcare.* Washington, DC: National Academies Press.

Smith, B., & Horne, S. (2007). Gay, lesbian, bisexual, and transgendered (GLBT) experiences with Earth-spirited faith. *Journal of Homosexuality, 52*(3–4), 235–248.

Smith, L. A., McCaslin, R., Chang, J., Martinez, P., & McGrew P. (2010). Assessing the needs of older gay, lesbian, bisexual and transgender people: A service learning and agency partnership approach. *Journal of Gerontological Social Work, 53*(5), 387–401.

Smyer, T., & Clark, M. C. (2011). A cultural paradox: Elder abuse in the Native American community. *Home Health Care Management Practice, 23*, 201–206.

Soumerai, S. B., Pierre-Jacques, M., Shang, F., Ross-Degnan, D., Adams, A. S., Gurwitz, J., . . . Safran, D. G. (2006). Cost-related medication non-adherence among elderly and disabled Medicare beneficiaries: A national survey 1 year before the Medicare drug benefit. *Archives of Internal Medicine, 166*, 1829–1835.

Spillman, B. C. (2004). Changes in elderly disability rates and the implications for health care utilization and cost. *Milbank Quarterly, 82*, 157–194.

Staley, M., Hussey, W., Roe, K., Harcourt, J., & Roe, K. (2001). In the shadow of the rainbow: Identifying and addressing health disparities in the lesbian, gay, bisexual and transgender population—a research and practice challenge. *Health Promotion Practice, 2,* 207–211.

States, R. A., Susman, W. M., Riquelme, L. F., Godwin, E. M., & Greer, E. (2006). Community health education: Reaching ethnically diverse elders. *Journal of Allied Health, 35*(4), 215–222.

Steen, R., Mogasale, V., Wi, T., Singh, A. K., Das, A., Daly, C., . . . Dallabetta, G. (2006). Pursuing scale and quality in STI interventions with sex workers: Initial results from Avahan India AIDS initiative. *Sexually Transmitted Infections, 82,* 381–385.

Steinberg, A., Brooks, J., & Remtulla, T. (2003). Youth hate crimes: Identification, prevention, and intervention. *American Journal of Psychiatry, 160,* 979–989.

Stevens, P., Carlson, L. M., & Hinman, J. M. (2004). An analysis of tobacco industry marketing to lesbian, gay, bisexual and transgender (LGBT) populations: Strategies for mainstream tobacco control and prevention. *Health Promotion Practice, 5,* 129S–34S.

Stevenson, J. S. (2005). Alcohol use, misuse, abuse, and dependence in later adulthood. *Annual Reviews of Nursing Research, 23,* 245–280.

Substance Abuse and Mental Health Services Administration (SAMHSA). (2003). *A provider's introduction to substance abuse treatment for lesbian, gay, bisexual, and transgender individuals.* Center for Substance Abuse Treatments. (DHHS Publication No. [SMA] 03-3819. NCADI Publication No. BKD392). Rockville, MD: U.S. Government Printing Office.

Sudore, R. L., Mehta, K. M., Simonsick, E. M., Harris, T. B., Newman, A. B., Satterfield, S., . . . Yaffee, K. (2006). Limited literacy in older people and disparities in health and healthcare access. *Journal of the American Geriatrics Society, 54*(5), 770–776.

Sullivan, M. (Ed.). (2003). *Sexual minorities: Discrimination, challenges and development in America.* New York: Haworth Press.

Svihula, J., & Estes, C. L. (2007). Social Security politics: Ideology and reform. *Journal of Gerontology, Series B, Psychological Sciences and Social Sciences, 62B,* S79–S89.

Sykes, J. T. (2006). Global aging aspirations confront cultural and regional realities. *Gerontologist, 46,* 555–558.

Szczepura, A. (2005). Access to healthcare for ethnic minority populations. *Postgraduate Medical Journal, 81,* 141–147.

Teaster, P. B., & Roberto, K. A. (2004). Sexual abuse of older adults: APS cases and outcomes. *Gerontologist, 44*(6), 788–796.

Thompson, E. H. (2006). Being women, then lesbians, then old: Femininities, sexualities, and aging. *Gerontologist, 46*(2), 300–305.

Tomaka, J., Thomson, S., & Palacios, R. (2006). The relation of social isolation, loneliness, and social support to disease outcomes in the elderly. *Journal of Aging and Health, 18,* 359–384.

Tozer, E. E., & Hayes, J. A. (2004). Why do individuals seek conversion therapy? The role of religiosity, internalized homonegativity, and identity development. *Counseling Psychologist, 32,* 716–740.

TranScience Longitudinal Aging Research Study. (2007). Retrieved from www.tran science.org/

Tucker, E. W., & Potocky-Tripodi, M. (2006). Changing heterosexuals' attitudes towards homosexuals: A systematic review of the empirical literature. *Research on Social Work Practice, 16,* 176–190.

Turra, C. M., & Goldman, N. (2007). Socioeconomic differences in mortality among U.S. adults: Insights into the Hispanic paradox. *Journal of Gerontology, Series B, Psychological Sciences and Social Sciences, 62B*(3), S184–S192.

Ulrich, L. (2011). *Bisexual invisibility: Impacts and recommendations.* Retrieved from www.sf-hrc.org/Modules/ShowDocument.aspx?documentid=989

Umberson, D., Brosnoe, R., & Reczek, C. (2010). Social relationships and health behavior across the life course. *Annual Review of Sociology, 36,* 139 – 157.

United Nations. (2001). *Reducing disparities: Balanced development of urban and rural areas and regions within the counties of Asia and the Pacific.* Bangkok, Thailand: UN Economic and Social Commission for Asia and the Pacific, 2001. Retrieved from www.unescap.org/huset/disparities/title.pdf

U.S. House Select Committee on Aging, Subcommittee on Health and Long-Term Care. (1990). *Elder abuse: A decade of shame and inaction.* Washington, DC: Government Printing Office.

Van Baarsen, B. (2002). Theories of coping with loss: The impact of social support and self-esteem on adjustment to emotional and social loneliness following a partner's death in later life. *Journal of Gerontology, Series B, Psychological Sciences and Social Sciences, 57B*(1), S33–S42.

Vance, D. E., Brennan, M., Enah, C., Smith, G. L., & Kaur, J. (2011). Religion, spirituality, and older adults with HIV: Critical personal and social resources for an aging epidemic. *Clinical Interventions in Aging, 6,* 101–109.

Velkoff, V. A., & Kinsella, K. (1998). Gender stereotypes: Data needs for ageing research. *Aging International, 24*(4), 18–38.

Victoria, C. G. (2006). The challenge of reducing health inequalities. *American Journal of Public Health, 96*(1), 10–11.

Wallace, S. P., Cochran, S. D., Durazo, E. M., & Ford, C. L. (2011). The health of aging lesbian, gay and bisexual adults in California. *Policy Brief CLA Center for Health Policy Research* (PB2011-2), 1–8.

Walsh, C. A., Ploeg, J., Lohfeld, L., Horne, J., MacMillan, H., & Lai, D. (2007). Violence across the lifespan: Interconnections among forms of abuse as described by marginalized Canadian elders and their care-givers. *British Journal of Social Work, 37,* 491–514.

Wamala, S. P., Merlo J., Boström, G., Hogstedt, C. (2007a). Perceived discrimination, socioeconomic disadvantage and refraining from seeking medical treatment in Sweden. *Journal of Epidemiology and Community Health, 61,* 409–415.

Wamala, S., Merlo, J., Boström, G., Hogstedt, C., & Agren, G. (2007b). Socioeconomic disadvantage and primary non-adherence with medication in Sweden. *International Journal for Quality in Health Care, 19,* 134–140.

Wang, J., Noel, J. M., Zuckerman, I. H., Miller, N. A., Shaya, F. T., & Mullins, C. D. (2006). Disparities in access to essential new prescription drugs between non-Hispanic whites, non-Hispanic blacks, and Hispanic whites. *Medical Care Research and Review, 63,* 742–763.

Ward, R., Vass, A. A., Aggarwal, N., Garfield, C., & Cybyk, B. (2005). A kiss is still a kiss? The construction of sexuality in dementia care. *Dementia, 4,* 49–72.

Warner, J., McKeown, E., Griffin, M., Johnson, K., Ramsay, A., Cort, C., & King, M. (2004). Rates and predictors of mental illness in gay men, lesbians and bisexual men and women: Results from a survey based in England and Wales. *British Journal of Psychiatry, 185,* 479–485.

Wasson, J. H., & Benjamin, R. (2006). Postscript: Health disparity and collaborative care. *Journal of Ambulatory Care Management, 29*(3), 233–234.

Waysdorf, S. L. (2002). The aging of the AIDS epidemic: Emerging legal and public health issues for elderly persons living with HIV/AIDS. *Elder Law Journal, 10*(1), 47–89.

Weber, S. (2010). A stigma identification framework for family nurses working with parents who are lesbian, gay, bisexual, or transgendered and their families. *Journal of Family Nursing, 16*(4), 378–393.

Wei, W., Akincigil, A., Crystal, S., & Sambamoorthi, U. (2006). Gender differences in out-of-pocket prescription drug expenditures among the elderly. *Research on Aging, 28,* 427–453.

Wen, X. (2004). Trends in the prevalence of disability and chronic conditions among the older population: Implications for survey design and measurement of disability. *Australasian Journal on Ageing, 23*(1), 3–6.

Wilcox, M. M. (2002). When Sheila's a lesbian: Religious individualism among lesbian, gay, bisexual and transgender Christians. *Sociology of Religion, 63*(4), 497–513.

Willging, C. E., Salvador, M., & Kano, M. (2006). Unequal treatment: Mental health care for sexual and gender minority groups in a rural state. *Psychiatric Services, 57*(6), 867–870.

Williams, D. (2005). The health of US racial and ethnic populations [Special issue 2]. *Journal of Gerontology, Series B, Psychological Sciences and Social Sciences, 60B,* 53–62.

Wilson, R. S., Krueger, K. R., Arnold, S. E., Schneider, J. A., Kelly, J. F., Barnes, L. L., . . . Bennett, D. A. (2007). Loneliness and risk of Alzheimer disease. *Archives of General Psychiatry, 64,* 234–240.

Witten, T. M. (2003). Transgender aging: An emerging population and an emerging need. *Review Sexologies, 12*(4), 15–20.

Witten, T. M. (2004). Life course analysis. The courage to search for something more: Middle adulthood issues in the transgender and intersex community. *Journal of Human Behavior in the Social Environment, 8*(3–4), 189–224.

Witten, T. M. (2005). Birth sex is not gender: Comments on "Efforts to address gender inequalities must begin at home." *Lancet, 366*(9496), 1505. Retrieved from www.thelancet.com/journals/lancet/article/PIIS0140673605676052/comments ?action=view&totalComments=1

Witten, T. M. (2008). Transgender bodies, identities, and healthcare: Effects of perceived and actual violence and abuse. In J. J. Kronenfeld (Ed.), *Research in the sociology of healthcare: Inequalities and disparities in health care and health— concerns of patients.* (Vol. 25, pp. 225–249). Oxford: Elsevier JAI.

Witten, T. M. (2009). Graceful exits: III. Intersections of aging, transgender identities and the family/community. *Journal of GLBT Family Studies, 5,* 36–63. doi:10 .1080/15504280802595378.

Witten, T. M. (2011). Results from the Trans MetLife Survey.

Witten, T. M., & Eyler, A. E. (1999). Hate crimes and violence against the transgendered. *Peace Review, 11*(3), 461–468.

Witten, T. M., & Whittle, S. P. (2004). TransPanthers: The graying of transgender and the law. *Deakin Law Review, 9*(2), 503–522.

Wong, M. D., Shapiro, M. F., Boscardin, W. J., & Ettner, S. L. (2002). Contribution of major diseases to disparities in mortality. *New England Journal of Medicine, 347,* 1585–1592.

World Health Organization. (2002). *Missing voices: Views of older persons on elder abuse.* Geneva: World Health Organization. Retrieved from whqlibdoc.who.int /hq/2002/WHO_NMH_VIP_02.1.pdf

World Health Organization. (2007a). *Aging and life course.* Retrieved from www.who .int/ageing/projects/en/

World Health Organization. (2007b). *More oral health care needed for ageing populations.* Retrieved from www.who.int/bulletin/volumes/83/9/infocus0905/en/index .html

World Health Organization. (2007c). *Missing voices. View of older persons on elder abuse: A study from eight countries—Argentina, Austria, Brazil, Canada, India, Kenya, Lebanon and Sweden.* Retrieved from www.who.int/ageing/projects/elder _abuse/missing_voices/en/index.html

Worthington, R. L., Savoy, H. B., Dillon, F. R., & Vernaglia, E. R. (2002). Heterosexual identity development: A multi-dimensional model of individual and social identity. *Counseling Psychologist, 40,* 496–531.

Wright, N. M. J., Tompkins, C. N. E., Oldham, N. S., & Kay, D. J. (2004). Homelessness and health: What can be done in general practice? *Journal of the Royal Society of Medicine, 97,* 170–173.

Wu, L.-T., & Blazer, D. G. (2011). Illicit and nonmedical drug use among older adults: A review. *Journal of Aging and Health, 23,* 481–504.

Xu, K. T. (2003). Financial disparities in prescription drug use between elderly and nonelderly Americans. *Health Affairs, 22,* 210–221.

Yagoda, L. (2005). Older adults and health disparities: The impact on access to care. *InterSections in Practice NASW, 4,* 6–9.

Young, R. M., & Meyer, I. H. (2005). The trouble with "MSM" and "WSW": Erasure of the sexual minority person in public health discourse. *American Journal of Public Health, 95,* 1144–1149.

Zack, M. M., Moriarty, D. G., Stroup, D. F., Ford, E. S., & Mokdad, A. H. (2004). Worsening trends in adult health-rated quality of life and self-rated health, United States, 1993–2001. *Public Health Report, 119*(5), 493–505.

CHAPTER TWO

Informal Caregiving in the LGBT Communities

KAREN I. FREDRIKSEN-GOLDSEN, PH.D., M.S.W.

Equity in health is critical to society given its ethical and social justice implications. Despite tremendous advancements in medicine and improved health for many Americans, historically disadvantaged communities continue to bear higher levels of illness, disability, and premature death. The National Institutes of Health (2010) affirm a commitment to "reducing health disparities impacting racial and ethnic minority populations and other disadvantaged populations across the nation." Although lesbian, gay male, bisexual, and transgender (LGTB) persons encounter social inequalities, such as discrimination, that result in health disparities, sexual orientation and gender identity have largely been neglected as potential risk factors in the public and scientific discourse (Fredriksen-Goldsen, Hyun-Jun, Muraco, & Mincer, 2009; Fredriksen-Goldsen & Muraco, 2010; Institute of Medicine [IOM], 2011; Thompson, 2008). In addition to these factors, aging also affects health in critical ways. When we juxtapose sexual orientation and gender identity with differences in health by aging, we find multiple challenges lacking any targeted response from the health care and elder care professions.

The acronym LGBT will be used here to refer to those who self-identify as lesbian, gay, bisexual, or transgender. In most contexts, differing amounts of research have been conducted with these subpopulations (Fredriksen-Goldsen, Kim, & Goldsen, 2011; IOM, 2011). The available data regarding caregiving, for example, have generally been collected from research participants who self-identify as lesbians or gay men. Nonetheless, LGBT will be used for inclusiveness and to maintain awareness of the need for further research on behalf of each of these underrepresented groups.

Existing research suggests that health disparities exist across a variety of indicators, reflecting differences in access to health care, the prevalence of disease, and health outcomes. For example, certain segments of LGBT communities have been found to be at higher risk of financial barriers to care, victimization, smoking, obesity, suicide, alcohol and drug use, and infection with HIV/AIDS (Fredriksen-Goldsen et al., 2011; IOM, 2011). A study using area probability sampling found that, in one major urban area, lesbian and bisexual women, as compared with heterosexual women, had more limited access to health care and used fewer health screening services (Bowen et al., 2004). However, these differences did not exist across all indicators. For example, the two groups did not differ significantly in smoking rates, fat intake, or mammography screenings. More recent research illustrates differences in health indicators and health-related quality of life among lesbian and bisexual women, demonstrating the heterogeneity of the LGBT community (Fredriksen-Goldsen, Hyun-Jun, Barkan, Balsam, & Mincer, 2010).

Disparities in health care often result from differences in access, coverage, and quality of care and may increase reliance on informal caregivers to meet health-related needs. Within most medical and social services, the needs of LGBT elders are largely unmet. For example, Feldman and Bockting (2003) report that as many as 30% to 40% of transgender persons in the United States do not have a regular physician and often rely on emergency room and urgent care physicians for immediate health care needs. Fredriksen-Goldsen et al. (2011) found that 22% of transgender older adults needed to see a doctor but could not because of cost. Anecdotal evidence, along with studies of Witten and Eyler (discussed in the chapter 6, "Transgender and Aging"), point to many potential reasons for this lack of primary care.

Caregiving is a critical aging concern, influenced by health disparities that affect LGBT elders. In this chapter, I will explore the confluence of sexual orientation and gender identity as they intersect with aging and the changing nature of caregiving supports. I will also examine the prevalence of caregiving responsibilities and explore the unique structural issues that may impact caregiving in these communities. Factors that place these caregivers and those that receive care at risk for negative outcomes, as well as protective factors that may assist them in meeting the challenges they face, will be discussed. I will examine current federal and state laws and policies that may increase the vulnerability of LGBT caregivers and exacerbate existing health disparities. In conclusion, I will outline the necessary next steps in service delivery, public policy, and research to address the unique needs of these caregivers and those receiving care.

CAREGIVING

Caregiving is defined as unpaid assistance, provided by family members, friends, and neighbors, to help ill and disabled individuals remain in the community (Fredriksen-Goldsen & Scharlach, 2001). Factors such as the changing nature of the American family and the aging of the U.S. population significantly influence the extent and nature of caregiving. While the nuclear family is still normative, it no longer predominates as the normative family type; family caregiving is being provided in a variety of arrangements. Members of LGBT communities serve as primary caregivers, providing the majority of assistance to their loved ones when needed (Brotman, Ryan, & Cormier, 2003; Brotman et al., 2007; Fredriksen, 1999; MetLife, 2010).

The older LGBT population is projected to grow from approximately 2 million to more than 6 million by 2030 (Cahill, South, & Spade, 2000; Fredriksen-Goldsen & Muraco, 2010). Most long-term care for older adults is not provided in nursing homes but is given informally, at little or no public cost, within private homes or other community-based settings (National Academy on an Aging Society, 2000; Stone, 2000; Tennstedt, 1999). If informal supports such as these were not available, the long-term care costs would more than double (Arno, Levine, & Memmott, 1999). Informal care to elders is now typically more time intensive and technologically demanding, of longer duration, and provided to multiple family members at the same time (Bengtson, 2001). Current state and federal pressure to reduce health care costs, including shortened hospital stays and reduced funding to the Medicare and Medicaid programs, places even greater demands on informal caregivers.

As a result of their history of disadvantage, marginalization, and invisibility, LGBT individuals can encounter numerous obstacles in giving and receiving caregiving support, including discrimination in health care and long-term care settings, limited access to supportive services, and lack of legal protection for their partners and other loved ones. These unique and often challenging circumstances suggest that LGBT persons may be at especially high risk for negative health and caregiving outcomes. For example, because of inadequate health care and insurance coverage, transgender people of color are often at high risk because of compounding sources of stigmatization and discrimination related to racism, transphobia, and poverty (Xavier, 2004). Among LGBT persons with limited income, particularly low-income persons of color and immigrants, financial barriers are acute and often further limit access to formal supports.

Prevalence and Types of Caregiving

As members of historically disadvantaged groups, LGBT caregivers and those receiving care illustrate the diversity of needs, care arrangements, and effective informal and formal supports. Although an accurate assessment is difficult, given the ambiguities of defining sexual orientation and gender identity as well as the reluctance of research participants to self-disclose, estimates of the proportion of the population who are lesbian, gay, or bisexual range from as low as 2% to as high as 20% (Cahill et al., 2000; Sell, Wells, & Wypij, 1995; Tanfer, 1993). Michael, Gagnon, Lauman, and Kolata (1994) found, in one of the first representative data sets available, that 5% of males (although this figure rose to 10.9% of male respondents by age 50 years) and 4% of females reported having engaged in homosexual sex since age 18; 3% of males and 1.5% of females in the sample self-identified as homosexual. An analysis of the 2000 U.S. Census data found that 594,391 households self-identified as same-sex unmarried partners, representing nearly 1.2 million gay and lesbian partnered adults (Bradford, Barrett, & Honnold, 2002). The 2010 U.S. Census only asked for information about same-sex partners and spouses, not LGBT individuals (http://2010.census.gov/partners/pdf/factSheet_General_LGBT.pdf).

There are currently no reliable population estimates for transgender individuals, although in 1996, it was reported that more than 25,000 persons had obtained sex reassignment surgery and more than 60,000 planned to do so (Goldberg, 1996). Witten (2003; see also chapter 6, "Transgender and Aging") estimates that the 65 years and older transgender population in the United States may constitute 350,000 to 1 million individuals. The LGBT population is tremendously diverse with respect to age, ethnicity, education, income, geographic location, partnership status, living arrangement, and other familial relationships. For many LGBT persons, their families encompass both family of origin and family of choice, including partners, children, grandchildren, parents, grandparents, and other relatives, as well as intimate friends and other extended family members.

Thus, LGBT persons may be involved in caregiving through a variety of relationships: they may be caring for partners, friends, parents, children, and grandparents, as well as neighbors. Older LGBT persons also receive care, a trend that will likely increase with the aging of the population.

Caregivers who are LGBT, like other caregivers, assist individuals with a wide variety of illnesses and conditions and provide a range of caregiving assistance, including help with activities inside and outside the home (e.g., transportation, meal preparation, and housework), personal care (e.g., bathing, feeding, and dressing), emotional support, and mediating with formal service providers and agencies (Fredriksen, 1999; Hash, 2001; Hash & Cramer, 2003). The first national study on gay and lesbian caregiving across the life span documented extensive family care responsibilities in these communities. In this study, Fredriksen (1999) found that 32% of gay men and lesbians in the study were providing some type of caregiving, ranging from the care of children to the care of adults with serious illness or disability. Among the 27% who were providing adult care, 23% were assisting someone 18 to 64 years old and 8% were assisting someone 65 years or older. Among caregivers providing care for ill and disabled adults, most care recipients were friends (61%), followed by parents (16%), partners (13%), and other family members (10%). When comparing lesbians caring for ill and disabled adults with lesbians not providing such care, Fredriksen (1999) found caregivers to be older, less educated, and more likely to be partnered. Gay male caregivers, compared with their non-caregiving peers, were more likely to be older and out of the labor force.

In a large cross-sectional work site survey at a major university, Fredriksen (1996) found that 13% of the sample respondents who cared for a disabled or sick partner or spouse were in same-sex relationships. In another study of LGBT caregivers aged 50 years and older, 45% were currently providing care, including those caring for a partner or friend (23%), another family member—usually a parent—(18%), or both (4%) (Cahill, Ellen, & Tobias, 2002). Not surprisingly, these LGBT caregivers needed the same support as other caregivers, including respite, information and referral, backup services, and support groups. A recent study of LGBT caregivers aged 45 to 64 found that survey respondents were slightly more likely (21%) to engage in caregiving of another adult, relative to the heterosexual comparison group (17%) (MetLife, 2010); gay, bisexual, and transgender men were nearly as likely as women to be providing such care. However, LGBT respondents were less likely to be providing care to children and youth.

Kinship and Gender Effects in LGBT Caregiving

Unique structural issues differentiate LGBT caregiving from other types of care, including differing types of kinship relations and gender effects. In the general caregiving literature, kinship ties have been found to be related to the extent and pattern of care received. Among those in the general population, more than 50% of older adults who need assistance and live outside institutional settings rely primarily on spouses or adult children to help with their care (National Academy on an Aging Society, 2000). Among LGBT persons 50 years of age and older, most report that they would go to their partners first for assistance; among those without partners, the majority would seek assistance from friends (Cahill et al., 2002). The importance of friends in the lives of LGBT older adults has been demonstrated repeatedly (deVries, 2010; deVries & Megathlin, 2009; MetLife, 2010; Muraco, 2006; Muraco & Fredriksen-Goldsen, 2011).

Within gay and lesbian communities, it is common for intimate friends to form chosen family networks and to play significant roles in one another's lives (Muraco & Fredriksen-Goldsen, 2011). In addition, LGBT persons often have fewer children to provide assistance in old age, as compared with their heterosexual peers. Cahill et al. (2002) found that 80% of the New York City LGBT elders in their study did not have children. In a recent national study, three quarters of LGBT elders did not have children, with men significantly more likely not to have children as compared with women (Fredriksen-Goldsen et al., 2011). In the MetLife (2010) study of LGBT adults (aged 45–64), 1 household in 10 contained at least one child or adolescent under age 18, compared with 2 households in 10 in the heterosexual comparison group.

Significant gender differences in caregiving in the general population may not be reflected among LGBT populations. Nationwide, women provide the majority of family caregiving assistance, caring for dependent children, disabled working-age adults, and elderly persons (Fredriksen-Goldsen & Scharlach, 2001; Mitchell, 2000). In one study of lesbian and gay male caregivers, resource availability differed by gender (Fredriksen, 1999); gay male caregivers were more likely to have higher incomes, while lesbian caregivers were more likely to have a partner with whom they shared their family care tasks and responsibilities. In a recent study (MetLife, 2010), LGBT caregivers were similar to those in the general population in terms of caring for parents, partners, or spouses, but substantially more likely (21% compared with 6%) to be caring for friends. This study also found that men who identified as gay, bisexual, or transgender were substantially more likely than their heterosexual peers to be in significant caregiving roles. Additional research is needed to explore how gender transition and differing gender identities may impact caregiving and receiving care for transgender individuals and their families.

Risk Factors Impacting LGBT Caregiving

Several factors can place LGBT caregivers at risk for negative health and caregiving outcomes. These include stigma, harassment, nondisclosure, limited support and access to formal services, and lack of legal protection for loved ones.

Stigma

Stigma affects not only the attitudes of family members, friends, and helping professionals but also the help-seeking behaviors of LGBT persons and available formal services and family-based public policies (Fredriksen-Goldsen, 2007a). For example, differences in gender identity and gender nonconformity continue to be severely stigmatized and are still sometimes regarded as mental disorders (American Psychiatric Association, 2000). This type of severe stigmatization, as well as the historical context and negative attitudes toward LGBT persons, likely influences the strain on informal caregivers and those receiving care.

Discrimination, Harassment, and Hate Crimes

Discrimination and prejudice create several significant risk factors for LGBT individuals and their communities (Herek, 1990, 2000). In a study conducted in 1990, as many as 94% of lesbians and gay men reported some type of harassment or discrimination related to the perception of their sexual orientation (National Gay and Lesbian Task Force, 1990), and these types of experiences appear to influence the health of LGBT older adults and their caregivers (Fredriksen-Goldsen et al., 2009). Gay and lesbian caregivers report encountering several types of harassment and abuse, which include verbal (93%), emotional (46%), physical (14%), and sexual (8%) (Fredriksen, 1999). Violence, harassment, and discrimination are also common experiences among transgender people (Fredriksen-Goldsen et al., 2011; Lombardi, 2001; Xavier, 2004), setting the stage for particular challenges for caregivers and those receiving care.

According to the Federal Bureau of Investigation, 7,783 hate crimes were reported in 2008 of which 1,297 (17%) were based on sexual orientation (www.hrc .org/documents/FBI_Hate_Crime_stats_2008.pdf). This figure is likely extremely low since an estimated 80% or more of hate crimes based on sexual orientation are unreported—most often because of fear of being openly identified as LGB

(National Organization for Women, 2003). However, legal protections for sexual and gender minority persons have recently improved. Public Law No. 111-84, the Matthew Shepard and James Byrd, Jr. Hate Crimes Prevention Act (HCPA; www.hrc.org/laws_and_elections/5660.htm) signed into law by President Obama on October 28, 2009, expanded the demographic groups covered by hate crime legislation and the U.S. Department of Justice now has the power to investigate and prosecute violent crimes based on the victim's actual or perceived race, color, national origin, religion, gender, gender identity, sexual orientation, or disability. Furthermore, the FBI is now required to keep hate crime statistics based on such demographic characteristics.

Disclosure

Unlike some other minority groups, most LGBT persons are not readily identifiable; thus, as caregivers and those receiving care, they must manage disclosure of their sexual orientation or gender identity. For transgender individuals, the public nature of a gender transition may result in increased exposure to unwelcome comments and reactions from others (Cook-Daniels, 2006). The extent of self-disclosure determines the nature and depth of one's support system, and a high degree of social support available to a caregiver has been found to be associated with positive caregiving outcomes (Magana, 1999). Ironically, disclosure can also expose an individual to hostility from others.

Potential Lack of Traditional Sources of Support

Family members are usually a primary source of support for caregivers. However, LGBT caregivers may receive less support than they need, from their own or the care recipient's family of origin. They may be expected to provide high levels of caregiving assistance within their families of origin, yet also be denied support when caring for seriously ill or disabled partners, friends, or other persons in their extended family networks. Members of one's family of origin may treat "chosen families" as "temporary and not important" or as a cohabiting arrangement rather than as a stable family (Erera & Fredriksen, 1999).

Family members may perceive members of these groups to be "single" and less place-bound, with the availability to provide care to ill or ailing parents or to other family members. Prejudice and a lack of recognition of primary relationships and extended family networks likely fuel this process. It has long been suggested that lesbians and gay men may be expected, and more likely, to assume a primary caregiving role within the family of origin (Kimmel, 1992).

Among gay men and lesbians caring for a partner or friend, 7% reported receiving no support of any kind from their family of origin, 68% received at least *some* support, and another 25% reported that their entire family supported them (Fredriksen, 1999). Although supportive, family members may not be actively involved in helping them meet their day-to-day caregiving responsibilities. Other studies have examined the roles of LGB older adults within families of origin and the level of support received (reviewed in Fredriksen-Goldsen & Muraco, 2010); this remains an ongoing area of research interest.

In a review of bisexuality and aging, Dworkin (2006) reports that bisexual persons in the United States are more likely than gay men or lesbians to have been married and to have had children. The MetLife Study of Lesbian, Gay, Bisexual, and Transgender Baby Boomers (MetLife, 2010) found that the experiences of bisexual women and men were different from their lesbian and gay peers. Bisexual survey respondents were more likely to be guarded about their sexual orientation and less likely to be out; they were also less likely to have strong friendship networks and families accepting of their sexual orientation.

Workplace discrimination and hostility also places LGBT caregivers at higher risk for caregiving stress by denying them the day-to-day emotional support and access to workplace benefits accorded to other families in similar situations. Unsupportive workplaces discourage LGBT persons from being honest about themselves and their lives and can foster denial of their personal identities, the legitimacy of their relationships, and their care responsibilities.

Lack of Access to Supportive Services

In the general caregiving literature, it has long been reported that caregivers experiencing diminished access to formal support systems face significantly more physical, psychological, emotional, social, and financial risks than those who receive this assistance (George & Gwyther, 1986). Unfortunately, many LGBT persons are reluctant to disclose their sexual orientation or transgender identity and their primary relationships in formal care settings because of real or expected harassment and discrimination from professionals and institutions.

Service providers sometimes fail to acknowledge relationships within LGBT families or openly disregard them and discredit the role of these caregivers. Furthermore, some agencies and institutions have such entrenched biases that they openly deny access to services to LGBT persons and their families. For reasons such as these, many LGBT caregivers and those receiving care may not seek out supplementary support or formal services, even when it is understood that there is a need for specialized care (Fredriksen-Goldsen et al., 2011; IOM, 2011; Tully, 1989).

Patients receive a higher quality of care, and more thorough care, when they are able to be honest and open with their health care and social service providers (Lambda Legal, 2003; Robertson, 2003). Support services developed within the LGBT community are most likely to be used by individuals who openly identify as members of these groups. Conversely, those that conceal their sexual orientation or gender identity may be less likely to use formal support services, even though they may be the most isolated and in need of assistance.

Lack of Legal Protection

Many federal and state laws and policies that provide family-based benefits use legal and structural forms inherently biased against LGBT caregivers and those that receive care. The regulatory policies intended to support families in times of need are often not accessible to LGBT families and, in many cases, raise additional barriers to receiving help. The range of institutional inequities includes allowing discrimination in employment, housing, and public accommodations, and denying same-sex partners health care benefits, family leave benefits, equivalent Medicaid spend-downs, Social Security benefits, and bereavement leave. Managed care and insurance policies are also often discriminatory (Garnets, Hancock, Cochran, Goodchilds, & Peplau, 1991; Kauth, Hartwig, & Kalichman, 2000; Phillips & Fischer, 1998; Winegarten, Cassie, Markowski, Kozlowski, & Yoder, 1994). If extensive legal planning is not completed in advance, LGBT caregivers and care recipients can be left highly vulnerable to the conflicting desires of members of the biological family, even if they have not been involved in the life of the LGBT individual for many years.

Discrimination in employment, housing, and public accommodation. In 2011, 21 states and the District of Columbia have laws banning employment discrimination based on sexual orientation; 16 of these states plus the District of Columbia also prohibit employment discrimination based on gender identity (www.hrc.org /documents/Employment_Laws_and_Policies.pdf). Housing discrimination is prohibited in 20 states based on sexual orientation and 16 states based on gender identity, and federal regulations prohibiting discrimination in HUD-administered housing programs are under consideration (ibid.). Some local ordinances banning discrimination are also in effect; however, millions of Americans still lack these basic protections.

Lack of protection from discrimination in employment leaves LGBT caregivers and those receiving care highly vulnerable to economic insecurity. In one study, gay and lesbian caregivers were more likely to report an increased likelihood of job termination as a result of their care responsibilities than were their heterosexual peers (Fredriksen, 1999). Furthermore, since discrimination in housing and public accommodations is generally not prohibited, LGBT caregivers and their care recipients may be openly discriminated against in many settings, including retirement and long-term care settings.

Lack of legal recognition of same-sex couples. The current lack of legal protection for same-sex couples raises significant barriers for LGBT caregivers caring for disabled partners. Although domestic partnership benefits are often perceived as providing rights equivalent to marriage, most are but a pale shadow. Legally recognized marriages bestow hundreds of rights, responsibilities, and benefits on married couples, many at the federal level. According to the General Accounting Office, there are more than 1,000 benefits, protections, and responsibilities automatically conferred on the legally married (Cahill et al., 2000). As of August, 2011, six states and the District of Columbia recognize full legal marriage for same-sex couples; seven states allow civil unions or domestic partnership providing most state-level spousal rights, and three states offer more limited domestic partnerships, which provide access to some state benefits. Two states have passed civil union statutes that will take effect on January 1, 2012. Civil unions and domestic partnerships do not provide any federal protections or benefits and are usually not "portable" to other states; that is, they are not legally recognized in other states and confer no specific benefits outside the home state, unless both states provide civil union or same-sex marriage recognition. Interestingly, one state that does not allow same-sex marriages, civil unions, or domestic partnerships recognizes same-sex marriages from other states. (www.hrc.org/resources/entry/maps-of-state-laws-policies/Relationship_Recognition_Laws_Map.pdf). In contrast, other sex marriages are recognized reciprocally throughout the United States and in other countries.

Numerous city and county governments offer some sort of domestic partnership recognition. Domestic partnership benefits vary widely between different states and municipalities, ranging from health care benefits to simple registration for same-sex couples without explicit benefits (Human Rights Campaign, 2003). Health benefits are most typical, followed by dental benefits, bereavement and sick leave, and, in a few cases, retirement benefits, death benefits, and long-term care and life insurance benefits (Cahill et al., 2002).

The federal Defense of Marriage Act (DOMA), passed in 1996, defines marriage as "a legal union between one man and one woman as husband and wife" and affirms that no state is required to honor same-sex marriages performed in another state. In 2004, the Federal Marriage Amendment, which would have amended the U.S. Constitution with the DOMA definition, failed in the U.S. Senate by a 50 to 48 vote. Many states have passed a state-level version of DOMA, which explicitly prohibits the recognition of same-sex couples, or have passed constitutional amendments banning gay marriage. Some states have passed broader antigay family measures that ban other forms of partner recognition in addition to marriage (such as domestic partnership and civil unions) (Jacobs, 2006; National Gay and Lesbian Task Force, 2007). However, on February 23, 2011, the Obama administration announced that the U.S. Department of Justice would no longer defend DOMA, and legislation that would repeal DOMA, the Respect for Marriage Act of 2011, is currently under consideration (H.R. 1116, S. 598). Although the outcome of this struggle remains uncertain, LGBT older adults commonly express the need for legal marriage. In the MetLife survey (2010) 26% of partnered LGBT older adults were married, despite the fact that only five states offered marriage licenses at that time. Many more said that they would be "very" or "fairly" likely to marry if marriage was legal at the federal (63%) or state (55%) level.

Legal recognition and protection are especially important in the event of a health emergency or other crisis to ensure recognition and economic security of LGBT family members. One important benefit of marriage is "next of kin" status. When a heterosexual couple marries, each automatically becomes the legal next of kin. The rights that are bestowed with the next-of-kin status include the right to make health care decisions on behalf of an incapacitated spouse and the uncontested inheritance of both real and personal property (Ettelbrick, 1996). If a LGBT person becomes incapacitated and has not executed a legal durable power of attorney for health care, many state laws mandate that a married spouse or legally recognized family member be appointed to manage affairs and make decisions, regardless of the disabled person's wishes (Epstein, 2003). In one study of caregivers for gay men with AIDS, more than 60% did not have a will, a living will, or a durable power of attorney for health care (Fredriksen-Goldsen, 2003).

Although legally recognized family members and legally married spouses have the right to see their loved ones in a medical emergency, hospital staff have at times barred LGBT partners and others from visiting. For example, a Baltimore jury ruled in favor of a hospital that prevented a gay man from visiting his dying lover because the longtime partner was not considered "family" (Epstein,

2003). By the time the partner was allowed to visit, the patient was unconscious and unable to say goodbye. However, effective January 18, 2011, new federal regulations were enacted which prohibit discrimination in visitation based on sexual orientation and gender identity by hospitals participating in Medicare and Medicaid programs (Center for Medicare and Medicaid Services, 42 C.F.R.).

Family and Medical Leave Act. Family leave has been endorsed by employees as the workplace policy most likely to help them manage their family caregiving and work responsibilities (Fredriksen-Goldsen & Scharlach, 2001). Under the federal Family and Medical Leave Act (FMLA) of 1993, employers with more than 50 employees are required to allow 12 weeks of unpaid leave during a 12-month period for employees to care for ill family members or new children or to attend to personal illness. Employers must continue health care coverage during leaves and restore employees to their jobs or equivalent positions on their return. Although individual companies may extend family leave benefits to employees in same-sex partnerships, FMLA does not include domestic partners or same-sex couples. In 2011, nine states and the District of Columbia include same-sex spouses and domestic partners in state-level family and medical leave laws. The Family Medical Leave Inclusion Act would broaden the scope of FMLA benefits and would include domestic partners and same-sex spouses. It is under consideration currently, but its future is uncertain (www.hrc.org/resources/entry/maps-of-state-laws-policies).

Supplemental Security Income and Social Security Disability Insurance. Cahill et al. (2000) suggest that "Social Security's treatment of same-sex couples is perhaps the most blatant and costly example of institutionalized heterosexism in federal policy." While legally married couples and their children are entitled to survivor's benefits, same-sex couples are not, and only in those states that recognize second-parent adoption can surviving children receive Social Security benefits. Spousal benefits allow the surviving partner in a legally recognized marriage to collect the partner's benefit amount if that amount is greater than their own, based on their lifetime work history. Denial of spousal benefits to elder lesbian and gay couples robs them of about $124 million per year in survivors' benefits (Cahill et al., 2000). Based on 2000 U.S. Census figures, the average loss in Social Security income by the surviving same-sex spouse is $5,528 per year (Human Rights Campaign, 2004).

The inequality of benefits for same-sex partners also extends to Social Security Disability Insurance. If a working-age adult becomes disabled, in addition to his or her own disability benefit, the legally married spouse also receives one-half of the monthly benefit of the disabled spouse. For same-sex couples, there is no recognition of the relationship and, hence, no second benefit. Because of such discriminatory policies, caregivers and those receiving care in same-sex relationships often have fewer financial resources available to meet their caregiving needs.

Medicaid. Another arena in which caregivers and those receiving care in same-sex couples are discriminated against is the joint federally and state administered Medicaid spend-down program. Medicare will usually cover expenses for the first 100 days in a nursing home or skilled nursing facility, when care is needed for recuperation and rehabilitation after surgery or acute illness. However, Medicaid usually pays for long-term stays (more than 100 days) in nursing homes for disabled individuals who lack substantial financial resources.

For those who require nursing-home care but cannot afford it, Medicaid will pay for long-term care and home health care through the Medicaid spend-down program. The spend-down program has strict eligibility requirements for income and assets and depends on marital status. When a husband or wife in a heterosexual marriage enters a nursing home with Medicaid benefits, federal law allows the spouse to remain in their joint residence; he or she need not sell the home to "spend down" to a minimum level of assets to pay for care. Since same-sex relationships are not recognized at the federal level, this protection is absent. The couple may be forced to choose between keeping the home and Medicaid eligibility to pay for the nursing home care (Human Rights Campaign, 2004).

Another aspect of the Medicaid spend-down program that affects LGBT caregivers in same-sex couples is the estate recovery process. This program allows for the recovery of Medicaid expenditures from the estate of the deceased person, typically through the sale of the home or other assets. For legally married heterosexual couples, the state will generally not begin recovery proceedings (e.g., forced real property sale) from the estate until the surviving spouse has also died. This allows the survivor to remain in the home, without fear of impoverishment or homelessness. This benefit does not extend to couples whose relationships lack legal recognition. After the death of the loved one, a surviving partner may be forced to sell the home (if jointly owned) that they have shared and surrender half of the proceeds to the state (Cahill et al., 2000; WAGS, 2003). Such policies are intended to help families in need but clearly discriminate against families with caregivers and care recipients in same-sex relationships, thereby increasing their economic insecurity and emotional stress (Human Rights Campaign, 2004).

CAREGIVING OUTCOMES

General caregiving studies suggest that informal care of a relative with disabilities often results in negative consequences for caregivers and their families (Owens, 2001; Polen & Green, 2001). In the general caregiving research, caregiving strain has repeatedly been associated with decreased physical and psychological health among caregivers, including increased levels of caregiver burden (Braithwaite, 2000), role strain, fatigue (Polen & Green, 2001), anxiety (Cochrane, Goering, & Rogers, 1997; Polen & Green, 2001), depression (Berg-Weger, Rubio, & Tebb, 2000; Han & Haley, 1999), and poor health outcomes over time (Beach, Schulz, Yee, & Jackson, 2000).

The majority of research that has examined LGBT caregiving has focused on HIV/AIDS-related caregiving outcomes. Among caregivers assisting gay men with AIDS, several risks have been found: family and employment conflicts, social isolation, depression, sleep disturbance, physical ailments, and relationship pressures (Folkman, Chesney, & Christopher-Richards, 1994; Fredriksen-Goldsen, 2003; Turner, Catania, & Gagnon, 1994). Caregiver distress has been described as the secondary epidemic associated with the AIDS crisis (Rait, 1991), adversely affecting the psychological well-being of informal caregivers (Irving, Bor, & Catalan, 1995; Pearlin, Mullan, Aneshensel, Wadlaw, & Harrington, 1994; Tolliver, 2001) and resulting in the restriction of social opportunities and an increase in economic problems (Callery, 2000; Clipp, Adinolfi, Forrest, & Bennett, 1995; Raveis & Siegal, 1991; Turner et al., 1994; Wight, 2000).

Less is known about the physical or psychological health of LGBT caregivers outside the context of AIDS care, though information is increasing (Fredriksen-Goldsen, 2010; Fredriksen-Goldsen et al., 2011; MetLife, 2010). Hash (2001) reported an increased risk of physical and psychological strain, poor nutrition, and financial problems among gay and lesbian caregivers. In addition, a few community-based surveys have documented high levels of care responsibilities, with many caregivers experiencing physical, financial, and emotional strain (Fredriksen, 1999; Hoctel, 2002; Shippy, Cantor, & Brennan, 2001). In one study comparing outcomes among caregivers assisting ill and disabled partners in same-sex versus other-sex couples, those caring for ill or disabled same-sex partners were providing significantly more hours of care and higher levels of assistance and were experiencing higher levels of role strain and increased likelihood of job termination as a result of their care responsibilities (Fredriksen, 1996). The MetLife (2010) study found that gay, bisexual, and transgender men engaged in adult caregiving reported investing the greatest time commitment of any of the study groups (41 hours weekly as compared to 26–29 hours weekly).

Available research also demonstrates a high level of resilience among many of these caregivers and those receiving care, in part because of the capacities and skills they have developed through surmounting obstacles as members of disadvantaged and disenfranchised groups (Clunis et al., 2005; Fredriksen-Goldsen, 2003; Fredriksen-Goldsen & Muraco, 2010). Their skill in adapting to adverse circumstances and gender role flexibility likely assist them in meeting caregiving demands.

NEXT STEPS TO ASSIST LGBT CAREGIVERS

Several steps are needed to assist LGBT caregivers and those needing care. These include ensuring access to appropriate services, increasing social support, developing culturally appropriate caregiving interventions, advocating for equitable public policies, and conducting methodologically sound and rigorous research aimed at fully understanding the caregiving needs, strengths, and experiences within these diverse communities.

Educational materials, support groups, and even simply interacting with other LGBT elders and their families have been shown to be efficacious in helping family members and friends address concerns regarding sexual orientation. These interventions can help family members confront their own biases as well as counter social stigma, isolation, and feelings of inadequacy, grief, and loss. It is important for LGBT persons to communicate the significance and meaning of their relationships to their families of origin, who may not understand the significance of these committed relationships.

Support services and organizations need to address discriminatory practices in access and delivery of services (Coon, 2003; Fredriksen-Goldsen, 2007b). It is imperative that service agencies evaluate the ability of their employees to serve LGBT clients professionally and compassionately and provide training if they do not. Agency forms and assessment instruments should be reviewed to ensure that they are culturally sensitive and relevant to the lives of LGBT persons.

Training can help professionals to understand the multifaceted nature of individual identity and the impact of other factors such as age, ethnicity, income, geographic location, and ability as they relate to the caregiving experience. Educational efforts should include the use of gender- and sexuality-inclusive language and should address the inherent dangers of making unwarranted assumptions about relationship status, gender identity, sexual orientation, and other related factors.

When assured of privacy and offered a safe and welcoming environment, caregivers and those receiving care are more likely to disclose crucial information that can influence the services they receive. Formal service providers should acknowledge the central role of extended families and friendship networks in providing needed support to LGBT caregivers and those receiving care (Bonuck, 1993; Fredriksen, 1999; Weston, 1991). Service providers should also become familiar with the culturally competent professionals and available resources within LGBT communities. When agencies fail to adopt culturally appropriate and nondiscriminatory policies, LGBT caregivers and those receiving care should be referred to knowledgeable and supportive providers. As new services are developed, LGBT community involvement and feedback will be important. By including input from the community, more relevant services can be developed, and these, in turn, can promote a deeper understanding of aging and caregiving within LGBT communities.

Legal professionals, service providers, caregivers, and care recipients can benefit from training and education in navigating existing public policies. Until full social equality is achieved, assisting LGBT clients in legal planning will remain the best means of ensuring economic security for all members of LGBT families. It is vital that estate planning documents, wills, revocable trusts, and durable powers of attorney for property, finances, and health care, as well as advance directives, all be in place before they are needed. Although legal documents can be challenged, caregivers in same-sex couples should, at minimum, have a durable health care power of attorney that specifies the following for the partner: first priority for visitation in hospitals, release of information about a partner's condition, authorization of medical treatment if incapacitated, authorization of release of bodily remains from a hospital, and provisions for services and last requests (Epstein, 2003). In addition, an understanding of Medicaid eligibility and requirements are necessary, because the recovery of Medicaid-paid expenses from the deceased's estate can seriously affect surviving partners, as can the disallowance of death and property tax reassessment exemptions (Human Rights Campaign, 2004; Wenzel, 2002). This cannot be remedied under the current federal policies but must be considered in family financial and legal planning.

PUBLIC POLICY ISSUES

For LGBT caregivers and their relationships to be wholly accepted and respected, both attitudes and policies of government institutions and the larger society must change. A first step is the evaluation of policies that discriminate against unmarried or same-sex couples, such as family medical leave and health care benefits for same-sex and other-sex partners. Service providers should also become familiar with existing policies at the local, state, and federal levels, and the ways in which these can negatively affect both caregiving and the larger social context within which LGBT persons live their lives. The primary policy goal is to promote respect and equality for LGBT caregivers and those receiving care. Well-informed caregivers, care recipients, service providers, and health care professionals can work toward revising public policies, such as the Family and Medical Leave Act, Social Security, and Medicaid spend-down requirements.

Additional LGBT caregiving research that emphasizes theoretical and methodological rigor is strongly needed. Research would be strengthened by examining variations in caregiving needs, experiences, and outcomes as they relate to values and norms among historically disadvantaged populations. One significant limitation in existing LGBT research is that most studies have focused on the experiences of young and healthy individuals, without attending to the experiences of older adults with functional disabilities and in need of care (Fredriksen & Muraco, 2010).

Additional research is needed to explore more fully the requirements and experiences of LGBT caregivers and those receiving care, focusing on the vast diversity within these communities. Important variables that warrant further attention include age, ethnicity, education, income, physical ability, religion, geographical location, and generational and historical cohort differences, as well as differing relationship and familial arrangements. All health and social science research should include information on sexual orientation and gender identity as important structural characteristics that influence health and caregiving outcomes.

Future research should examine long-term plans and decision-making processes guiding LGBT caregivers and those receiving care, the interrelationship between both informal and formal supports, and the effectiveness of interventions to serve these communities. For example, as gay men and lesbians often have fewer children than their heterosexual peers, and rely heavily on friends for caregiving assistance, it will be important to examine the experiences of the oldest-old members of these population groups, who may have few surviving same-age peers to provide assistance (Fredriksen-Goldsen & Muraco, 2010). In these cases, research is needed to more thoroughly explore the provision of informal and formal care and whether other intergenerational relations are instrumental in providing ongoing assistance.

Although some areas of inquiry have sought to understand how people stay healthy despite serious adversity, the field of caregiving generally has not addressed this question. Future research on behalf of LGBT caregivers and those receiving care should examine factors that may serve as protective mechanisms and support them in their caregiving and aging experiences, and result in positive health and caregiving outcomes. In addition, most LGBT research participants are those who most readily self-disclose personal identity, whereas those least likely to participate may be the most isolated and the most in need of supportive services. Thus, additional effort is necessary to ensure broader representation in future studies. Longitudinal studies are also needed to explore more fully the ways in which family processes and development can impact LGBT caregiving over time.

MOVING FORWARD

The interplay of prejudice and shame, combined with institutional and legal discrimination, differentiates LGBT caregiving from the experience of most caregivers and can place these families at increased risk for poor health. Contrary to popular perception, LGBT persons often have extensive caregiving responsibilities (Fredriksen, 1999; Fredriksen-Goldsen et al., 2011; MetLife, 2010), which will likely increase as the population ages. We must respond to the risk factors impacting LGBT caregivers and those receiving care and explore the strengths and resilience that these individuals and families bring to aging and caring for one another.

REFERENCES

American Psychiatric Association. (2000). *Diagnostic and statistical manual of mental disorders* (4th ed., text rev.). Washington, DC: Author.

Arno, P. S., Levine, C., & Memmott, M. M. (1999). The economic value of informal caregiving. *Health Affairs, 18*(2), 182–188.

Beach, S., Schulz, R., Yee, J., & Jackson, S. (2000). Negative and positive health effects of caring for a disabled spouse: Longitudinal findings from the Caregiver Health Effects Study. *Psychology and Aging, 15*(2), 259–271.

Bengtson, V. L. (2001). Beyond the nuclear family: The increasing importance of multigenerational bonds. *Journal of Marriage and the Family, 63*(1), 1–16.

Berger, R. M. (1996). *Gay and gray: The older homosexual man* (2nd ed.). Binghamton, NY: Haworth Press.

Berg-Weger, M., Rubio, D. M., & Tebb, S. S. (2000). Depression as a mediator: Viewing caregiver well-being and strain in a different light. *Families in Society, 81*(2), 162–173.

Bowen, D. J., Bradford, J. B., Powers, D., McMorrow, P., Linde, R., Cody Murphy, B., . . . Ellis, J. (2004). Comparing women of differing sexual orientations using population-based sampling. *Women & Health, 40*(3), 19–34.

Bradford, J., Barrett, K., & Honnold, J. A. (2002). *The 2000 census and same-sex households: A user's guide.* New York: Policy Institute of the National Gay and Lesbian Task Force, the Survey and Evaluation Research Laboratory, and the Fenway Institute.

Braithwaite, V. (2000). Contextual or general stress outcomes: Making choices through caregiving appraisals. *Gerontologist, 40*(6), 706–717.

Brotman, S., Ryan, B., Collins, S., Chamberland, L., Cormier, R., Julien, D., & Richard, B. (2007). Coming out to care: Caregivers of gay and lesbian seniors in Canada. *Gerontologist, 47*, 490–503.

Brotman, S., Ryan, B., & Cormier, R. (2003). The health and social service needs of gay and lesbian elders and their families in Canada. *Gerontologist, 43*(2), 192.

Cahill, S., Ellen, M., & Tobias, S. (2002). *Family policy: Issues affecting gay, lesbian, bisexual, and transgender families.* New York: Policy Institute of the National Gay and Lesbian Task Force.

Cahill, S., South, K., & Spade, J. (2000). *Outing age: Public policy issues affecting gay, lesbian, bisexual, and transgender elders* [Policy report]. New York: Policy Institute of the National Gay and Lesbian Task Force.

Callery, K. E. (2000). The role of stigma and psycho-social factors on perceived caregiver burden in HIV/AIDS gay male caregivers. *Dissertation Abstracts International: Section B. The Sciences and Engineering, 61*(5B), 2469.

Clipp, E. C., Adinolfi, A. J., Forrest, L., & Bennett, C. L. (1995). Informal caregivers of persons with AIDS. *Journal of Palliative Care, 11*(2), 10–18.

Clunis, M., Fredriksen-Goldsen, K. I., Freeman, P., & Nystrom, N. (2005). *Looking back, looking forward: The lives of lesbian elders.* Binghamton, NY: Haworth Press.

Cochrane, J. J., Goering, P. N., & Rogers, J. M. (1997). The mental health of informal caregivers in Ontario: An epidemiological survey. *American Journal of Public Health, 87*(2), 2002–2007.

Cook-Daniels, L. (2006). Trans aging. In D. C. Kimmel, T. Rose, & S. David (Eds.), *Lesbian, gay, bisexual, and transgender aging: Research and clinical perspectives* (pp. 20–35). New York: Columbia University Press.

Coon, D. W. (2003). *Lesbian, gay, bisexual, and transgender (LGBT) issues and family caregiving.* San Francisco: Family Caregiver Alliance National Center on Caregiving.

deVries, B. (2010, Winter). Friendship and family: The company we keep. *Transition, 2010,* 1–4.

deVries, B., & Megathlin, D. (2009). The meaning of friendship for gay men and lesbians in the second half of life. *Journal GLBT Family Studies, 5*(1–2), 82–98.

Dworkin, S. H. (2006). The aging bisexual: The invisible of the invisible minority. In D. C. Kimmel, T. Rose, & S. David (Eds.). (2006). *Lesbian, gay, bisexual, and transgender aging: Research and clinical perspectives* (pp. 36–52). New York: Columbia University Press.

Epstein, A. (2003, December 19). Gay basics: Partner medical rights documentation. *Gay Financial News.*

Erera, P. I., & Fredriksen, K. I. (1999). Lesbian stepfamilies: A unique family structure. *Families in Society, 80*(3), 263–270.

Ettelbrick, P. L. (1996). Legal issues in health care for lesbians and gay men. *Journal of Gay and Lesbian Social Services, 5*(1), 93–109.

Federal Bureau of Investigation. (2003). *Hate crime statistics: 2002* (Uniform Crime Reporting Program). Washington, DC: Author.

Feinberg, L. F. (2001). *Systems development for family caregiver support services.* San Francisco: Family Caregiver Alliance.

Folkman, S., Chesney, M. A., & Christopher-Richards, A. (1994). Stress and coping in caregiving partners of men with AIDS. *Psychiatric Clinics of North America, 17*(1), 35–53.

Fredriksen, K. I. (1996). *Lesbian and gay caregiving.* Paper presented at the 18th Annual National Lesbian and Gay Health Conference, Seattle, WA.

Fredriksen, K. I. (1999). Family caregiving responsibilities among lesbians and gay men. *Social Work, 44*(2), 142–155.

Fredriksen-Goldsen, K. I. (2007a). *Caregiving with pride.* Binghamton, NY: Haworth Press.

Fredriksen-Goldsen, K. I. (2007b). HIV//AIDS caregiving: Predictors of well-being and distress. *Journal of Gay and Lesbian Social Services, 18*(3/4), 53–73.

Fredriksen-Goldsen, K. I., Hyun-Jun, K., Barkan, S. E., Balsam, K. F., & Mincer, S. L. (2010). Disparities in health-related quality of life: A comparison of lesbians and bisexual women. *American Journal of Public Health, 100,* 2255–2261.

Fredriksen-Goldsen, K. I., Hyun-Jun, K., & Goldsen, J. (2011). *The health report: Resilience and disparities among lesbian, gay, bisexual and transgender older adults— preliminary findings.* Seattle, WA: Institute for Multigenerational Health.

Fredriksen-Goldsen, K. I., Hyun-Jun, K., Muraco, A., & Mincer, S. (2009). Chronically ill midlife and older lesbians, gay men, and bisexuals and their informal caregivers: The impact of social context. *Sexuality Research & Social Policy, 6*(4), 52–64.

Fredriksen-Goldsen, K. I., & Muraco, A. (2010). Aging and sexual orientation: A 25-year review of the literature. *Research on Aging, 32,* 372–413.

Fredriksen-Goldsen, K. I., & Scharlach, A. E. (2001). *Families and work: New directions in the twenty-first century.* New York: Oxford University Press.

Garnets, L., Hancock, K., Cochran, S., Goodchilds, J., & Peplau, L. (1991). Issues in psychotherapy with lesbians and gay men: A survey of psychologists. *American Psychologist, 46*(9), 964–972.

Gender Public Advocacy Coalition. (2007). Four more states ban gender identity /expression discrimination. Retrieved from www.gpac.org/workplace/news.html ?cmd=view&archive=news&msgnum=0678

George, L. K., & Gwyther, L. P. (1986). Caregiver well-being: A multidimensional examination of family caregivers of demented adults. *Gerontologist, 26*(3), 253–259.

Goldberg, C. (1996, September 8). He and she, they fight for respect. *New York Times*, p. 10.

Han, B., & Haley, W. E. (1999). Family caregiving for patients with stroke: Review and analysis. *Stroke, 30*(7), 1478–1485.

Hancock, K. A. (2000). Lesbian, gay, and bisexual lives: Basic issues in psychotherapy training and practice. In B. Green & G. L. Croom (Eds.), *Education, research, and practice in lesbian, gay, bisexual, and transgendered psychology* (pp. 91–130). Thousand Oaks, CA: Sage.

Hash, K. M. (2001). Preliminary study of caregiving and post-caregiving experiences of older gay men and lesbians. *Journal of Gay and Lesbian Social Services, 13*(4), 87–94.

Hash, K. M., & Cramer, E. P. (2003). Empowering gay and lesbian caregivers and uncovering their unique experiences through the use of qualitative methods. *Journal of Gay and Lesbian Social Services, 15*(1/2), 47–63.

Herek, G. M. (1990). The context of anti-gay violence: Notes on cultural and psychological heterosexism. *Journal of Interpersonal Violence, 5*(3), 316–333.

Herek, G. M. (2000). The psychology of sexual prejudice. *Current Directions in Psychological Science, 9*(1), 19–22.

Hoctel, P. D. (2002). Community assessments show service gaps for LGBT elders. *Aging Today, 23*(1), 5–6.

Human Rights Campaign. (2003). *States banning workplace discrimination based on sexual orientation.* Washington, DC: Author.

Human Rights Campaign. (2004). *The cost of marriage inequality to gay, lesbian and bisexual seniors.* Washington, DC: Author.

Human Rights Campaign. (2007). *Hate crimes amendment removed from Department of Defense conference report.* Retrieved from www.hrc.org/8435.htm

Institute of Medicine (IOM). (2011). *The health of lesbian, gay, bisexual, and transgender people: Building a foundation for better understanding.* Washington, DC: National Academies Press.

Intersex Society of North America (ISNA). (2006). *Frequently asked questions: What is intersex? How common is intersex?* Retrieved from www.isna.org/faq

Irving, G., Bor, R., & Catalan, J. (1995). Psychological distress among gay men supporting a lover or partner with AIDS: A pilot study. *AIDS Care, 7*(5), 605–617.

Jacobs, S. (2006, May 17). Georgia's gay marriage ban voided. *Atlanta Journal-Constitution.* Retrieved from www.hrc.org

Kauth, M. R., Hartwig, M. J., & Kalichman, S. C. (2000). Health behavior relevant to psychotherapy with lesbian, gay, and bisexual clients. In R. Perez, K. A. DeBord, & K. J. Bieschke (Eds.), *Handbook of counseling and psychotherapy with lesbian, gay, and bisexual clients* (pp. 435–446). Washington, DC: American Psychological Association.

Kimmel, D. C. (1992). The families of older gay men and lesbians. *Generations, 16*(3), 37–38.

Lambda Legal. (2003). *Brooklyn Housing v. Lynch: New case!* Washington, DC: Author.

Lombardi, E. (2001). Enhancing transgender health care. *American Journal of Public Health*, 91(6), 869–872.

Magana, S. M. (1999). Puerto Rican families caring for an adult with mental retardation: Role of familialism. *American Journal on Mental Retardation*, 104(5), 466–482.

MetLife. (2010). *Still out, still aging: The MetLife Study of Lesbian, Gay, Bisexual, and Transgender Baby Boomers*. Westport, CT: MetLife Mature Market Institute.

Michael, R., Gagnon, J., Lauman, E., & Kolata, G. (1994). *Sex in America*. Boston: Little, Brown.

Mitchell, V. (2000). The bloom is on the rose: The impact of midlife on the lesbian couple. *Journal of Gay and Lesbian Social Services*, 11(2/3), 33–48.

Muraco, A. (2006). Intentional families: Fictive kin ties between cross-gender, different sexual orientation friends. *Journal of Marriage and Family*, 68, 1313–1325.

Muraco, A., & Fredriksen-Goldsen, K. I. (in press). "That's what friends do": Informal caregiving for chronically ill midlife and older lesbian, gay and bisexual adults. *Journal of Social & Personal Relationships*.

National Academy on an Aging Society. (2000). *Helping the elderly with activity limitations*. Paper presented at Caregiving No. 7, Washington, DC.

National Coalition of Anti-Violence Programs. (2005). *Anti-lesbian, gay, bisexual and transgender violence in 2004: A report of the National Coalition of Anti-Violence Programs*. Washington, DC: Author.

National Gay and Lesbian Task Force. (1990). *Anti-gay violence, victimization, and defamation in 1989*. Washington, DC: Author.

National Gay and Lesbian Task Force. (2007a). *Anti-gay marriage measures in the U.S.* Washington, DC: Author.

National Gay and Lesbian Task Force. (2007b). *Hate crime laws in the U.S. as of November 2007*. Washington, DC: Author. Retrieved from http://thetaskforce.org/downloads/reports/issue_maps/hatenon_crimes_11_07_color.pdf

National Gay and Lesbian Task Force. (2007c). *State non-discrimination laws in the U.S. (as of September 17, 2007)*. Washington, DC: Author. Retrieved from http://thetaskforce.org/downloads/reports/issue_maps/non_discrimination_09_07_color.pdf

National Institutes of Health. (2010). *Biennial report of the director, National Institutes of Health, fiscal years 2008 and 2009*. Washington, DC: Author.

National Organization for Women. (2003). Statistics about homophobia: Did you know? In *New York Gay and Lesbian Anti-Violence Project annual report, 1996*. New York: Author.

Owens, S. D. (2001). African American female elder caregivers: An analysis of the psychosocial correlates of their stress level, alcohol use and psychological well-being. *Dissertation Abstracts International: Section A. Humanities and Social Sciences*, 62(1), 332A–333A.

Pearlin, L. I., Mullan, J. T., Aneshensel, C. S., Wadlaw, L., & Harrington, C. (1994). The structure and functions of AIDS caregiving relationships. *Psychosocial Rehabilitation Journal*, 17(4), 52–67.

Phillips, J., & Fischer, A. (1998). Graduate students' training experiences with lesbian, gay, and bisexual issues. *Counseling Psychologist, 26*(5), 712–734.

Polen, M. R., & Green, C. A. (2001). Caregiving, alcohol use and mental health symptoms among HMO members. *Journal of Community Health, 26*(4), 285–301.

Rait, D. S. (1991). The family context of AIDS. *Psychiatric Medicine, 9*(3), 423–439.

Raveis, V. H., & Siegal, K. (1991). The impact of caregiving on informal family caregivers. *AIDS Patient Care, 5*(1), 39–43.

Robertson, P. A. (2003). Offering high-quality OB/GYN care to lesbian patients. *Contemporary Ob/Gyn, 48*(9), 49–56.

Sell, R. L., Wells, J. A., & Wypij, D. (1995). The prevalence of homosexual behavior and attraction in the United States, the United Kingdom, and France: Results of a national population-based sample. *Archives of Sexual Behavior, 24*(3), 235–248.

Shippy, R. A., Cantor, M. H., & Brennan, M. (2001, November). *Patterns of support for lesbians and gay men as they age.* In M. H. Cantor (Chair), *Social support networks.* Symposium held at the 54th annual scientific meeting of the Gerontological Society of America.

Stone, R. I. (2000). *Long-term care for the elderly with disabilities: Current policy, emerging trends, and implications for the twenty-first century.* New York: Milbank Memorial Fund.

Tanfer, K. (1993). National survey of men: Design and execution. *Family Planning Perspectives, 25*(2), 83–86.

Tennstedt, S. (1999). *Family caregivers in an aging society.* Baltimore: U.S. Administration on Aging Symposium on Longevity in the New American Century.

Thompson, E. H. (2008). Do we intend to keep this closeted? *Gerontologist, 48,* 130–132.

Tolliver, D. E. (2001). African American female caregivers of family members living with AIDS. *Families in Society: The Journal of Contemporary Human Services, 82*(2), 145–156.

Tully, C. T. (1989). What do midlife lesbians view as important? *Journal of Gay and Lesbian Psychotherapy, 1*(1), 87–103.

Turner, H. A., Catania, J. A., & Gagnon, J. (1994). The prevalence of informal caregiving to persons with AIDS in the United States: Caregiver characteristics and their implications. *Social Science and Medicine, 38*(11), 1543–1552.

U.S. Census Bureau. (2003). *Percent childless and births per 1,000 women in the last year: Selected years, 1976 to present* (Current Population Survey Reports: Fertility of American Women). Washington, DC: U.S. Department of Commerce.

Washington Alaska Group Services (WAGS). (2003). *Medicaid.* Retrieved from www.wagsltc.com/medicaid/

Wenzel, H. V. (2002). *Fact sheet: Legal issues for LGBT caregivers.* San Francisco: Family Caregiver Alliance.

Weston, K. (1991). *Families we choose.* New York: Columbia University Press.

Wight, R. G. (2000). Precursive depression among HIV infected AIDS caregivers over a time. *Social Science and Medicine, 51*(5), 759–770.

Winegarten, B., Cassie, N., Markowski, K., Kozlowski, J., & Yoder, J. (1994). *Aversive heterosexism: Exploring unconscious bias toward lesbian psychotherapy clients.* Paper presented at the 102nd annual convention of the American Psychological Association, Los Angeles, CA.

Witten, T. M. (2003). Transgender aging: An emerging population and an emerging need. *Review Sexologies,* 10(4), 15–20.

Witten, T. M., Eyler, A. E., & Weigel, C. (2004). Trans issues in aging: Information for health care providers. *Outword.*

Xavier, J. (2000). *The Washington, D.C. Transgender Needs Assessment Survey: Final report for phase two.* Washington, DC: Gender Education and Advocacy.

CHAPTER THREE

Aging in the Gay Community

BRIAN DE VRIES, PH.D., AND GIL HERDT, PH.D.

The combination of *aging* and *gay*, key words in the title of this chapter, brings together two constructs and two divergent ideas variously and ambiguously defined, rendering their conjoint use both fascinating and problematic. By "aging," we typically mean to characterize those who are already over a "certain age" and might already be defined as "old," notwithstanding the developmental or action orientation of the term. Numerically, this "certain age" has most frequently been designated as age 65—itself a problematic number in that it was chosen, rather arbitrarily, by Bismarck in 1882 as the age for retirement (at a time when the average life expectancy of a person was about 50 years) and enshrined in the United States in the Social Security Act of 1935. Clearly, these decisions did not use the most empirical methods for establishing a threshold that has come to carry such heavy political weight.

The term *gay* fares no better; it probably evolved into a cultural reference to homosexuality during the mid- to late twentieth century, allegedly originating with an ambiguous reference by Gertrude Stein in 1922 and a more pointed reference by Noel Coward in 1929. The word became politicized in the 1960s and has since characterized men more exclusively, while remaining an overly simplistic, binary representation of what is increasingly appreciated as a more fluid and dynamic consideration—sexuality—with *queer* as the latest and most unstable of these identity meanings. On their own, the terms *aging* and *gay* merit deeper consideration; together, their referents are at once exacerbated and more readily scrutinized.*

Not long ago these two terms were thought to be at best incongruous and at worst incompatible. The incongruity derived from ageist notions of homosexual culture; the incompatibility derived from linking AIDS with homosexuality, in which the presence of the disease precluded a future (Jacobson & Grossman, 1996). Doug Kimmel, a well-known name to those who study gay aging, made a similar comment in his 1985 presidential address to members of the American Psychological Association's Division 44 (Society for the Psychological Study of Lesbian, Gay, and Bisexual Issues) during which he was told that his interests in aging and gay men were "optimistic."

Still, an impressive if incomplete body of literature has developed around aging in gay men (even if much of the literature is not accurately characterized as optimistic in nature; Cahill, South, & Spade, 2000). More recently framed as "LGBT aging," it is nonetheless gay men who have received the disproportionate share of attention.[†] This is an interesting fact perhaps attributable to an extension of social science androcentrism into the study of disenfranchised persons or more simply the study of those most visible or with the greatest physical presence in developing countercultures. For whatever reason, this literature forms the basis of the text that follows. We have supplemented this literature review with interviews we conducted with several dozen older gay men; their statements annotate the discussion and give voice to those whose experiences we describe. These interviews and focus groups were conducted with AIDS caregivers and members of community groups in San Francisco and older community residents in Chicago. The focus of these interviews and focus groups ranged from housing and health care issues to friendships and social support to later-life reflections.

Some general interrelated statements about the literature reviewed in this chapter merit attention for the context within which this literature should be seen. First, this literature has developed in both size and complexity over the past 25 years. The recent Institute of Medicine report (IOM, 2011) makes this point

---

*The terms used reflect both political values and cohort experiences; *homosexuality* connotes the older, "disease state" notion, *gay* is the baby-boomer identity, and *queer* is the newer expression— some would argue now that queer destabilizes the hetero-/homo-binary in ways that merit attention.

[†] A sizable number of studies and articles have included both gay men and lesbians; given the topic of this chapter, only the former is highlighted herein unless specific contrasts or comparisons merit further discussion.

most clearly. Early publications were largely anecdotal, clinical, or both, describing (older) homosexual men (and women) as socially isolated, depressed, sexually frustrated, and unhappy, among a series of negative characteristics (Berger, 1996; Friend, 1989; Kehoe, 1988; Kimmel, 1978, 1979; Vacha, 1985; Weinberg & Williams, 1974). As the field grew, publications became increasingly empirical, although still based on small samples, most of which were self-selected and recruited through sexual minority organizations (Barker, 2004). Many studies of aging in gay male communities actually have been based on work with younger adults (Hostetler, 2004). Recent studies have struggled to overcome these sample-based limitations, and a few have met with some success. Still, the extent to which there can be a representative sample of men (and women) manifesting characteristics (or representing terms and constructs) in flux remains problematic.

Second, and embedded in the previous discussion, is the pervasive ageism alleged and reported (Bergling, 2004) in gay culture (Herdt, 1992). This ageism, as culturally inflected and thus psychologically internalized by many and perhaps by most gay men, is certainly implied by the relative paucity of older men in studies of gay male aging (or their clinical presentation) and explicitly scrutinized in some accounts (reported next). Blando (2001, p. 87) has noted the "twice hidden" nature of older gay (and lesbian) lives—invisible in contemporary communities and invisible in gay (and lesbian) communities. As context, however, this ageism has the grave potential to shape the experience of aging—in ways that have not typically been considered.

Third, the study of older gay men analyzes a cohort of textbook clarity. Gerontologists have long discussed cohorts, referring to groups of people bound by time of birth, life experience, or both. They have proposed, for example, that comparing individuals of different ages at a single point in time (cross-sectionally) may ultimately reveal more about the different contexts in which these individuals were reared and socialized than anything directly attributable to age, which may be best understood through longitudinal research. The literature on gay and lesbian older adults almost uniformly comments on the marked cohort effects in communities of homosexuals and how the lives of gay men and lesbians have been shaped "in important ways by the historical period in which they have grown and developed, lived, and worked" (Reid, 1995, p. 217). Indeed, since the time of the Stonewall riots in 1969, much has happened to transform the social and psychological understanding of same-sex relations and lives. AIDS has certainly shaped the experiences of gay men whose "coming out" and "coming of age" have taken place since Stonewall (e.g., Herdt, 1997). AIDS has destroyed communities while simultaneously increasing the visibility of gays (and lesbians) and facilitated the creation of well-developed communities by gays and lesbians themselves, including community service organizations, publications, and various professional and social associations (Herdt & Boxer, 1992). Large numbers of gay men have come out and come of age and are facing later life with little historical experience or cultural expectations to guide them. There exists little literature from which to draw comparisons with previous cohorts of older gay men, and even if such literature existed, the accounts and interpretations of such times are historically broken from the present along the Stonewall lines previously described.

Thus, this chapter is an attempt to describe these relatively "uncharted lives" (Siegel & Lowe, 1995) and this unique juncture of history and biography. In congruence with other chapters in this book, this description is organized around the following areas: psychological issues (including mental health and social science); biomedical issues (including AIDS and the broader biomedical context of male aging); social issues (including social support and those on whom an individual might call in times of need); sexual issues; socioeconomic and legal issues (including those derived from the denial of marriage and full citizenship in American society); and services, programs, and agencies that have developed to address the unique and common needs of an aging gay population. Many studies have focused exclusively on gay men; several have combined gay men and lesbians (and often bisexual and transgender persons) into a single category (LGBT) for analyses. Whenever possible, the data relating to gay men are highlighted or called out, although some findings will by necessity refer to these (often marginalized) sexual groups as a whole.

PSYCHOLOGICAL ISSUES AND GAY MALE AGING

In relative contrast to the modest research into the physical well-being of older gay men, dozens of reports address the psychological and emotional well-being of this population. Much of this research has emerged in refutation of the pervasive negative stereotypes and cultural myths that have characterized older homosexual men (and women) as depressed, hidden, and bitter (Berger, 1996; Friend, 1989; Kehoe, 1988; Kimmel, 1978, 1979; Vacha, 1985; Weinberg & Williams, 1974). In a review of almost 60 studies on gay men and aging, Wahler and Gabbay (1997) concluded that the negative stereotypes about older gay men are largely unwarranted. A similar conclusion may be reached by way of the recent IOM report, as well as the review of literature by Fredriksen-Goldsen and Muraco (2010). Recent authors note that happiness and successful adaptation to aging are commonly reported by older gay men (and most LGBT persons in general, see IOM, 2011), perhaps because of coping skills and competencies unique to aging homosexuals. Berger (1996) went further and suggested that well-being among gay men may actually increase with age. Three key features merit elaboration in this context: (1) depression and psychological distress, (2) the role of "coming out," and (3) the role of aging.

Depression. As described earlier, depression is often assumed to be a hallmark of the experience of the older gay male. Interestingly, depression may be either overdiagnosed (or assumed) or underdiagnosed in gay men; with overdiagnosis, behaviors more common among gay men may be heteronormatively pathologized; with underdiagnosis, depression may be believed to be attributable to one's homosexuality (Kantor, 1999), implicitly engaging homophobia. Depression, however, is one of the few dimensions noted in previous negative characterizations of older gay men that has some empirical validity.

Many reasons exist to support higher rates of depression among gay men, including living in a homophobic culture, threatened or actual exclusion or rejection by families of origin, state-based discounting of love relationships, and other cues of disenfranchisement. (It is worth recalling, however, that mental health encompasses significantly more than depression, and several studies assessing the mental health status of homosexuals find that most gay men [and lesbians] enjoy high levels of psychological adaptation, although very few studies have compared the mental health status of homosexuals with that of heterosexuals; see Sandfort, de Graaf, Bilj, & Schnabel, 2001, for an exception.) Nonetheless, some researchers have found that, as compared with members of the general population, gay men and lesbians may be susceptible to higher rates of depression (Paul et al., 2002) as well as suicidal thoughts and beliefs (Herrell et. al., 1999; Paul et al., 2002) and mental disorders (Cochran & Mays, 2000). Mills et al. (2004) found a rate of depression of 17% among men over the age of 50 who have sex with men; 31% of the LGBT persons in the very recent study by Fredriksen-Goldsen, Kim, and Goldsen (2011) were depressed; data separated by sex or gender orientation were not provided. D'Augelli and Grossman (2001) found that 13% of their sample of LGB older adults had attempted suicide, with men reporting significantly greater suicidality related to their sexual orientation than women. Significantly, however, the incidence of these stress-related disorders is increasingly identified by the American Psychological Association and many U.S. mental health professionals as a result of discrimination and the legacy of homophobia (Herdt & Ketzner, 2006).

"Coming out." The foregoing implication of culture may also have more "local" interpretations. That is, in addition to the national context of greater acceptance

of (actual or presumed) homosexuality is the community context of personal disclosure. To whom, when, and how an individual identifies himself often depends on his "position" in history (i.e., whether he identifies himself as homosexual, gay, or queer), and the response he receives has multiple and interactive influences on his social environment, including health care, and thus influences his psychological well-being. For example, several men in our focus groups and interviews commented that they had to actively decide whether to "out" themselves to new people they meet in almost every professional and personal situation. One man commented that he chose not to go to his 45th class reunion; as he put it, he didn't want to "out" himself to "people he didn't have much to say to 50 years ago and still doesn't." Others reminded us that sexual encounters and self-identification as gay are not synonymous and simultaneous. For example, one man described his adolescence and early adulthood when he was dating women at the same time he was having sexual experiences with men, all along considering himself as an "exploring" and "curious" heterosexual.

Rawls (2004) analyzed data relevant to this topic from a study of gay men in several large cities initiated at the University of California, San Francisco, in the late 1990s (the Urban Men's Health Study [UMHS]; Catania et al., 2001). The study created a probability sample* from New York, Los Angeles, Chicago, and San Francisco. These data show that the age of first attraction began for these men before age 10, supporting the hypothesis that sexual development occurs before "puberty" (actually between adrenarche and gonadarche; see Herdt & McClintock, 2000). As compared with heterosexual men, there is a slightly earlier sexual developmental onset (Laumann et al., 1994). A second critical factor was also discovered: The sample naturally divided into "gender atypical" and "gender typical" self-described respondents, as has been reported in other studies (Bailey & Oberschneider, 1997). When this factor is controlled, gender atypicality predicts earlier sexual attraction, while typical gender behavior is associated with a statistically significant later development of sexual attraction as well as depression and psychological distress (Paul et al., 2002; Rawls, 2004). The role of age and cohort remains to be fully explored.

Homophobia represents a life theme in the sexual development of these men. Overall, half of the San Francisco respondents in the UMHS reported that they were harassed multiple times before the age of 16, because they were gay (presumably for reasons of gender nonconformity). Childhood harassment is strongly related to age and birth cohort; 60% of respondents in their 20s and 30s reported

---

* This sample comprised 2,881 men aged 18 and older.

that they were harassed (because they were gay) four or more times before the age of 16, whereas under half of respondents in their 40s reported this level of harassment, and only 28% of the respondents over age 50 reported comparable levels of harassment. These data have relevance to current discussions about bullying in childhood and adolescence based on (presumed or actual) sexual orientation.

Harassment is not restricted to childhood and adolescence, as Fredriksen-Goldsen and colleagues (2011) report. They found that older LGBT adults identified an average of four incidents of victimization and discrimination over the course of their lives attributable to their sexual orientation or gender identity; these experiences typically took the form of verbal insults (65%) and physical violence (40%). The rates were significantly higher for men than for women.

Still, it is largely believed that disclosure of one's homosexuality is associated with positive psychological adaptation and well-being. Rawls (2004) points out that this has become the default statement, with a wide variety of studies supporting the association between well-being and indices of disclosure defined as acceptance of one's homosexuality, commitment to homosexuality, having a positive homosexual identity, or being a member of homosexual social groups (Bell & Weinberg, 1978; Jacobs & Tedford, 1980; Schmitt & Kurdek, 1987). However, not all studies have found significant effects of "being out" on mental health (as addressed later); more and sophisticated research is clearly needed.

That is, associations between well-being and disclosure indices are correlational such that involvement with others, group membership, positive identity, and commitment may be as equally predictive of the degree of being "out" as they are predicted by measures of "outness" (Rawls, 2004). Equally important is the ongoing caveat that most studies have relied on self-selected convenience samples of (younger) gay men, usually recruited through public (e.g., street fairs) and semipublic (e.g., bars) venues and often personal networks (Boxer & Cohler, 1989). It is impossible to discern whether these socially active men benefit more from their social involvement, their "outness," or both. Moreover, age is often masked, hidden, or obscured in those analyses (Cohler, 2004). It does appear that coming out later in life has little influence on overall depression scores (Rawls, 2004), although McDonald (1982) described greater variability in milestones identified by respondents who reported coming out later in life.

Research has typically identified coming out as a process, occurring in one's mid-20s and over the course of 10 or 11 years (e.g., Herdt, 1989; McDonald, 1982; Rawls, 2004). For example, in a study of 5 cohorts, the oldest being ages 55 and older, Grov and colleagues (2006) found that women and men in the youngest cohort (aged 18–24 years) reported coming out to themselves at younger ages than women and men in the older cohort; in addition, the average age of coming out was younger for men than for women, especially among the older cohort.

Finally, it is worth commenting on the terms used in gay men's self-identification, that is, as *what*, exactly, are these men coming out? Although the developmental flow of the three most frequently used terms (i.e., homosexual, gay, and queer) has not yet been studied, several studies suggest that older gay men (and lesbians) use different terms in self-description than do younger gay men (and lesbians). Adelman, Gurevitch, de Vries, and Blando (2006), for example, report that when given a variety of terms from which to choose (including, homosexual, gay, and queer), older men were significantly more likely to use the first of these identities, whereas younger men were significantly more likely to use either of the latter two terms, a finding echoed by Rawls (2004). These alleged cohort differences are intriguing, with potential intergenerational implications (Russell & Bohan, 2005).

Age and adaptation. The previous discussion implies the context in which older gay men were socialized. In the interviews we conducted, we have heard accounts of the guarded manner in which interactions and life transpired. For example, one 83-year-old gay man reported, "We would go to this bar in North Beach; the lights were dim and men would dance with drinks in hand. When someone unknown to the door man would approach the club, he would turn the lights brighter and everyone adopted a neutral standing position, as if engaged in conversation. When the approaching person either was cleared for or dissuaded from entry, the lights would again dim and festivities would continue."

Public social interactions were pursued with great caution; recall that these gay men lived lives declared to be "sick by doctors, immoral by clergy, unfit by the military and a menace by the police" (Kochman, 1997, p. 2). Many of those who survived adopted a stance along the lines of "that which doesn't kill or hurt us will ultimately make us stronger."

That perspective has found its way into popular gay culture as well into the nascent empirical literature. A poignant example of this perspective in popular culture may be noted in a line from Harvey Fierstein's *Torch Song Trilogy,* in which Fierstein's character, Arnold, speaking with his mother, says that he can cook a meal, sew a shirt, hammer a nail—whatever it takes to get through—he can do it himself. He has had to defend and create himself throughout his life, and this experience has afforded him the skills to continue to do so.

Such skills have been noted in a variety of reports. For example, Kimmel (1979) has suggested older gay men (and lesbians) may be better suited to cope with age-related changes as a result of having survived all that is entailed in being homosexual in a homophobic society (e.g., Rawls, 2004), a term he coined as "crisis competence." Other researchers have similarly proposed that older homosexuals may have successful coping strategies or skills that allow them to enter old age at an advantage, relative to their heterosexual peers (Berger, 1982, 1996; Berger & Kelly, 1986; Weeks, 1983).

Many of the men we interviewed have largely believed that the circumstances of their lives have made them more aware of life. They believed, for example, that "because of what gay men have gone through, they could move home or move next door—they are equipped." Another man, making reference to both a popular song of the disco era performed by Gloria Gaynor and the San Francisco city supervisor slain in 1978, proclaimed that earlier in his life he was "afraid, he was petrified." He now reports: "I'm not afraid and I'm not petrified. If I walk out that door, I know I will survive. Thank you, Harvey Milk."

Such discussions bear remarkable resemblance to the literature on successful aging. Early gerontological research tended to focus on aging in terms of decline and loss, not an unreasonable focus given that so much research originated in institutional settings with patients as subjects. As the study of aging expanded to include community settings as well, however, the focus also expanded to include the "well elderly" (de Vries & Blando, 2004). This expanded focus led to comparisons between these two groups and further to distinctions among the well elderly, leading to the identification of "usual" and "successful" aging as nonpathological states (Rowe & Kahn, 1998). This distinction was intended to identify two groups of "nondiseased" older persons—(1) those without pathology but at risk (the usual agers) and (2) those without pathology and not at risk (the successful agers).

The term *successful aging* has enjoyed wide and popular appeal in recent gerontological literature with applications to physical (e.g., Garfein & Herzog, 1995), cognitive (e.g., Baltes & Baltes, 1990), and psychological and social functioning (e.g., Wong & Watt, 1991). This broader use of the term and its application to a variety of outcome measures has led to deservedly greater scrutiny. Some critics have charged that the adoption of terms such as *successful aging* represents the capitalist takeover of aging (Cole, 1984) and fails to account for the effects of history and culture, as well as gender, class, and social circumstances. In contrast, it may be argued that purely subjective definitions of success render the concept ineffectual or that successful aging is an oxymoron in that successful aging implies not aging at all (Baltes & Carstensen, 1996). A variation on this theme is that all aging is successful given the alternative (de Vries & Blando, 2004).

Several authors have commented that gay men and lesbians may be more likely than comparably aged heterosexuals to be prepared overall for aging, given their socialization and early experiences with stress (e.g., Brown, Alley, Sarosy, Quarto, & Cook, 2001). For example, in the recent MetLife (2010) survey of LGBT boomers, 74% of the more than 1,200 respondents reported that being LGBT has helped prepare them for aging; importantly, almost half (54%) similarly noted that being LGBT has made aging more difficult. Friend (1991) has offered a theory of successful aging as applied to older lesbians and gay men, primarily based on "crisis competence" and confronting rigid gender roles and ageist assumptions—perhaps specific forms of "meaning making." Friend suggests that being freed (or forced) from the relative bounds of traditional gender role definitions has afforded gay men and lesbians the opportunity to engage in behaviors throughout their lives that heterosexuals rarely confront until the death of a spouse (Lund, Caserta, Dimond, & Shaffer, 1989).

Lee (1987, 1991), however, cautions that proposals of "extraordinary aging" may be misleading because such a perspective might lead researchers to overlook the yet unknown, but less desirable, realities of aging among persons who have remained hidden to social research (Rawls, 2004). Further, Lee (1987) found in his research on older gay Canadian men that those who remain closeted were happier than those with higher rates of disclosure. He further reported that older gay men with higher rates of disclosure had a higher lifetime prevalence of stressful events and were more likely to experience lower levels of psychological well-being in old age, a finding similar to Adelman's (1991) among her sample of older gay men in San Francisco. This complexity mirrors the findings of the MetLife (2010) report.

The experience of aging is further complicated by the purported emphasis on youth in gay male culture (e.g., Bergling, 2004; Herdt, 1989; Weinberg and Williams, 1974). Concomitantly, several authors have referred to accelerated aging among gay men—the idea that gay men are considered by self and others to be in midlife or elderly at earlier ages than are heterosexual men (Friend, 1980; Kelly, 1977, 1980). AIDS may have added to this effect by exaggerating burdens of care and loss prematurely, as well as by creating a sexual distance between older and younger gay men (Herdt 1997; Levine, Gagnon, & Nardi, 1997). The evidence is equivocal with respect to the presence of accelerated aging among gay men. Kelly (1977, 1980) reported that age-status norms for middle and old age were earlier than those reported by Neugarten, Moore, and Lowe (1965), whose earlier work introduced this notion to gerontology. In contrast, Minnigerorde (1976) and Laner (1978) found no such differences, and both reported that their data contradicted suggestions of accelerated aging. Bennett and Thompson (1991) suggest that this discrepancy may be understood by the referents used by gay men. That is, in their study, they found that gay men saw their own middle age as beginning at about the same age as did heterosexual men; in contrast, though, these same men believed that other gay men saw midlife and old age as beginning earlier: the self was seen as an exception to the general principle. More research on these phenomena is needed to address the extent to which such effects continue.

Older gay men in social science theory. Gerontology, in general, appears to have disinherited theory: Bengtson, Burgess, and Parrott (1997) lament that fewer than 20% of published articles in leading social gerontology journals mentioned or used theoretical formulations in interpreting or explaining results. Amid this paucity, the theoretical orientation most frequently cited was the life course perspective, and within this perspective, Erikson's life course theory was most frequently cited (e.g., Erikson, 1982; Erikson, Erikson, & Kivnick, 1986). (A minority stress perspective [e.g., Meyer, 2003] has been profitably engaged in studies of LGBT lives, positing that sexual and gender minorities experience chronic stress as a result of their stigmatization; its application to the later years has great potential, only beginning to be explored.)

Erikson's theory holds that later stages of the life course may be characterized by the psychosocial developmental conflicts of generativity and stagnation, and integrity and despair. Integrity has most often been framed in terms of life review and, as such, is accompanied by many other theories proclaiming the later years as prime time for such reflection (Birren & Hedlund, 1987; Bulter, 1963; Lowenthal, Thurnher, & Chiriboga, 1975). Generativity is seen in the acts of creativity among those in the middle years and beyond and is often manifested in parenting. There have been several efforts attempting to locate gay men in these theoretical frameworks (e.g., Cornett & Hudson, 1987).

In the context of life review, for example, several books (Berube, 1990; Farnham & Marshall, 1989; Nardi & Sanders, 1994; Vacha, 1985) have addressed the stories of life as told by older gay men. These men naturally looked to the older gay men who came before, thought of those who will follow, and spoke of their own experiences in contrast to both. In our own research, some men believed that "older gay men have references that younger gay men don't; they have seen friends murdered and police not even investigate it." One man believed that the use of the word *queer* was a slap in the face to older gay men who helped pave the way for greater acceptance. He believed that older gay men "have done the struggle and younger gay people don't get it." He thought that the AIDS struggle in youth is not the same.

Others believed that "kids don't have the thrill of discovery. Things had to find me when I was young; I was so naïve," as one older gay men reported. "My first sex with a man was when I was 21. At that time, gay life was unsavory; people feared exposure. People were closeted." Another said, and his statement represented many others, "You literally had to back into bars so as to be vigilant not to be seen. You would pass the bar several times before entering and this influences you; it gives you another perspective."

The search for community and the care of community was a frequently repeated theme and reflection in the lives of the gay men we interviewed. The men referred to their chosen family and the important role that friendship plays in their lives. They spoke of the loyalty and camaraderie that existed in their relationships. Implicit in many of their comments is the complex role of "generativity" in the lives of these gay men. Generativity is rightfully credited as the term introduced by Erik Erikson as the hallmark of midlife; McAdams (1993, p. 227) refers to it as the "legacy of the self . . . generated and offered up to others as the middle-aged adult comes to realize, in the words of Erik Erikson, that 'I am what survives me.'" Generativity has frequently been interpreted by researchers, clinicians, and the popular press in terms of childbearing and child rearing. In the lives of gays and lesbians, however, generativity may assume a wide array of forms—multiple manifestations that have been explored by a few authors (Cohler, Hostetler, & Boxer, 1998; Cornett & Hudson, 1987; de Vries & Herdt, 2000; Isay, 1996). Childbearing and child rearing are activities not restricted to heterosexuals. Perhaps the tendency to "take care of what one truly cares for" (as Erikson has referred to generativity) may be seen in career choices (e.g., social service and teaching professionals), artistic endeavors (i.e., the activities of creation), and even political activism. Generativity, in this context, may be interpreted as change-making agents in the service of creating for the self and others a better place to be (de Vries & Blando, 2004).

Many men in our focus groups were or had previously been caregivers for a partner or friend with AIDS. In fact, the recent MetLife (2010) survey reveals the high frequency with which midlife and older gay men have served, and continue to serve, as caregivers to others in their social networks. Gay and bisexual men were almost as likely as lesbians and bisexual women to have provided care in the past six months, according to the MetLife (2010) survey, and much more likely than heterosexual men. Just over one-fifth of the sample of gay and bisexual men reported that they were or continue to be caregivers. Moreover, gay and bisexual men provided significantly more hours of care than women, of any sexual orientation, and heterosexual men. Fourteen percent of the men indicated that they were full-time caregivers, compared with 3% of the lesbian and 2% of the bisexual sample. The care recipients, for all LGBT groups, were disproportionately parents, spouses, and friends.

Almost all of the gay men in our interview and focus group research pointed to their caregiving experiences as periods of growth and development; these men ultimately expressed gratitude for their caregiving experiences. One man said that, although he recalls stress and burdens as a caregiver, he feels "honored that they feel that he's that much of a friend to be a caregiver." Another group member poignantly commented that "it is like a gift to be with someone who is dying. I can't have children and can't give life, but being with someone at the end of their life is a gift." Generativity may be found in a variety of life choices, beliefs, and commitments, ranging from childbearing and child rearing, certainly, to vocation/occupation, professional activities, volunteer activities, social group memberships, friendships, and even leisure pursuits. These latter areas of vocation, recreation, and social participation, particularly, remain relatively unexplored in the midlife and in the older life of gay (and lesbian) adults, with the notable exception of some of the work of McAdams and his colleagues (McAdams, 1993; McAdams & de St. Aubin, 1992; McAdams, Ruetzel, & Foley, 1986).

BIOMEDICAL ISSUES AND GAY MALE AGING

The prevalence of chronic conditions and functional deficits increases markedly beginning in midlife (Merrill & Verbrugge, 1999; National Academy on an Aging Society, 1999) as witnessed by the onset or exacerbation of various chronic conditions (Kane et al., 1999; National Academy of Aging Society, 1999). Many of these common conditions result in significant functional impairment (Trupin & Rice, 1995) and the need for either temporary or permanent care of older gay men, or by older gay men as reported earlier (see Barker, Herdt, & de Vries, 2006)—itself an important issue to an aging population in general and the aging LGBT population in particular (see chapter 2).

HIV/AIDS. There is little empirical literature addressing physical health issues and gay male aging per se, except the voluminous literature on HIV/AIDS. A Federal Interagency Forum on Aging and Related Statistics (2000) report revealed that about 16% of men older than age 65 and 25% of women of comparable age had a chronic disability. In recent work, we found numbers in the LGBT population in excess of these: approximately one-third of our sample of more than 300 older gay men and lesbians reported some self-identified form of chronic illness or disability (Adelman et al., 2006). Interestingly, this proportion was consistent across life span age groups for gay men. Dramatically, the recent national community-based survey conducted by Fredriksen-Goldsen and colleagues (2011) found that 43% of their large sample of gay men over 50 reported that they had a disability.

HIV/AIDS is a likely factor in reporting illness and disability; among LGBT communities, gay men have been disproportionately affected by HIV/AIDS, particularly gay men in their middle and later years (Linsk, 2000). As reported in the recent IOM report (2011), about 29% of people living with AIDS in the United States are currently aged 50 and over; however, 70% of people with HIV in the United States are at least 40 years of age. Aging with HIV/AIDS will necessarily become a health issue of some significance in the years to come (CDC, 2007). The percentage of gay men included in these estimates is not clear; however, as noted in the IOM report, the percentage can be assumed to be large given that more than half of all new HIV infections in the United States occur among men who have sex with men (CDC, 2010).

Symptoms of HIV may be misunderstood as manifestations of aging and associated with costly delays in treatment; similarly, symptoms of common age-related illnesses and conditions may be misrepresented as HIV-related and associated with interventions potentially more harmful than helpful to a body already under assault (Shippy, 2004). High et al. (2008) report that some evidence suggests that HIV compresses the aging process, possibly accelerating the development of morbidities and frailty. Moreover, being HIV-positive does not protect against the common age-associated illnesses. Problems are likely to be complicated by drug interactions and the effects of antiretroviral drugs on drugs used to treat diseases that affect the elderly and vice versa, as are the particular ways in which common diseases of later life manifest in those already combating HIV (Ernst, 2004).

Broader concerns. HIV/AIDS is, of course, only part of the broader issue of health and aging among gay men. Pfizer (2003) reported on diseases and conditions of particular importance to men in general. Heart disease ranks first among these; almost 48% of deaths in men are from cardiovascular disease (Daviglus et al., 1998). Men are at higher risk of death due to cardiovascular disease than are women (Roger et al., 2011) and are more likely to experience a first heart attack at an earlier age than are women. Men are also at higher risk for developing the constellation of cardiovascular risks known as "metabolic syndrome" (Roger et al., 2011), although, for many cardiovascular risk factors such as hypertension and diabetes, age, race, and other factors are more predictive of prevalence differences than is gender. The Gay and Lesbian Medical Association adds that gay men and men who have sex with men should also discuss with their health care provider their risks of sexually transmitted infections, including HIV/AIDS and hepatitis, some cancers, and substance abuse, as well as psychological and mental health issues.

Exposure to some illnesses and conditions that may place gay men at some disadvantage relative to comparably aged heterosexuals may be extrinsically rather than intrinsically determined; that is, many gay men may not have access to health care insurance coverage (given patterns of potential underemployment and absence of same-sex partner employer-sponsored benefits). Other social factors also influence the health status of older gay men. Rates of substance use in general and alcohol use in particular (Gruskin et al., 2007), for example, are reportedly higher among older gay men (and lesbians) than among comparably aged heterosexuals. Grossman and colleagues (2001) found that gay men had significantly higher levels of alcohol use and problem drinking than lesbians.

Much of the research in this area is not without critics, many of whom comment that such findings are overstated given typical convenience samples that may overrepresent heavy users (often drawing from bars; e.g., Hughes, 2003). Moreover, recent reports suggest that such age-related behaviors are diminishing, given levels of societal acceptance, educational interventions, and increasing social outlets (Crosby et al., 1998). However, studies have revealed that drinking rates among gay men (and lesbians) do not decrease as rapidly with age as they appear to among heterosexual populations (Dean et al., 2000).

The legacy of discrimination and harassment endured by many of these older gay men and lesbians should not be underestimated (de Vries, 2006), along the lines of the minority stress theory, as introduced earlier. Its effects may be most pronounced in health care settings, influenced by institutionalized heterosexism (Brotman, Ryan, & Cormier, 2003; Cahill, 2002). As de Vries (2006) has noted, the associated feelings of shame and guilt (Kaufman & Raphael, 1996) and internalized homophobia (Cohler, 2004), compounded by ageism and feelings of invisibility within gay and lesbian community contexts (even more pronounced within African-American communities, see David & Knight, 2008), have reportedly led older gay men (and older lesbians) to seek out health care services less frequently than their heterosexual peers (Harrison & Silenzio, 1996; see IOM, 2011). The

Movement Advancement Project (2010) noted that LGBT adults of all ages are much more likely than heterosexual adults to delay or not to seek medical care. They reported that 30% of transgender adults, 29% of LGB adults, and 17% of heterosexual adults delayed or did not seek care.

This is particularly problematic given the reported tendencies of men in general not to seek medical help in timely ways (Addis & Mahalik, 2003; Mansfield, Syzdek, Green, & Addis, 2008). The few and localized settings in which gay and lesbian support and services are available are associated with more frequent use (in comparison with the use of general senior services available to all; Quam & Whitford, 1992) and are evaluated more positively (Jacobs, Rasmussen, & Hohman, 1999).

Dean et al. (2000) identify the multilayered framework within which the health of sexual minorities and older members of these minorities in particular must be considered. That is, for gay men, in addition to the health risk factors associated with age, there are gay male sexual-specific risk factors, including an array of sexually transmitted infections, such as HIV/AIDS, hepatitis A and B, enteritis, and anal cancer. There also are cultural-specific health factors, including those associated with body culture (e.g., eating disorders), socialization through bars, drugs, and alcohol use, as well as gender polarity in the dominant culture. There are factors associated with disclosing sexual orientation, including related psychological adjustment, interpersonal conflicts, and perhaps physical dislocation, just as there are factors associated with concealing sexual identity, such as reluctance to seek preventive care, the delay of medical treatment, or the provision of an incomplete medical history (concealing sexually related complications, for example). Finally, there are factors associated with prejudice and discrimination, such as healthcare provider bias, limited access to care or insurance coverage (due to the absence of partner benefits), and violence (Dean et al., 2000). A clear and proactive approach to health would necessarily includes all of these factors and dimensions in the context within which they occur.

SOCIAL ISSUES AND GAY MALE AGING

Social support has been a valuable avenue for gerontological theory and research, with strong and mounting evidence proclaiming its positive effects on the physical and psychological well-being of older persons (Antonucci, Sherman, & Akiyama, 1996; Barker et al., 2006). This research has both explored social support as a construct, as well as defined the particular relationships believed to offer support to individuals. That is, gerontologists have studied family ties (e.g.,

Connidis, 2001), marital relations (e.g., Umberson & Williams, 2005), friendship ties (e.g., de Vries, 1996; de Vries & Megathlin, 2009), as well as variations and loss of these important ties (e.g., de Vries & Johnson, 2002). As these terms suggest, research has largely accounted for the experiences of presumably heterosexual older adults; more recent research has attempted to expand the study of important relationships in the lives of older gay men (and lesbians).

Grossman, D'Augelli, and Hershberger (2000) posit that the positive contributions of support networks to individual well-being should be even more powerfully noted in the lives of older gay men and lesbians, given that this social support from peers "can serve a unique function in mitigating the impact of stigmatization" (p. 171). Adelman et al. (2006) asked more than 1,300 LGBT respondents ranging in age from 18 to 92 to whom they would turn in a crisis. They reported that more than 20% of gay men and just under 10% of lesbians said they would turn exclusively to their friends, with an additional 25% of gay men and more than 40% of lesbians including friends in combination with others. Partners were mentioned by fewer gay men (10%) than by lesbians (17%); siblings, exclusively, were mentioned significantly more frequently by gay men (about 15%) than by lesbians (2%). Together, these findings identify the gendered membership of the social networks of these respondents and their potential sources of support and care. An important point tempering these findings, however, is that almost 14% of gay men and just less than 10% of lesbians reported that they did not know to whom they would turn in a crisis. Along comparable lines, a national sample of 1,000 LGBT midlife persons (MetLife 2010) reported that an average of 15% of the sample could not identify a primary caregiver when the need arose, higher among gay and bisexual men than among lesbians and bisexual women. In the more recent MetLife survey (2010), about one quarter of LGBT boomers reported that they had "no one" to whom they could turn for care during periods of ill health.

Similar data have guided much of the modest literature aiming to understand the unique roles and functions of others in the lives of older gay men. In the following sections, this support is examined around particular relationships (family, partners, and friends), the circumstances of the single, older gay man and the experiences of loss.

Family. Much research in gerontology contrasts support from friends with support from family (e.g., de Vries, 1996; Johnson, 1983). This distinction, however, is blurry and ambiguous in the lives of older gay men and lesbians (de Vries & Hoctel, 2007), with frequent mention of "families of choice" (Weston, 1991) and their "extended families" (Herdt & Koff, 2000). The notion of a "chosen" family is often linked with an alleged alienation from or abandonment by biological kin of gay men and lesbians. Such comments were common among the older gay men we interviewed.

Emphasizing the conservative social, political, and religious climate in which they were socialized, many gay men we interviewed described early experiences of disconnectedness and feeling different. "I always felt different" was probably the most frequently repeated comment. One participant said that he felt "molded by what he hated in the town" in which he grew up; others reported feeling remote and isolated. This disconnectedness was described as pervasive—from place and especially from family. For example, one man described growing up in the South, "in a small town he tries to forget and rarely mentions." Another lived in a small town that "only had edges" (e.g., divisions and borders), and he felt empty. The men uniformly reported that they felt like they "didn't fit in" their community or even in their family.

At the same time, these older men commented on the importance of "family values" and the role that those values had played in their lives. It was not uncommon to hear comments such as, "What is consistent in life is loyalties." One man added that he "has long-term friendships because of his grandmother" and what she taught him. "All of it helps, my family background, etc. Today, kids don't have those things." Several men added that regardless of their criticisms of their upbringing, they are in a better position than "younger people [who] don't know how to fashion a stable world. Their baby boomer parents have not prepared them." Even though they had felt alienated, different, and divorced from their histories, the men felt that the values instilled in them helped carry them through their lives, and at least at some level, they appreciated this foundation.

Families of choice. In addition to the complex roles of traditional families in the lives of older gay men are the creative (and often complex) experiences of chosen families born out of exchanges of "trust and loyalty to individuals in their ever-expanding concentric circles of friends, acquaintances, and lovers" (Siegel & Lowe, 1995, p. 40). Many popular accounts chronicle the "chosen families" of older gays and lesbians, what Maupin (2007) has cleverly termed as the "logical kin" as contrast to biological kin. Manasse and Swallow (1995), for example, in photographs and essays characterizing 24 gay families, report that friendships exist at the core, as evidenced in the following (p. 153): "The way a lot of gay men and lesbians come out in the world is very alienating. For many of us, building families of linkage and connection is very healing. It's important for us to feel that love and connection because it's the antithesis of the alienation of homophobia. It's important for us to say, 'This is the innermost circle.'"

The presence of such families has been noted in empirical accounts as well. Beeler, Rawls, Herdt, and Cohler (1999), for example, report that two-thirds of their sample of middle-aged and older gay men and lesbians held that they had a family of choice—about the same proportion as in the MetLife (2010) study of more than 1,200 LGBT boomers. De Vries and Hoctel (2007) report in their in-depth qualitative study of gay men and lesbians over age 65 that all but one considered their friends to be their family in some manner.

Such discussions of family of choice reveal the primacy of the family as an organizing construct and its complexity in gay and lesbian contexts. Weston (1991) reported that many gay men and lesbians have fought the creation of "chosen family," opposing its attempt to achieve heterosexual ideals and, they believe, to encourage oppression. Weinstock (2000) referenced this complexity in the pattern of friends as family she identified in her sample: friends as substitute family members, friends as a challenge to the core structure of the family, and friends as in-laws.

Families of choice are also noted in the categories of "family" identified by the older gay men and lesbians in the de Vries and Hoctel (2007) study. Respondents engaged several strategies in their conceptualization and representation of family. Just under one-third of respondents reported, simply, that "our friends are like a family to us" or "this inner circle I call family." Other responses were somewhat more qualified. About one quarter of the participants felt that their friends were like family yet different: "I consider them like an alternative family," or "I do consider my friends as family, but not in the same way as my blood family; it's like my second family." A similar number viewed their friends as family by default. Representative statements of this category included, "They're all I have left" to "I see my friends as my family, because I don't have any connections with my birth family." Finally, about 20% saw their friends as greater than, or superior to, their family. They expressed such sentiments as "I feel closer to them than to my own family" or "To my family of choice, I am a whole person" or "They [friends] provide the sustenance that you ordinarily would want a family to provide."

More than half of respondents also believed that friendships were more important to gays and lesbians than they were to heterosexuals, perhaps a view often based on a sense of mutual dependence. For example, one man said that "gay people have to make their friends their family. If my brother and sister-in-law's friends fell away, they'd still have their family. If my friends fell away, I would have nothing." For those for whom friendships are not seen as more important, respondents adopted a time-sensitive perspective, expressing the belief that "although friendships were probably more important to gays and lesbians in the past, when you had to have that certain thing with people to be protected," this was no longer the case because it was so easy to be out, or they adopted a normative model, expressing sentiments such as "We're all social beings regardless of our sexual orientation" or "Friendships are important to everyone."

Friends. Much of the literature in this nascent area of the meaning of friendship among gay men is colloquial and inferential, often presented, as previously mentioned, in compilations of personal narratives (e.g., Adelman, 1986; Farnham & Marshall, 1989; Vacha, 1985). The few empirical attempts at examining the importance of friendship among gay men and lesbians, particularly in later life, include Nardi's (1999) study of gay men, representing a broad age range; Quam and Whitford's (1992) study of gay men and lesbians over age 50 and de Vries and Hoctel's (2007) and de Vries and Megathlin's (2009) studies of the same age range; Weinstock's (2000) analysis of the friendships of lesbians at midlife and later; and Beeler, Rawls, Herdt, and Cohler's (1999) study of midlife and later-life gay men and lesbians in Chicago.

De Vries and Megathlin (2009) compared the meaning of friendship for gay men and lesbians over age 50 with comparably aged heterosexuals; they used a framework proposed by Adams, Blieszner, and de Vries (2000). De Vries and Megathlin (2009) reported that, relative to the heterosexual group, gay men and lesbians were more likely to define friends using cognitive dimensions (e.g., expressions of loyalty, commitment, and trust) and affective processes (e.g., expressions of love and care) and less likely to engage behavioral (e.g., shared activities) and structural (e.g., group membership) dimensions. Similar to the interpretations offered by de Vries and Hoctel (2007) in their more limited study, de Vries and Megathlin (2009) comment on the importance of friends in the context of having a community as underlying the high percentage of lesbians and gay men, describing friends in cognitive terms, particularly in the realms of trust and shared interests and values. Feeling welcomed and included in this community and within a circle of friends may account for the higher frequency of affective terms. In both cases, these issues are less commonly assumed (and found) in the accounts of friends among heterosexuals, for whom family typically and presumably fulfills these roles. That behavioral processes were less frequently mentioned may be interpreted along those same lines: it is less what people do together and more how they feel and think about one another that matters: friendship as a safe haven.

In sum, these definitions suggest a cultural specificity about the ways in which older gay men and lesbians consider their friends and the potential role that these friends may play in their lives. That is, the friends of older gay men and lesbians are defined in ways that one might expect would be applied to kin among heterosexual adults. This finding reinforces the high frequency with which these respondents identified their friends as their family and begs the question of their perceived place in their lives—a return to the discussion of chosen families. The differences in these experiences for older gay men and lesbians remain to be seen.

Relationship status. A number of studies describe the psychological and physical health benefits of romantic heterosexual partnerships (e.g., Gove, Styles, & Hughes, 1990); comparable associations have been noted in the partnerships of gay men and lesbians of all ages (Bell & Weinberg, 1978; Peplau, Veniegas, & Campbell, 1996). In an extensive review of research on gay and lesbian partnerships (independent of age), Cohler and Galatzer-Levy (2000) reported many similarities between gay and lesbian couples and heterosexual couples on a number of dimensions, including partner selection, conflict and power, relationship satisfaction, and sexual expression. Even on measures of relationship longevity, Gottman and colleagues (2003) extrapolate from their 12-year study of gay and lesbian couples that the "divorce" rate is comparable to that of heterosexual couples. Comparable data were recently noted by Gates, Badgett, and Ho (2008) in their analysis of marriage registration and dissolution by same-sex couples in the United States.

The few differences to emerge among gay male couples as compared with heterosexual couples of similar age concerned a relatively more egalitarian division of labor (Blumstein & Schwartz, 1983; Kurdek, 1995; Peplau et al., 1996; Solomon, Rothblum, & Balsam, 2004), although this finding and interpretation have been called into question by Carrington (1999), and a relatively higher incidence of sexual nonmonogamy (Kurdek, 1994), although this too has been disputed (Niolon, 2006). Bell and Weinberg (1978) noted that gay men in couples were less likely to report "sexual problems" than were single gay men and expressed fewer symptoms of depression and greater well-being (O'Brien, 1992) and happiness (Kurdek, 1994). Gottman et al. (2003) also reported that gay couples were less likely to use negative communication styles during times of relational conflict than were heterosexual couples and that they adopted a more reality-based view of their partner. Solomon et al. (2004) reported that gay men (and lesbians) were more likely to receive support from friends than from family;

among those in civil unions, greater expressions of support from families were noted, attesting to the importance of cultural and societal recognition.

Recognition of same-sex couples has been noted to have a significant effect on plans for and anxieties about later life (de Vries, Mason, Quam, & Acquaviva, 2009). In their study of almost 800 lesbian, gay, and bisexual boomers (i.e., aged 40–61 years), they found patterns attributable to relationship status, state recognition, and the combination of these variables. That is, single respondents have greater fears of dying alone than do respondents who were part of a couple; single respondents also report a greater sense of urgency to get things accomplished and to get affairs in order. People who live in states that do not legally recognize same-sex couples are more likely to have prepared for the end of life by completing documents such as living wills and wills than people who live in states that do recognize these relationships. However, people who live in states that do not recognize same-sex couples are also more likely to have fears about their later life (e.g., dying in pain and facing discrimination). Single respondents living in states that do not recognize same-sex couples are more likely to report that they are not sure who will be their primary caregiver than are single respondents living in states recognizing such couples.

One strikingly consistent structural or demographic difference between samples of heterosexuals and homosexuals, however, has been the higher frequency of singlehood among the latter (Hostetler, 2004). For example, in (nonrepresentative) surveys, anywhere from 40% to 60% of gay men and 45% to 80% of lesbians are involved in committed relationships (Cohler & Galatzer-Levy, 2000). Such findings not only point to differences between heterosexual and homosexual persons but also identify the different social realities within which lesbians and gay men live.

A point embedded in the previous discussion, however, is definition: the lack of an acceptable definition of "same-sex couple" (Berger, 1992) or even "single" (Nardi, 1999). That is, just because two people live together does not mean that they are a "couple"; similarly, just because a person lives alone does not mean that he or she is "single" (Hostetler, 2004). The scrutiny of these terms and concepts has much to contribute to the understanding of the social experiences of gay men (and lesbians) and to social science generally (de Vries & Blando, 2004).

Previous heterosexual marriage. Heterosexual marriage and homosexuality are not independent, particularly among the current cohort of older gay men. Almost one-third of the men older than 55 we interviewed reported a previous marriage to a woman. This percentage is comparable to that found in the meager body of relevant research (e.g., Herdt, Beeler, & Rawls, 1997). For many of these men, a heterosexual marriage was seen as evidence of adherence to conventional norms. This reason is not necessarily the dominant one, however. Several men confided that they truly loved the women they married; others suggested that they were either unaware or unwilling to accept their homosexuality. Interestingly, homosexuality was not always given as the cause for the marriage's end. We heard several accounts of men reporting irreconcilable differences that they did not attribute to their homosexuality.

Whatever led these men into and out of these marriages, the outcome was consistent: having been in long-term marriages and then coming out as gay, several participants said that they felt out of synchrony with age-appropriate social and developmental tasks experienced by their peers. Having come out later in life, these men often found themselves struggling with life tasks more typically associated with late adolescence. As one participant said, "I'm doing what most people do at 23." Another man described his energy as being focused on "learning the gay thing." All participants portrayed their current, postdivorce experience as a time of experimenting, learning about a new "world," and meeting new people. Even after having made same-age gay friends, they complain that these others do not "share" their struggles with coming out because of their divergent histories. In the words of one participant, "for my gay friends who have been out most of their lives, coming out is ancient history."

Single gay male. Across a wide array of samples of gay men in the second half of life, approximately one half describe themselves as single (Hostetler, 2004). This number is larger than that of comparably aged heterosexual men and that of comparably aged lesbians. Describing oneself as single remains a unique feature of the aging gay male, the notations of which have variously been credited as fueling the negative images and portrayals of older gay men as alone and lonely (Laner, 1978) or furthering the evidence of the "crisis competence," or resilience, that these men have developed over their lives (e.g., Kimmel, 1979).

Hostetler and Cohler (1997) comment that the single gay male largely has been ignored in the growing body of gay and lesbian literature and that research samples have focused instead on the smaller, partnered proportions of gay men. Hostetler (2004) and Carrington (1999) wonder whether such neglect, active or otherwise, might not be associated with the desire of gay or lesbian authors to provide respectable images and find common venues to redress the marginalization and disenfranchisement that has characterized the treatment and presentation of gay men and lesbians (e.g., Warner, 1999). For whatever reason, significantly less is known about this population, leaving open the idealized and perhaps inaccurate interpretations suggested earlier.

When the single gay male has come into focus, the image unveiled is of course less unidimensional. For example, Hostetler (2004) reports that rather than an experience of isolation, loneliness, and aloneness, the single gay male may feel a greater sense of community-belongingness than do partnered gay males, given the centrality of bars and other singles-oriented gathering spaces; age, however, may serve to undermine this sense of community. Perhaps the crucial piece of this puzzle derives from the path into singlehood as experienced by the gay man. Hostetler (2004) found that roughly half of the gay men he interviewed (with a mean age of 52 years) could be identified as either "loners" (a single status reflecting long-standing dispositional or temperamental characteristic) or "aloners" (a single status derived also from dispositional characteristics and exacerbated by age-related social isolation). The developmental pattern, or particular age basis of this typology, remains to be determined.

Grief and bereavement. Understanding the experiences of older gay men, similar to understanding social relationships in general, is incomplete without attention to the experiences of loss (de Vries, 2008). Contemporary gay men of the middle years and beyond have suffered the loss through AIDS of countless members of their social networks; these experiences reveal themselves in the nature of the ties that endure and in their experiences of intimacy (de Vries, 2001). Several authors have proposed that the study of grief in all populations is ultimately "the study of people and their most intimate relationships" (Deck & Folta, 1989, p. 80). An oddly clearer meaning of relationships—the self, the other, the community— may be found in the experience and expression of grief.

Not all grief is equal, however. Doka (1989), for example, has discussed "disenfranchised grievers" and "disenfranchised deaths," two constructs within which gay men and lesbians figure prominently—as do friends, colleagues, and others outside the American heteronormative family system. Disenfranchised grief occurs in relationships with no recognizable kin ties and when loss is not socially defined as significant; disenfranchised deaths are those that are socially unsanctioned and perhaps shameful such as death from AIDS (Levine et al., 1997). Those who are disenfranchised from grief and death systems lack the support and social structure through which their grief might be addressed, an experience that may be both debilitating and freeing (de Vries & Blando, 2004). In the process, new languages and systems may be created. The NAMES Project AIDS Memorial Quilt is one such example; the quilt allows the expression of grief, both individually and as part of a larger community of loss (Corless, 1995). This creative expression of grief, both individually and communally, now extends beyond the gay community.

The same might be said of obituaries posted by surviving gay men and their friends. Richards, Wrubel, and Folkman (2000) found that 38% of bereft partners of those who died from AIDS-related illness posted obituary announcements, and often, the announcement was written and published for two audiences. One was written for a primarily gay audience and was submitted to one of San Francisco's gay community newspapers. The other was a tailored obituary, written for the hometown paper of the kin of the deceased. That two such venues exist reveals the complexity of grief and the social context within which the loss has occurred.

Several studies have sought to examine the effect on gay men of cumulative grief from multiple losses. Martin and Dean (1993) compare the AIDS-loss experience to "previously studied stressors, such as the experiences of concentration camp survivors and soldiers in combat . . . wherein survivors experience unremitting death of fellow companions" (p. 323). Across a wide number of settings and countries (e.g., Biller & Rice, 1990; Carmack, 1992; Martin, 1988; Viney, Henry, Walker, & Crooks, 1992), researchers suggest that "for gay men, old beliefs about how the world functions are no longer valid; reality is no longer what it was. A sense of personal invulnerability, a belief that one has control over one's actions . . . are no longer viable for gay men to hold" (Schwartzberg, 1992, p. 427).

In an interview with a 53-year-old gay man, we heard of an interaction with his elderly mother in which she had commented that she had lost all of her friends and siblings and that he (the son) just "didn't know." Incensed, this man sent her a letter with the names of all of the people that had died in his life; his mother called him back and apologized. Such accounts highlight the unexpected parallel between the lives of gay men and older persons in general; both groups of individuals have seen the dissolution of their social networks through death. One man, for example, wonders whether he is going to be "the only one left to turn out the lights when everyone is gone." With each subsequent loss, previous losses are reviewed and relived, and consequently, the world changes (de Vries & Blando, 2004). Moss and Moss (1989) have referred to this re-experience as the "personal pool of grief" that persists and intensifies with subsequent losses. Along similar lines, years earlier Kastenbaum (1969) proposed "bereavement overload," proposing that the experience of multiple losses and their cumulative effect lead the surviving individuals to be "particularly vulnerable to the psychological effects of loss" (p. 47).

This "personal pool of grief" likely describes the experiences of many midlife and older gay men; moreover, those who survived are now preparing for a second wave of loss as they and their survivor colleagues approach the later years and a more normative expectation of mortality. Does a past so full of loss prepare an individual for a future of the same? How does the timing of such losses contribute to their experience? Although efforts have begun to explore these areas (Shernoff, 1997), much remains to be learned.

SEXUAL ISSUES AND AGING

Sexuality, sexual development, and sexual behavior in the later life course provide an important context for understanding the aging of gay men; little research exists in this area, however. Gay men's lives offer an interesting contrast to heterosexuals' lives (de Vries & Blando, 2004). The Academy Award–winning film *Brokeback Mountain* tells a realistic story of two young men who meet in the summer of 1963, have sex, fall in love, and continue a long-distance relationship for two decades, without ever knowing how to name or label their relationship or how to incorporate their feelings into the otherwise heteronormative lives they have developed for themselves. Heteronormativity, the sense that only heterosexuality is normal and natural, as compared with the historical idea of homosexuality as a disease, dominated the lives of such men for decades and is still salient today in the lives of older gay men (Herdt, 1997). Culture, the formation of sexual identity, and the social regulation of relationships frame the sexual behavior of homosexual men who "pass" as heterosexual and of gay men who are "out" (Cohler & Galatzer-Levy, 2000).

Two apparently mutually inconsistent stereotypes operate in gay men's sexuality. On the one hand, older persons are in general perceived as asexual (and perhaps women more so than men); on the other hand, gay men in general are perceived as sexually promiscuous, and older gay men have been seen as sexual perverts and predators (e.g., Kelly, 1977) according to the discriminatory cultural prejudices of an earlier era. This heritage of homophobia surrounds the self-perception of middle-aged gay men in the United States, Western Europe, Canada, and Australia, who grew up and came to accept the stigma and social oppression they felt as members of a sexual minority (e.g., Herek, 2004; Meyer 1995; recently reviewed in Herdt & Ketzner, 2006). Although such contradictory stereotypes may free individuals from certain normative role constraints such as the pressure to marry (e.g., Friend, 1991), they nonetheless continue to burden the self and sexual development and frame the way in which these individuals are perceived. These stereotypes also may restrict access to prospective sex partners and, by extension, influence personal beliefs and self-concept (Cohler, 2004). As outlined in the next section, the new marriage rights movement is changing the normative role requirements of gay men and lesbians (Herdt & Ketzner, 2006).

The first generation of studies on gay aging was focused primarily on whether elder gay men and lesbians fit the stereotypes of being depressed, socially isolated, alone, or with low self-esteem. This focus dissolved with the demonstration of the diverse patterns of aging (Kimmel, 2004). The subsequent emergence of the AIDS pandemic further burdened the understanding of gay men's sexual behavior as a research area (Levine et al., 1997) and of older gay men's sexuality in particular (Gorman & Nelson, 2004). New research questions are now being entertained: How do individuals sustain gay or lesbian identities in relation to their well-being and gay and lesbian community involvement? How is this well-being related to their sexual behavior? Such questions are based in part on the changing cultural and social context (Gagnon, 2004; Laumann, Gagnon, Michael, & Michaels, 1994). Among these later studies, the significant gap between desire, identity, and behavior has been critical to understanding gay men's sexuality in the United States. For example, while the percentage of men who engage in same-sex *behavior* over time is relatively low, the percentage of those who have same-sex *desire* is much higher (Laumann et al., 1994). Age-related differences in these percentages remain to be fully explored, as do the implications of such findings. These general population data also do not fully address the previous questions, nor address the larger issue of how sexual prejudice may influence the sexual behavior of older gay men.

Since the time of Kinsey et al. (1948) up to the present, it has been questioned whether rural versus urban centers have functioned to influence the expression of gay men's sexual behavior. Michaels (1996) argued persuasively that the estimate of 10% of the U.S. population being homosexual was actually a function of migration over time to the more anonymous and tolerant environment of larger cities (Herdt, 1989; Murray, 1995). Thus, since World War II, gay men have been attracted to cities as places to live their lives, especially to find prospective sexual partners; and their numbers vary between 8% and 12% in these environments. Given the larger incidence of gay men in larger American cities, it is understandable that, as the HIV epidemic advanced in the 1980s, this population would be the hardest hit (Brown, 1997; Levine et al., 1997). This historical cohort of men, now coming into midlife and beyond, constitute the core of urban gay male populations in the United States in cities such as San Francisco, New York, and Chicago.

A review of studies related to gay men's capacity to form committed relation-ships, whether they lived together or not, as well as their ability to support mu-tual and intimate long-term bonds with other men, suggests that older gay men are equally able to enter into successful intimate relationships despite the legacy of discrimination and marriage denial (Herdt & Kertzner, 2006). Unfortunately, there have been few comprehensive population-based studies of gay men's sexu-ality, but the previously cited UMHS study reveals that 38.5% of older men expe-rienced sexual difficulties in the year preceding the study (Rawls, 2004). Of this group, about two-thirds attributed their sexual difficulties to medical health or medications, and the rest attributed their difficulties to psychological explana-tions. Rawls remarks that more than one-fourth of these men described the issue as related to distress, depression, or both—higher than among the general popu-lation. At present, we do not know the extent to which such a finding is generaliz-able, but we ought to take seriously the continuing challenges of social support and minority stress as these men age.

SOCIOECONOMIC AND LEGAL ISSUES AND GAY MALE AGING

Most gay men and lesbians in the United States experience denial of full person-hood and citizenship, as defined by their ability to fully disclose their sexual ori-entation in public or in civil society, to engage in mutually consenting relation-ships with peers as supported by the state through marriage, and to receive the social benefits associated with marriage (Herdt & Kertzner, 2006). The denial of full personhood and citizenship raises fundamental questions about the socio-economic status and legal and political rights of gay men, who, according to the recent surveys, are in the more than 400,000 households of same-sex male part-ners (Gates, 2006), 53% of the total number of same-sex households. While a comprehensive study of personhood denied has not yet been undertaken in the United States, some research, including census data, sheds light on this popula-tion at large.

Gay men and lesbians are generally well educated and frequently more highly educated than their heterosexual counterparts as noted in U.S. Census and Gen-eral Social Survey data sets (Black, Gates, Sanders, & Taylor, 2000), as well as a variety of community-based surveys (de Vries, 2006). In contrast to the well-cited link between education and income, however, these levels of educational attain-ment do not translate into higher levels of personal or household income, a sur-prising finding, given the prevalence and hardiness of the myth of wealthy gay men (and lesbians) as members of an affluent North American elite. In a critical and comprehensive review of methodologically rigorous large-scale surveys, Badget (1998) found that "lesbian, gay, and bisexual people are spread throughout the range of household income distribution, just as heterosexual people are" (p. 15). Badgett (2004) has also shown that the benefits of marriage generally support heterosexual couples, both in the United States and in Western Europe, and denial of these benefits creates economic burdens on gays and lesbians.

The recent reviews of the literature by Herdt and Kertzner (2006) and Herek (2006) have established that the long-term impact of marriage denial may harm the mental health of gay men and lesbians in the United States. Although marriage is not for everyone and, indeed, there exists the risk of restigmatization of those who choose to remain single (Hostetler, 2004), compelling mental health evidence suggests the need to extend to those gay men (and lesbians) who do wish to marry the right to do so, affirming not only their partnerships but their children and extended families.

Marriage brings a host of tangible and intangible benefits to heterosexual couples, as decades of social and psychological studies have shown, including a slight economic advantage (Waite & Gallagher, 2000; Williams, 2003). Marriage influences income taxation; the right to welfare, medical, death benefits; and the right to adopt and foster children (Johnson, 2002). The mental health benefits are considerable (Brim, Ryff, & Kessler, 2004; Herek, 2006) and include personal growth, a sense of purpose in life, and engagement in life challenges. Equally impressive, however, are the economic and social support benefits. These institutional effects include spousal benefits, such as Social Security and public pensions, income tax benefits, inheritance, insurance, and survivorship rights, including estate tax benefits and health insurance in spouses' group plans; the right to sue for wrongful death of a spouse; and the power to make medical decisions on behalf of a spouse (Rutter & Schwartz, 1996). Most insured Americans receive health care through their employer or their spouses' employer or other family member (Badgett, 2004). This places gay men and lesbians who are not able to marry legally at an even greater economic disadvantage relative to their heterosexual peers.

De Vries (2006), in reviewing a range of community-based needs surveys of older LGBT persons, found that legal concerns were frequently raised. This is especially relevant for couples who do not have access to spousal benefits. Several studies asked about preparations for late life, including wills and powers of attorney for health care and related concerns. Up to half of the older respondents, in as few as one-fourth of the studies in which such questions were asked, affirmed that these preparations had been made. De Vries et al. (2008) found in their national sample of LGBT boomers that less than half of their respondents had completed a will, a living will, or a durable power of attorney; the proportions of those who had completed such documents varied with state recognition of same-sex relationships. The comparable numbers of LGBT boomers in the recent MetLife (2010) survey who had completed such documents was less than 40%; data separated by gender were not available. Clearly more work is needed to assist LGBT persons in preparing more fully for later life.

A large number of lesbians and gay men have expressed an interest in being legally married, if this option were available to them (Henry J. Kaiser Family Foundation, 2001; MetLife 2010). Marriage remains the strongly preferred choice among types of relationship recognition (Gates et al., 2008). This interest, or deep cultural wish, to marry should be understood in the historical context of American culture, which connects aspirations of the self to legitimate intimate connection through marriage (Bellah et al., 1985). In its denial of marriage for lesbians and gay men, "civil society can be conceptualized as a heterosexual construction that serves to make entry into the public realm," for example, and makes being elected to political office "very difficult for those whose sexual lives are judged 'immoral'" (Hubbard, 2001, p. 55). Here, older stereotypes of homosexuality as mentally abnormal, a disease, or a sin render gay men and lesbians *partial citizens* (Richardson, 1998), excluded from marital entitlements, yet expected to pay the taxes that support those entitlements. As the marriage rights movement gains support in the polls and in LGBT communities, it remains to be seen how this critical arena of social support and politics will impact the lives of older gay men. The vicious cycle might be broken in which gay men are denied the right to marry, accused of being promiscuous and unfit for marriage or parenting, and then in turn denied the legitimacy of their relationships because they are perceived to be unfit (Herdt & Kertzner, 2006). This debate may help to define the social, legal, moral, and political dimension of the lives of gay men baby boomers as they move into their retirement years.

PROGRAMS AND ORGANIZATIONS FOR AN AGING GAY POPULATION

Organized support and services for gay and lesbian seniors remain rare in American cities. When available, such services are more frequently used in comparison with generic senior services (Quam & Whitford, 1992) and are evaluated more positively (Jacobs et al., 1999). The absence of LGBT services is associated with a decreased likelihood to seek out health care services, compared with similarly aged heterosexual women and men (Harrison & Silenzio, 1996).

Housing has become a flashpoint for the needs and concerns of older gay men and lesbians (Adelman et al., 2006). Sad and distressing accounts depict gay men and lesbians who "find themselves having to go back into hiding when they begin to require health-care services" (Brotman et al., 2003, p. 193). Cahill (2002) suggests that the need for supportive housing may assume different forms, including developing housing with a particular LGBT focus or rendering existing housing LGBT friendly—what some have termed the "queering of the elder housing and care environment" (de Vries, 2006, p. 65).

LGBT communities have become more cognizant of the issues affecting their elders, resulting in dozens of surveys of the needs of older LGBT individuals in general, often framed around housing and future health care needs. These surveys have recently been reviewed (de Vries, 2006) and reveal the unique resources and challenges of these individuals and communities and a valuable compilation of regionally contextualized data. The surveys reported include 13 completed studies from across the United States, all but two of which have been conducted within the past 5 to 10 years.

Several reliable themes emerge from these reports that speak to the social context and the housing and care needs of older LGBT adults. Findings include higher levels of education and comparable levels of income relative to heterosexuals of similar ages, duplicating the patterns previously reported. The most dramatic demographic findings, relative to issues of care and support, which are consistent with some of the previously cited literature, concerned relationship status (i.e., greater likelihood of being single) and living arrangements (i.e., greater likelihood of living alone). In both cases, these proportions were frequently higher for gay men than for lesbians, with both groups demographically different than older heterosexuals. In addition to the economic issues of being single and living alone are significant social, health, and caregiving implications (as previously suggested).

In a similar context, most older gay men and lesbians (roughly two-thirds of those surveyed and again disproportionately including gay men) did *not* have children (as compared with the estimated 10% of older, presumably heterosexual, Americans with no children). For example, Adelman et al. (2006) found that 72% of gay men and 43% of lesbians over age 65 reported having no children. In the absence of a partner, children, or both, on whom are these older gay men and lesbians likely to call for support in a health or other crisis? Such a question was frequently posed in the surveys. Friends emerged as likely sources of support, although vague norms governing friendship interaction and complex and clear norms governing family interactions compromise the availability and manifestation of this form of support (de Vries, 2005). Several studies noted sizable numbers of respondents unable to identify someone on whom they might call; these estimates ranged from 10% to almost 25%, as reviewed previously. Notably, almost 20% of respondents in the MetLife survey reported their greatest fear about growing older as an LGBT person is "being or dying alone." While such concerns are common within the general aging population, they may take on even greater significance for LGBT boomers whose chosen families lack social or legal sanction.

Social services were sometimes mentioned instead, yet many respondents commented on previous negative interactions with such services attributable to sexual-orientation insensitivity by service providers (18% in one study). In addition, as many as 25% of respondents reported not being "out" to their providers or rarely discussing sexual orientation with their provider. In the MetLife (2010) study of LGBT boomers, more than 30% cited their greatest concern about aging was discrimination due to their sexual orientation; further, almost 20% of the respondents reported little or no confidence that medical personnel would treat them with dignity and respect as LGBT persons in old age.

Services for older gay men. In recent years, services and organizations for older gay men and lesbians in many major urban communities across the country have become more available, although the exact number of such organizations remains difficult to determine in the absence of an overarching, umbrella agency. A couple of agencies do offer overview services, however. The LGBT Community Centers listing (www.lgbtcenters.org/Centers/find-a-center.aspx), through CenterLink, is one such option. Based in Fort Lauderdale, Florida, CenterLink works with other national organizations to provide LGBT community centers with information and analysis of key issues. They serve more than 200 LGBT community across the country (in 46 states and the District of Columbia); they help strengthen existing LGBT centers, through networking opportunities for center leaders, peer-based technical assistance and training, and a variety of capacity-building services. Interestingly, noted on its website is that 40% of LGBT centers provide direct health care and 10% of these centers exclusively serve LGBT communities of color, youth, seniors, or women—often with modest budgets and no full-time staff.

Similarly, SAGE (Services and Advocacy for LGBT Elders, formerly Senior Action in a Gay Environment) is a New York–based social-service organization dedicated to serving the needs of the senior LGBT population. It recently has become the lead agency in the National Resource Center on LGBT Aging (www.lgbtagingcenter.org/). The National Resource Center on LGBT Aging is a technical assistance resource center aimed at improving the quality of services and supports offered to LGBT older adults. It was established in 2010 through a federal grant from the U.S. Department of Health and Human Services; it provides training, technical assistance, and educational resources to aging providers, LGBT organizations, and LGBT older adults.

SAGE is heralded as the world's largest and oldest organization serving LGBT elders, having celebrated its 30th anniversary in the fall of 2008. SAGE affiliates are proliferating, attesting to both the desire to offer services for LGBT elders in local communities as well as the recognition of SAGE as an organization. Some services offered include crisis intervention and counseling, support groups, and individual assistance (such as home care and some medical and legal services), caregiver-support programs, as well as recreational groups. In addition, SAGE offers educational and organizational services that extend well beyond its geographic location; for example, SAGE has hosted several national conferences on gay and lesbian aging, attracting hundreds of LGBT seniors, their caregivers, and those who work with this population.

Efforts are dramatically accelerating in programs and services for LGBT elders in general. A recent survey of the 30 largest U.S. and 15 largest Canadian cities revealed a total or 27 LGBT community centers, 13 of which provided senior-specific programming (de Vries, Croghan, & Worman, 2006). Many programs offered through these centers are the general services needed by older adults; some are targeted to LGBT concerns, including legal aid and insurance assistance as well as intergenerational programs, such as one-on-one matching of gay youth and older adults. Several cities have local chapters of PrimeTimers (and Old Lesbians Organizing for Change) as well as independent groups advocating for LGBT elders, such as the LGBT Aging Project in Boston, Rainbow Train in Seattle, and Gay and Gray in Denver (see de Vries et al., 2006).

Moreover, across North America in both formal and informal ways, collaboratives and networks are emerging to share information on LGBT aging issues (de Vries et al., 2006). The overarching goal of these collaboratives is to ensure that LGBT older adults have access to services, that their needs are represented on the agendas of both LGBT-focused service providers as well as providers in more heteronormative contexts, and that they are offered opportunities to make a difference in their communities. Most important, the catalyst for such collaborations and partnerships sometimes arises from the traditional aging network organizations. Whatever the route into these associations, the desired outcome is a sensitive, more focused outreach and service provision to LGBT elders. An extension of these efforts might include activities specifically designed to include and support older gay men.

Outreach and social networking groups already exist in some cities and communities. PrimeTimers is one example. PrimeTimers is designed as a social organization for older gay and bisexual people with more than 73 chapters around the world, primarily in the United States. Other, similar groups exist, although no formal listing is available. For example, the Golden Rainbow Center, in Palm Springs, California, has a weekly men's chat group; comparable groups exist within various community centers around the country.

Housing initiatives. Housing has become a focal point for the efforts of several communities and local organizations. As Adelman et al. (2006) have pointed out, several of these initiatives were formed in the 1970s and 1980s. The AIDS crisis arrested these efforts as the community dealt with significant loss of life and struggled to develop support services and to demand needed resources. An earnest revisiting of these efforts took place in the late 1990s, leading to several projects now under way, two of which are reviewed next. These endeavors have worked to create open and LGBT-supportive housing while adhering to the federal Fair Housing Act. The response has been the development of exemplary policies of nondiscrimination that include age, gender identity, sexual orientation, and spousal affiliation. Three examples of such projects follow.

RainbowVision (www.rainbowvisionprop.com) is the first retirement community specifically created for LGBT older adults. It is located on 13 acres in Santa Fe, New Mexico. It offers condominiums for purchase, independent living in leased residences with access to meal services and other amenities, and assisted living with access to health care and support services. RainbowVision offers a series of educational and social programs as well as health maintenance, recreational, and housekeeping and supportive services. An affiliated development in Vancouver, British Columbia, is planned.

In Los Angeles, the nonprofit Gay and Lesbian Elder Housing (www.gleh.org) is now a fully occupied rental apartment facility, in the Hollywood district, for LGBT older adults of limited income who are capable of independent living. Residents have access to support services, housekeeping, transportation, and related services, as well as at least one meal per day. In addition, an affiliated adult recreational and social service agency will be built on city-owned land with a grant from the Aging with Dignity Initiative, initially sponsored by the State of California in 2001.

The openhouse (openhouse-sf.org) is a San Francisco-based nonprofit organization dedicated to creating and sustaining senior housing (with services) that welcomes all seniors and that honors LGBT people. Formerly known as Rainbow Adult Community Housing, or RACH, this organization has been in existence since 1998 and is planning to build a sizable new affordable senior housing facility expressly welcoming LGBT seniors. Recognizing the urgent need, however, openhouse is also creating a directory of affordable senior housing, reflecting the most current information on senior housing complexes in San Francisco, including pertinent information regarding waiting lists, rent range, income eligibility, meal provision, and degree of LGBT sensitivity. To ensure these housing sites are welcoming to LGBT seniors, openhouse volunteers have been visiting *each site* to tour the facility and interview the manager(s).

CONCLUSION

Older gay men share many concerns with their heterosexual peers yet face challenges unique to sexual minority persons and specific to this population. These include managing the legacy of homophobia and the effect of negative stereotypes about both homosexuals and older persons. Physical and emotional health and economic and social well-being are influenced by the life histories and experiences of this cohort of gay elders. Health and social service professionals will benefit from becoming familiar with the available scholarly literature and listening closely to the life stories and current concerns of the older gay persons they serve.

REFERENCES

Adams, R. G., Blieszner, R., & de Vries, B. (2000). Definitions of friendship in the third age: Age, gender, and study location effects. *Journal of Aging Studies, 14*, 117–133.

Adelman, M. (Ed.). (1986). *Long time passing: Lives of older lesbians.* Boston: Alyson.

Adelman, M. (1991). Stigma, gay lifestyles, and adjustment to aging: A study of later-life gay men and lesbians. *Journal of Homosexuality, 20*(3/4), 7–32.

Adelman, M., Gurevitch, J., de Vries, B., & Blando, J. (2006). Openhouse: Community building and research in the LGBT aging population. In D. Kimmel, T. Rose, & S. David (Eds.), *Lesbian, gay, bisexual, and transgender aging: Research and clinical perspectives* (pp. 247–264). New York: Columbia University Press.

American Heart Association. (2008). The heart profilers. Retrieved from www.americanheart.org/presenter.jhtml?identifier=3000416

Antonucci, T. C., Sherman, A. M., & Akiyama, H. (1996). Social networks, support, and integration. In J. E. Birren (Ed.), *Encyclopedia of gerontology: Age, aging, and the aged* (pp. 505–515). New York: Academic Press.

Badget, L. (1998). *Income inflation: The myth of affluence among gay, lesbian, and bisexual Americans.* Washington, DC: Policy Institute of the National Gay and Lesbian Task Force and the Institute for Gay and Lesbian Strategic Studies. Retrieved from www.ngltf.org/downolads/income.pdf

Badgett, M. V. L. (2004). Will providing marriage rights to same-sex couples undermine heterosexual marriage? Evidence from Scandinavia and the Netherlands. *Journal of Sexuality Research and Social Policy*, 1, 1–10.

Bailey, J. M., & Oberschneider, M. (1997). Sexual orientation and professional dance. *Archives of Sexual Behavior*, 26(4), 433–444.

Baltes, M. M., & Carstensen, L. L. (1996). The process of successful aging. *Ageing and Society*, 16, 397–422.

Baltes, P. B., & Baltes, M. M. (1990). *Successful aging: Perspectives from the behavioral sciences*. New York: Cambridge University Press.

Barker, J., Herdt, G., & de Vries, B. (2006). Social support in the lives of gay men and lesbians at midlife and beyond. *Sexuality Research and Social Policy*, 3(2), 1–23.

Barker, J. C. (2004). Lesbian aging: An agenda for social research. In G. Herdt & B. de Vries (Eds.), *Gay and lesbian aging: Research and future directions* (pp. 29–72). New York: Sage.

Beeler, J. A., Rawls, T. D., Herdt, G., & Cohler, B. J. (1999). The needs of older lesbians and gay men in Chicago. *Journal of Gay and Lesbian Social Services*, 9(1), 31–49.

Bell, A. P., & Weinberg, M. S. (1978). *Homosexualities: A study of diversity among men and women*. New York: Simon and Schuster.

Bellah, R. N., Madsen, R., Sullivan, W. M., Swidler, A., & Tipton, S. M. (1985). *Habits of the heart: Individualism and commitment in American life*. Berkeley: University of California Press.

Bengtson, V. L., Burgess, E. O., & Parrott, T. M. (1997). Theory, explanation, and a third generation of theoretical development in social gerontology. *Journal of Gerontology, Series B, Psychological Sciences and Social Sciences*, 52B(2), S72–S88.

Bennett, K. C., & Thompson, N. L. (1991). Accelerated aging and male homosexuality: Australian evidence in a continuing debate. In J. A. Lee (Ed.), *Gay midlife and maturity* (pp. 65–75). New York: Haworth Press.

Berger, R. M. (1992). Research on older gay men: What we know, what we need to know. In N. J. Woodman (Ed.), *Lesbian and gay lifestyles: A guide for counseling and education* (pp. 217–234). New York: Irvington.

Berger, R. M. (1996). *Gay and gray: The older homosexual man* (2nd ed.). New York: Harrington Park Press.

Berger, R. M., & Kelly, J. J. (1986). Working with homosexuals of the older population. *Social Casework: The Journal of Contemporary Social Work*, 67, 203–210.

Bergling, T. (2004). *Reeling in the years: Gay men's perspectives on age and ageism*. New York: Harrington Park Press.

Berube, A. (1990). *Coming out under fire: The history of gay men and women in World War Two*. New York: Free Press.

Biller, R., & Rice, S. (1990). Experiencing multiple losses of persons with AIDS: Grief and bereavement. *Health and Social Work*, 15(4), 283–290.

Birren, J. E., & Hedlund, B. (1987). Contributions of autobiography to developmental psychology. In N. Isenberg (Ed.), *Contemporary topics in developmental psychology* (pp. 394–415). New York: Wiley.

Black, D., Gates, G., Sanders, S., & Taylor, L. (2000). Demographics of the gay and lesbian population in the United States: Evidence from available systematic data sources. *Demography, 37,* 139–154.

Blando, J. A. (2001). Twice hidden: Older gay and lesbian couples, friends, and intimacy. *Generations, 25*(2), 87–90.

Blumstein, P., & Schwartz, P. (1983). *American couples: Work, money, sex.* New York: Morrow.

Boxer, A., & Cohler, B. (1989). The life course of gay and lesbian youth: An immodest proposal for the study of lives. In G. Herdt (Ed.), *Gay and lesbian youth* (pp. 315–355). New York: Harrington Park Press.

Brim, O. G., Ryff, C. D., & Kessler, R. C. (2004). *How healthy are we? A national study of well-being at midlife.* Chicago: University of Chicago Press.

Brotman, S., Ryan, B., & Cormier, R. (2003). The health and social service needs of gay and lesbian elders and their families in Canada. *Gerontologist, 43,* 192–202.

Brown, L. B., Alley, G. R., Sarosy, S., Quarto, G., & Cook, T. (2001). Gay men: Aging well! *Journal of Gay and Lesbian Social Services, 13*(4), 41–54.

Brown, M. P. (1997). *Replacing citizenship: AIDS and radical activism.* New York: Guilford Press.

Butler, R. N. (1963). The life review: An interpretation of reminiscence in the aged. *Psychiatry, 26,* 65–76.

Cahill, S. (2002). Long-term care issues affecting gay, lesbian, bisexual, and transgender elders. *Geriatric Care Management Journal, 12,* 4–8.

Cahill, S., South, K., & Spade, J. (2000). *Outing age: Public policy issues affecting gay, lesbian, bisexual, and transgender elders.* Washington, DC: Policy Institute, National Gay and Lesbian Task Force.

Carmack, B. (1992). Balancing engagement/detachment in AIDS-related multiple losses. *Image: Journal of Nursing Scholarship, 24*(1), 9–14.

Carrington, C. (1999). *No place like home: Relationships and family among lesbians and gay men.* Chicago: University of Chicago Press.

Catania, J. A., Osmond, D., Stall, R. D., Pollack, L., Paul, J. P. Blower, . . . Coates, T. C. (2001). The continuing HIV epidemic among men who have sex with men. *American Journal of Public Health, 91*(6), 907–914.

Centers for Disease Control and Prevention. (2007). *Cases of HIV infection and AIDS in the United States and dependent areas, 2005.* Atlanta, GA: Author.

Centers for Disease Control and Prevention. (2010). *HIV and AIDS among gay and bisexual men.* Atlanta, GA: Author.

Cochran, S. D., & Mays, V. M. (2000). Lifetime prevalence of suicide symptoms and affective disorders among men reporting same-sex sexual partners: Results from NHANES III. *American Journal of Public Health, 90*(4), 573–578.

Cohler, B., & Galatzer-Levy, R. M. (2000). *The course of gay and lesbian lives*. Chicago: University of Chicago Press.

Cohler, B., Hostetler, A., & Boxer, A. (1998). Generativity, social context, and lived experience: Narratives of gay men in middle adulthood. In D. McAdams & E. de St. Aubin (Eds.), *Generativity and adult experience: Psychosocial perspectives on caring and contributing to the next generation* (pp. 265–309). Washington, DC: American Psychological Association Press.

Cohler, B. J. (2004). Saturday night at the Tubs: Age cohort and social life at the urban gay bath. In G. Herdt & B. de Vries (Eds.), *Gay and lesbian aging: Research and future directions* (pp. 211–234). New York: Springer.

Cole, T. R. (1984). Aging, meaning, and well-being: Musings of a cultural historian. *International Journal of Aging and Human Development, 19*, 329–336.

Connidis, I. A. (2001). *Family ties and aging*. New York: Sage.

Corless, I. B. (1995). Saying good-bye to tomorrow. In J. Kauffman (Ed.), *Awareness of mortality* (pp. 171–184). Amityville, NY: Baywood.

Cornett, C. W., & Hudson, R. A. (1987). Middle adulthood and the theories of Erikson, Gould, and Vaillant: Where does the gay man fit? *Journal of Gerontological Social Work, 10*(3/4), 61–73.

Crosby, M. G., Stall, R. D., Paul, J. P., & Barrett, D. C. (1998). Drug and alcohol and drug use have declined between generations of younger gay-bisexual men in San Francisco. *Alcohol Dependence, 52*, 177–182.

D'Augelli, A., & Grossman, A. (2001). Disclosure of sexual orientation, victimization, and mental health among lesbian, gay, and bisexual older adults. *Journal of Interpersonal Violence, 16*(10), 1008–1027.

David, S., & Knight, B. G. (2008). Stress and coping among gay men: Age and ethnic differences. *Psychology and Aging, 23*(1), 62–69.

Daviglus, M. L., Liu, K., Greenland, P., Dyer, A. R., Garside, D. B., Manheim, L., . . . Stamler, J. (1998). Benefit of a favorable cardiovasulcar risk factor profile in middle age with respect to Medicare costs. *New England Journal of Medicine, 339*, 1122–1129.

Dean, L., Meyer, I., Robinson, K., Sell, R., Sember, R., Silenzio, V., . . . Xavier, J. (2000). Lesbian, gay, bisexual, and transgender health: Findings and concerns. *Journal of the Gay and Lesbian Medical Association, 4*(3), 101–151.

Deck, E. S., & Folta, J. R. (1989). The friend-griever. In J. K. Doka (Ed.), *Disenfranchised grief: Recognizing hidden sorrow* (pp. 77–89). Lexington, MA: Lexington Books.

de Vries, B. (1996). The understanding of friendship: An adult life course perspective. In C. Magai & S. H. McFadden (Eds.), *Handbook of emotion, adult development, and aging* (pp. 249–268). New York: Academic Press.

de Vries, B. (2001). Grief: Intimacy's reflection. *Generations, 25*, 75–80.

de Vries, B. (2005). Making a case for friendship. *Healing Ministries, 12*, 25–28.

de Vries, B. (2006). Home at the end of the rainbow: Supportive housing for LGBT elders. *Generations, 29*, 64–69.

de Vries, B. (2008). Lesbian, gay, bisexual and transgender persons in later life. In D. Carr (Ed.), *Encyclopedia of the life course and human development* (pp. 161–165). Farmington Hills, MI: Gale Publishing.

de Vries, B., & Blando, J. A. (2004). The study of gay and lesbian lives: Lessons for social gerontology. In G. Herdt & B. de Vries (Eds.), *Gay and lesbian aging: Research and future directions* (pp. 3–28). New York: Springer.

de Vries, B., Croghan, C. F., & Worman, T. (2006). "Always independent, never alone": Serving the needs of gay and lesbian elders. *Journal of Active Aging, 4,* 45–52.

de Vries, B., & Herdt, G. (2000, November). Life stories and gay men: Life course pathways to gay identities. In J. W. Powell (Chair), *Sexuality, life stage, and life story: A symposium on narrative approaches to sexual identity.* Symposium conducted at the meeting of the Gerontological Society of America, Washington, DC.

de Vries, B., & Hoctel, P. (2007). The family friends of older gay men and lesbians. In N. Teunis & G. Herdt (Eds.), *Sexual inequalities and social justice* (pp. 213–232). Berkeley: University of California Press.

de Vries, B., & Johnson, C. L. (2002). The death of a friend in later life. *Advances in Life Course Research: New Frontiers in Socialization, 7,* 299–324.

de Vries, B., Mason, A., Quam, J., & Acquaviva, K. (2009). State recognition of same-sex relationships and preparations for end of life among lesbian and gay boomers. *Sexuality Research and Social Policy, 6*(1), 90–101.

de Vries, B., & Megathlin, D. (2009). The meaning of friends for gay men and lesbians in the second half of life. *Journal of GLBT Family Studies, 5,* 82–98.

Diaz, R. M. (1998). *Latino gay men and HIV.* New York: Routledge.

Doka, J. K. (Ed.). (1989). *Disenfranchised grief: Recognizing hidden sorrow.* Lexington, MA: Lexington Books.

Erikson, E. (1982). *The life-cycle completed.* New York: Norton.

Erikson, E. H., Erikson, J. M., & Kivnick, H. Q. (1986). *Vital involvement in old age: The experience of old age in our time.* New York: Norton.

Ernst, J. (2004). *It's always something: Medical complications of aging with HIV.* Acria update. Retrieved from www.thebody.com/cria/summer04/contents.html

Farnham, M., & Marshall, P. (Eds.). (1989). *Walking after midnight: Gay men's life stories.* New York: Routledge.

Federal Interagency Forum on Aging-Related Statistics. (2004, November). *Older Americans 2004: Key indicators of well-being.* Washington, DC: Government Printing Office.

Fredriksen-Goldsen, K. I., Kim, H.-J., & Goldsen, J. (2011). *The aging and health report: Disparities and resilience among lesbian, gay, bisexual, and transgender older adults.* Seattle, WA: Institute for Multigenerational Health.

Fredriksen-Goldsen, K. I., & Muraco, A. (2010). Aging and sexual orientation: A 25-year review of the literature. *Research on Aging, 32*(3), 372–413.

Friend, R. A. (1980). GAYging: Adjustment and the older gay male. *Alternative Lifestyles, 3,* 213–248.

Friend, R. A. (1989). Older lesbian and gay people: Responding to homophobia. *Marriage and Family Review, 14,* 241–263.

Friend, R. A. (1991). Older lesbian and gay people: A theory of successful aging. *Journal of Homosexuality, 20,* 99–118.

Gagnon, J. (2004). *An interpretation of desire: Essays in the study of sexuality.* Chicago: University of Chicago Press.

Garfein, A. J., & Herzog, A. R. (1995). Robust aging among the young-old, old-old, and oldest-old. *Journal of Gerontology, Series B, Psychological Sciences and Social Sciences, 50B,* S77–S87.

Gates, G. J. (2006). *Same-sex couples and the gay, lesbian, bisexual population: New estimates from the American Community Survey.* Los Angeles: Williams Institute.

Gates, G. J., Badgett, M. V. L., & Ho, D. (2008, July). *Marriage, registration, and dissolution by same-sex couples in the U.S.* Los Angeles, CA: The Williams Institute.

Gorman, E. M., & Nelson, K. (2004). From a far place: Social and cultural considerations about HIV among midlife and older gay men. In G. Herdt & B. de Vries (Ed.), *Gay and lesbian aging: Research and future directions* (pp. 73–93). New York: Springer.

Gottman, J. M., Levenson, R. W., Gross, J., Fredrickson, B. L., McCoy, K., Rosenthal, L., & Yoshimoto, D. (2003). Correlates of gay and lesbian couples' relationship satisfaction and relationship dissolution. *Journal of Homosexuality, 45*(1), 23–43.

Gove, W. R., Style, C. B., & Hughes, M. (1990). The effect of marriage on the well-being of adults: A theoretical analysis. *Journal of Family Issues, 11,* 4–35.

Grossman, A. H., D'Augelli, A. R., & Hershberger, S. L. (2000). Social support networks and lesbian, gay, and bisexual adults 60 years of age and older. *Journal of Gerontology, 55,* 171–179.

Grov, C., Bimbi, D. S., Nanin, J. E., & Parsons, J. T. (2006). Exploring racial and ethnic differences in recreational drug use among gay and bisexual men in New York City and Los Angeles. *Journal of Drug Education, 36*(2), 105–123.

Gruskin, E. P., Greenwood, G. L., Matevia, M., Pollack, L. M., & Bye, L. L. (2007). Disparities in smoking between the lesbian, gay, and bisexual population and the general population in California. *American Journal of Public Health, 97*(8), 1496–1502.

Harrison, A. E., & Silenzio, V. M. (1996). Comprehensive care of lesbian and gay patients and families. *Primary Care: Models of Ambulatory Care, 23,* 31–46.

Henry J. Kaiser Family Foundation. (2001). *Inside-OUT: A report on the experiences of lesbians, gays, and bisexuals in America and the public's views on issues and policies related to sexual orientation* (Publication No. 3195). Menlo Park, CA: Author. Retrieved from http://www.kff.org/kaiserpolls/loader.cfm?url=/commonspot/security/getfile.cfm&PageID=13873

Herdt, G. (1989). Introduction: Gay youth, emergent identities, and cultural scenes at home and abroad. In G. Herdt (Ed.), *Homosexuality and adolescence* (pp. 1–42). New York: Harrington Press.

Herdt, G. (Ed.). (1992). *Gay culture in America.* Boston: Beacon Press.

Herdt, G. (1997). *Same-sex, different cultures: Perspectives on gay and lesbian lives.* New York: Westview Press.

Herdt, G., Beeler, J., & Rawls, T. (1997). Life course diversity among older lesbians and gay men: A study in Chicago. *Journal of Gay, Lesbian, and Bisexual Identities, 2,* 231–247.

Herdt, G., & Boxer, A. (1992). Introduction: Culture, history, and life course of gay men. In G. Herdt (Ed.), *Gay culture in America* (pp. 1–28). Boston: Beacon Press.

Herdt, G., & Kertzner, R. (2006). I do, but I can't: The impact of marriage denial on the mental health and sexual citizenship of lesbians and gay men in the United States. *Sexuality Research and Social Policy: Journal of NSRC, 3*(1), 33–49.

Herdt, G., & Koff, B. (2000). *Something to tell you: The road families travel when a child is gay.* New York: Columbia University Press.

Herdt, G., & McClintock, M. (Eds.). (2000). Special issue on the development of sexual attraction. *Archives of Sexual Behavior, 29*(6).

Herek, G. M. (2004). Beyond "homophobia": Thinking about sexual stigma and prejudice in the twenty-first century. *Sexuality Research and Social Policy: Journal of NSRC, 1*(2), 6–24.

Herek, G. M. (2006). Legal recognition of same-sex relationships in the United States: A social science perspective. *American Psychologist, 61*(6), 607–621.

Herrell, R., Goldberg, J., True, W. R., Ramakrishnan, V., Lyons, M., Elsen, S., & Tsuang, M. T. (1999). Sexual orientation and suicidality: A co-twin control study is adult men. *Archives of General Psychiatry, 56,* 867–874.

High, K. P., Effros, R. B., Fletcher, C. V., Gebo, K., Halter, J. B., Hazzard, W. R., . . . Woolard, N. F. (2008). Workshop on HIV infection and aging: What is known and future research directions. *Clinical Infectious Diseases, 47*(4), 542–553.

Hostetler, A. J. (2004). Old, gay, and alone? The ecology of well-being among middle-aged and older single gay men. In G. Herdt & B. de Vries (Eds.), *Gay and lesbian aging: Research and future directions* (pp. 143–176). New York: Springer.

Hostetler, A. J., & Cohler, B. J. (1997). Partnership, singlehood, and the lesbian and gay life course: A research agenda. *Journal of Gay, Lesbian, and Bisexual Identity, 2,* 199–230.

Hubbard, P. (2001). Sex zones: Intimacy, citizenship, and public space. *Sexualities, 4,* 51–71.

Hughes, T. L. (2003). Lesbians' drinking patterns: Beyond the data. *Substance Use and Misuse, 38*(11–13), 1739–1758.

Institute of Medicine. (2011). *The health of lesbian, gay, bisexual, and transgender people: Building a foundation for better understanding.* Washington, DC: National Academies Press.

Isay, R. (1996). *Becoming gay: The journey to self-acceptance.* New York: Pantheon Books.

Jacobs, J. A., & Tedford, W. H. (1980). Factors affecting self-esteem of the homosexual individual. *Journal of Homosexuality, 5,* 373–382.

Jacobs, R., Rasmussen, L., & Hohman, M. (1999). The social support needs of older lesbian, gay men, and bisexuals. *Journal of Gay and Lesbian Social Services, 9,* 1–30.

Jacobson, S., & Grossman, A. H. (1996). Older lesbians and gay men: Old myths, new images, and future directions. In R. C. Savin-Williams & K. Cohen (Eds.), *The lives of lesbians, gays, and bisexuals: Children to adults* (pp. 345–373). Fort Worth, TX: Harcourt, Brace.

Johnson, C. (2002). Heteronormative citizenship and the politics of passing. *Sexualities, 5,* 317–336.

Johnson, C. L. (1983). Fairweather friends and rainy day kin: An anthropological analysis of old age friendships in the United States. *Urban Anthropology, 12,* 103–123.

Kantor, M. (1999). *Treating emotional disorder in gay men.* Westport, CT: Praeger.

Kastenbaum, R. (1969). Death and bereavement in later life. In A. J. Kutscher (Ed.), *Death and bereavement* (pp. 28–54). Springfield, IL: Charles C Thomas.

Kaufman, G., & Raphael, L. (1996). *Coming out of shame: Transforming gay and lesbian lives.* New York: Doubleday.

Kehoe, M. (1988). *Lesbians over 60 speak for themselves.* Binghamton, NY: Haworth Press.

Kelly, J. (1980). Homosexuality and aging. In J. Marmor (Ed.), *Homosexual behavior: A modern reappraisal* (pp. 176–193). New York: Basic Books.

Kelly, J. J. (1977). The aging male homosexual: Myth and reality. *Gerontologist, 17,* 328–332.

Kimmel, D. C. (1978). Adult development and aging: A gay perspective. *Journal of Social Issues, 34,* 113–130.

Kimmel, D. C. (1979). Life history interviews of aging gay men. *International Journal of Aging and Human Development, 10*(3), 239–248.

Kimmel, D. C. (2004). Issues to consider in studies of midlife and older sexual minorities. In G. Herdt & B. de Vries (Eds.), *Gay and lesbian aging: Research and future directions* (pp. 265–283). New York: Springer.

Kinsey, A. C., Pomeroy, W. B., & Martin, C. E. (1948). *Sexual behavior in the human male.* Bloomington: Indiana University Press.

Kochman, A. (1997). Gay and lesbian elderly: Historical overview and implications for social work practice. In J. Quam (Ed.), *Social services for senior gay men and lesbians* (pp. 1–25). New York: Haworth Press.

Kurdek, L. (1994). The nature and correlates of relationship quality in gay, lesbian, and heterosexual cohabiting couples: A test of the contextual, investment, and discrepancy models. In B. Greene & G. Herek (Eds.), *Lesbian and gay psychology: Theory, research, and clinical applications* (pp. 135–155). Thousand Oaks, CA: Sage.

Kurdek, L. (1995). Lesbian and gay couples. In A. R. D'Augelli & C. Patterson (Eds.), *Lesbian, gay, and bisexual identities over the lifespan: Psychological perspectives* (pp. 243–261). New York: Oxford University Press.

Laner, M. R. (1978). Growing older male: Heterosexual and homosexual. *Gerontologist, 18*, 496–501.

Laumann, E. O., Gagnon, J. H., Michael, R. T., & Michaels, S. (1994). *The social organization of sexuality: Sexual practices in the United States.* Chicago: University of Chicago Press.

Lee, J. A. (1987). The invisible lives of Canada's gray gays. In V. W. Marshall (Ed.), *Aging in Canada: Social perspectives* (pp. 138–155). Markham, Ontario: Fitzhenry & Whiteside.

Lee, J. A. (1991). Foreword. In J. A. Lee (Ed.), *Gay midlife and maturity.* New York: Haworth Press.

Levine, J., Gagnon, J., & Nardi, P. (1997). *In changing times.* Chicago: University of Chicago Press.

Linsk, N. L. (2000). HIV among older adults: Age-specific issues in prevention and treatment. *AIDS Reader, 10*(7), 430–444.

Lowenthal, M., Thurnher, M., & Chiriboga, D. (1975). *Four stages of life.* San Francisco: Jossey-Bass.

Lund, D. A., Caserta, M. S., Dimond, M. F., & Shaffer, S. K. (1989). Competencies: Tasks of daily living and adjustments to spousal bereavement in later life. In D. A. Lund (Ed.), *Older bereaved spouses: Research with practical applications* (pp. 135–156). Washington, DC: Taylor & Francis.

Manasse, G., & Swallow, J. (Eds.). (1995). *Making love visible: In celebration of gay and lesbian families.* Freedom, CA: Crossing Press.

Martin, J. L. (1988). Psychological consequences of AIDS-related bereavement among gay men. *Journal of Consulting and Clinical Psychology, 56*(6), 856–862.

Martin, J. L., & Dean, L. (1993). Bereavement following death from AIDS: Unique problems, reactions, and special needs. In M. S. Stroebe, W. Stroebe, & R. O. Hansson (Eds.), *Handbook of bereavement: Theory, research, and intervention* (pp. 315–330). New York: Cambridge University Press.

Maupin, A. (2007). *Michael Tolliver lives.* San Francisco: HarperCollins.

McAdams, D. (1993). *Stories we live by: Personal myths and the making of the self.* New York: William Morrow.

McAdams, D., & de St. Aubin, E. (1992). A theory of generativity and its assessment through self-report, behavioral acts and narrative themes in autobiography. *Journal of Personality and Social Psychology, 62*, 1003–1015.

McAdams, D., Ruetzel, K., & Foley, J. (1986). Complexity and generativity at midlife: Relations among social motives, ego development, and adults' plans for the future. *Journal of Personality and Social Psychology, 50*, 800–807.

McDonald, G. J. (1982). Individual differences in the coming out process for gay men: Implications for theoretical models. *Journal of Homosexuality, 8*, 47–60.

Merrill, S. S., & Verbrugge, L. M. (1999). Health and disease in midlife. In S. L. Willis & J. D. Reid (Eds.), *Life in the middle: Psychological and social development in middle age* (pp. 77–103). San Diego, CA: Academic Press.

MetLife (2010). *Still out, still aging: The MetLife Study of Lesbian, Gay, Bisexual, and Transgender Baby Boomers.* Westport, CT: MetLife Mature Market Institute.

Meyer, I. H. (1995). Minority stress and mental health in gay men. *Journal of Health and Social Behavior, 36*, 38–56.

Meyer, I. H. (2003). Minority stress and mental health in gay men. In L. D. Garnets & D. C. Kimmel (Eds.), *Psychological perspectives on lesbian, gay, and bisexual experiences* (2nd ed., pp. 699–731). New York: Columbia University Press.

Michaels, S. (1996). The prevalence of homosexuality in the United States. In R. P. Cabaj & T. Stein (Eds.), *Textbook of homosexuality and mental health* (pp. 43–63). Washington, DC: American Psychiatric Association Press.

Mills, T. C., Paul, J., Stall, R., Pollack, L., Canchola, J., Chang, Y. J., . . . , & Catania, J. A. (2004). Distress and depression in men who have sex with men: The Urban Men's Health Study. *American Journal of Psychiatry, 161*(2), 278–285.

Minnigerode, F. A. (1976). Age-status labeling in homosexual men. *Journal of Homosexuality, 1*(3), 273–275.

Moss, M., & Moss, S. (1989). The impact of death of elderly sibling: Some considerations of a normative loss. *American Behavioral Scientist, 33*, 94–106.

Movement Advancement Project and Services and Advocacy for Gay, Lesbian, Bisexual and Transgender Elders. (2010). *Improving the lives of LGBT older adults.* Retrieved May 13, 2011, from www.sageusa.org/uploads/Advancing%20Equality%20for%20LGBT%20Elders%20%5BFINAL%20COMPRESSED%5D.pdf

Murray, S. O. (1995). *American gay.* Chicago: University of Chicago Press.

Nardi, P. M. (1999). *Gay men's friendships: Invincible communities.* Chicago: University of Chicago Press.

Nardi, P. M., & Sanders, D. (1994). *Growing up before Stonewall: Life stories of some gay men.* London: Routledge.

National Academy on an Aging Society. (1999). *Chronic conditions: A challenge for the 21st century.* Washington, DC: National Academy Press.

Neugarten, B. L., Moore, J. W., & Lowe, J. C. (1965). Age norms, age constraints, and adult socialization. *American Journal of Sociology, 70*, 710–717.

Niolon, R. (2006). *Gay/lesbian resources: Stages of gay relationship development.* Retrieved from www.psychpage.com/gay/library/gay_lesbian_violence/stages_gay_relationships.html

O'Brien, K. (1992). Primary relationships affect the psychological health of homosexual men at risk for AIDS. *Psychological Reports, 71*, 147–153.

Paul, J. P., Catania, J., Pollack, L., Moskowitz, J., Canchola, J., Mills, T., . . . & Stall, R. (2002). Suicide attempts among gay and bisexual men: Lifetime prevalence and antecedents. *American Journal of Public Health, 92*, 1338–1345.

Peplau, L., Veniegas, R., & Campbell, S. (1996). Gay and lesbian relationships. In R. Savin-Williams & K. C. Cohen (Eds.), *The lives of lesbians, gays, and bisexuals: Children to adults* (pp. 250–273). New York: Harcourt Brace.

Quam, J., & Whitford, G. S. (1992). Adaptation and age-related expectations of older gay and lesbian adults. *Gerontologist, 32*, 367–374.

Rawls, T. (2004). Disclosure and depression among older gay and homosexual men: Findings from the Urban Men's Health Study. In G. Herdt & B. de Vries (Eds.), *Gay and lesbian aging: Research and future directions* (pp. 117–141). New York: Sage.

Reid, J. D. (1995). Development in later life: Older lesbian and gay lives. In A. R. D'Augelli & C. J. Patterson (Eds.), *Lesbian, gay and bisexual identities over the lifespan: Psychological perspectives* (pp. 215–242). New York: Oxford University Press.

Richards, T. A., Wrubel, J., & Folkman, S. (2000). Death rites in the San Francisco gay community: Cultural developments of the AIDS epidemic. *Omega, 40*(2), 335–350.

Richardson, D. (1998). Sexuality and citizenship. *Sociology, 32*(1), 83–100.

Roger, V. L., Go, A. S., Lloyd-Jones, D. M., Adams, R. J., Berry, J. D., Brown, T. M., . . . Wylie-Rosett, J.; American Heart Association Statistics Committee and Stroke Statistics Subcommittee. (2011). Heart disease and stroke statistics 2011 update: A report from the American Heart Association. *Circulation, 123*, e18–e209. doi:10.1161/CIR.0b013e3182009701.

Rowe, J. W., & Kahn, R. L. (1998). *Successful aging.* New York: Pantheon Books.

Russell, G. M., & Bohan, J. S. (2005). The gay generation gap: Communicating across the LGBT generational divide. *Policy Journal of the Institute for Gay and Lesbian Strategic Studies, 8*(1), 1–8.

Rutter, V., & Schwartz, P. (1996). Same-sex couples: Courtship, commitment, context. In A. E. Auhagen & M. von Salisch (Eds.), *The diversity of human relationships* (pp. 197–226). New York: Cambridge University Press.

Sandfort, T. G. M., de Graaf, R., Bijl, R. V., & Schnabel, P. (2001). Same-sex sexual behavior and psychiatric disorders: Findings from the Netherlands Mental Health Survey and Incidence Study (NEMESIS). *Archives of General Psychiatry, 58*(1), 85–91.

Schmitt, K. P., & Kurdek, L. H. (1987). Personality correlates of positive identity and relationship involvement in gay men. *Journal of Homosexuality, 13*(4), 101–109.

Schwartzberg, S. (1992). AIDS-related bereavement among gay men: The inadequacy of current theories of grief. *Psychotherapy, 29*, 422–429.

Shernoff, M. (Ed.), *Gay widowers: Life after the death of a partner.* New York: Harrington Press.

Shippy, A. (2004). *HIV and aging.* Acria update. Retrieved from www.thebody.com /cria/summer04/contents.html

Siegel, S., & Lowe, E. (1995). *Uncharted lives: Understanding the life passages of gay men.* New York: Plume.

Solomon, S. E., Rothblum, E. D., & Balsam, K. F. (2004). Pioneers in partnership: Lesbian and gay male couples in civil unions compared with those not in civil unions and married heterosexual siblings. *Journal of Family Psychology, 18*(2), 275–286.

Trupin, L., & Rice, D. (1995). *Health status, care use, and number of disabling condition in the United States* (Disability Statistics Abstract No. 9). Washington, DC: National Institute on Disability and Rehabilitation Research.

Umberson, D., & Williams, K. (2005). Marital quality, health, and aging: Gender equity? *Journal of Gerontology, Series B, Psychological Sciences and Social Sciences, 60B*, S109–S113.

Vacha, K. (1985). *Quiet fire: Memoirs of older gay men.* Trumansburg, NY: Crossing Press.

Viney, L., Henry, R., Walker, B., & Crooks, L. (1992). The psychosocial impact of multiple deaths from AIDS. *Omega: Journal of Death and Dying, 24*(2), 151–163.

Wahler, J., & Gabbay, S. G. (1997). Gay male aging: A review of the literature. *Journal of Gay and Lesbian Social Services, 6*(3), 1–20.

Waite, L. J., & Gallagher, M. (2000). *The case for marriage: Why married people are happier, healthier, and better off financially.* New York: Doubleday.

Warner, M. (1999). *The trouble with normal: Sex, politics, and the ethics of queer life.* Cambridge, MA: Harvard University Press.

Weeks, J. (1983). The problem of older homosexuals. In J. Hart & D. Richardson (Eds.), *The theory and practice of homosexuals* (pp. 177–185). London: Routledge Kegan Paul.

Weinberg, M. S., & Williams, C. J. (1974). *Male homosexuals: Their problems and adaptations.* New York: Oxford University Press.

Weinstock, J. S. (2000). Lesbian friendships at midlife: Patterns and possibilities for the 21st century. *Journal of Gay and Lesbian Social Services, 11*(2/3), 1–32.

Weston, K. (1991). *Families we choose: Lesbians, gays, kinship.* New York: Columbia University Press.

Williams, K. (2003). Has the future of marriage arrived? A contemporary examination of gender, marriage, and psychological well being. *Journal of Health and Social Behavior, 44,* 470–487.

Wong, P. T., & Watt, L. M. (1991). What types of reminiscence are associated with successful aging? *Psychology and Aging, 6,* 272–279.

CHAPTER FOUR

Aging in the Lesbian Community

NANCY M. NYSTROM, PH.D., M.S.W., L.I.C.S.W.,
AND TERESA C. JONES, PH.D., M.S.W.

The lives of older lesbians have rarely been the focus of research and scholarly writing. Much of the limited research base cited in current studies was developed in the 1970s, 1980s, and 1990s and originated in clinical, psychological settings. Many studies that include or are about lesbians have concentrated on relatively narrow areas of investigation, including sexual orientation and personal identity, mental health needs, and psychological adjustment (Adelman, 1990; Berger, 1986; Dorfman, Walters, Burke, & Hardin, 1995; Friend, 1990; Kehoe, 1988; Kimmel, 1978; McDougall, 1993; Parks, 1999; Rothblum, 1990; Trippet, 1994; West, 1983). In addition, some social science research has included comparisons of older lesbians and gay men (Berger, 1982, 1984; Dorfman et al., 1995; Gwenwald, 1983; Herdt, Beeler, & Rawls, 1997; Kimmel, 1992), comparisons of lesbians and heterosexual women (Tully, 1989), social supports (Slusher, Mayer, & Dunkle, 1996), and, more recently, lesbian parenting (Gartrell et al., 1999; Hare, 1994; Hequembourg & Farrell, 1999; Lott-Whitehead & Tully, 1993; Muzio, 1994).

Lesbian older adults have sometimes been included in more general studies of sexual minority aging. In their extensive review, Fredriksen-Goldsen and Muraco (2010) trace the evolution of research on LGB aging over time, from early studies that dismantled negative stereotypes about lesbian and gay older adults, to studies examining correlates of psychological adjustment and functioning, to identity development in the lives of LGB elders, to more recent research investigating "the social support and community-based needs and experiences of older LGB adults . . . the need for LGB-specific services in housing, health, caregiving and other human services . . . [and] the variation between and among individuals with respect to gender, aging bodies, relationships, family life, and social networks" (p. 402). In other words, older lesbians, and other LGBT older adults, have only very recently become the subjects of studies similar to the research conducted on behalf of the older members of the general society, rather than compared to preexisting negative stereotypes and assumed pathologies.

As members of a triply marginalized community (meaning the classifications of old, woman, and lesbian), the realities of older lesbians' lives have, until very recently, been overlooked by the scientific community as well as by heterosexual society and youth-oriented lesbian and gay communities. Negative images and stereotypes, although still popular within our society, are inaccurate reflections of the individuals who compose this population. Although frequently described as hidden or invisible (Berger, 1982; Fassinger, 1991; Kehoe, 1986a; Potter & Darty, 1981), older lesbians comprise a diverse, active, and vibrant facet of our society, a fact that is beginning to be reflected in some of the most recent literature (Institute of Medicine [IOM], 2011; MetLife, 2010).

In this chapter, terms used to refer to older persons in the lesbian community are taken from the existing geriatric and gerontologic literatures. Hooyman and Kiyak (2010) describe three distinct groups of elderly persons: the *young old*, who are between the ages of 65 and 74 years; the *old*, who are aged 75 to 84 years; and the *oldest old*, who are older than age 85 years. For those approaching Hooyman and Kiyak's first group, that is, persons in their mid-50s and early 60s, the term *aging* is used. Advocacy groups such as the Gray Panthers, Old Lesbians Organizing for Change (OLOC), Services and Advocacy for GLBT Elders (SAGE USA, formerly Senior Action in a Gay Environment), and others have not reached consensus regarding terminology describing the various levels of aging. Because of this lack of agreement, no system will appeal to all. OLOC refers to the old as those who are aged 60 years and older, choosing the word *old*—rather than *older* or *elderly*—as an empowering term, encouraging seniors to refer to themselves as "old" with pride. The authors wish to respect these varying views and have used the terms *old*, *elderly*, and *older* interchangeably when discussing all persons who would be classified in Hooyman and Kiyak's three groups.

THE AGING LESBIAN POPULATION

Reliable empirical evidence regarding the number of elderly lesbians in the United States is currently lacking. Extrapolations from U.S. Census data and other population studies suggest estimates of 1.0 to 2.8 million lesbian, gay, bisexual, and transgender (LGBT) elders, with this population estimated to grow to between 2 million and 6 million by 2030 (Cahill, South, & Spade, 2000; Gabbay & Wahler, 2002; O'Hanlan et al., 2004). Current estimates of the elderly lesbian population are between 350,000 and more than 1 million, with a projected growth to more than 3 million by 2030 (Gabbay & Wahler, 2002; O'Hanlan et al., 2004). Because women make up 60% of the population of older adults, it is likely that the same gender ratio applies within the LGBT population, although the premature death of many gay men during the early days of the HIV epidemic may tragically have affected this ratio somewhat. Nonetheless, the population of old lesbians may be larger than estimated, increasing to perhaps 4 million elders by 2030.

These estimates are based on existing data, using variations of percentile estimates of gay and lesbian people, which have been debated since the publication of the first Kinsey report in 1948 (Cahill et al., 2000). These percentile estimates of gay, lesbian, and bisexual persons range from a low of 1% to a high of 8% (Cahill et al., 2000). Within this range of estimates, it is difficult to determine actual numbers because of lack of reliable research in which questions about sexual orientation and gender identity are included. This situation, as well as reluctance on the part of elder lesbians to state their sexual orientation openly to researchers (IOM, 2011), has resulted in even less available information about aging and older lesbians, relative to some other minority groups (Cahill et al., 2000).

Reliable estimates of the actual size of this population will likely not be obtainable in the near future, because of the ongoing discrimination and hostility these women face, both within the general society and within the—still ageist—LGBT community. These circumstances limit lesbians' sense of safety, frequently forcing them to conceal their sexual orientation, thus making them a hidden population (Boxer, 1997; Herek, 1992; IOM, 2011). For these reasons, among others, many researchers conclude that the true population of LGBT people is probably substantially underreported (Cahill et al., 2000).

This reality has resulted in many studies of older persons failing to include old lesbians, creating a lack of knowledge of their unique issues and concerns, and contributing to their experience as a demographically invisible population (Boxer, 1997). Research has been more inclusive of older lesbians in recent years, but these efforts have not yet compensated for the exclusionary practices and scanty research efforts that were the norm for decades. Many existing research studies about lesbians were conducted with small, purposive samples, with qualitative research as the primary methodology. These have offered glimpses of the lesbian community and culture, yet none of these studies has been large enough to generalize its findings to the entire population.

Older lesbians not only have often been excluded from general studies about aging but also have been omitted from many studies of lesbian and gay life experiences and concerns. Frequently, methods used to recruit research study participants rely on contact with easily accessible groups whose members see the relevance of the research questions. For many older lesbians, fear of revealing their sexual orientation causes them to be isolated from typical social, community, and agency systems (IOM, 2011; Orel, 2006). Consequently, they may not be represented in the places where researchers are looking for participants. In addition, if the scope of the research is perceived to be either irrelevant or harmful, older lesbians will be much less inclined to participate. Because of this systematic exclusion from scholarly research, there is still much to learn about lesbian elders and their experiences and expectations as they age (Friend, 1990; Gabbay & Wahler, 2002).

Vignette I: General Aging Concerns

Susan is 76, and Linda is 58. They have been partners for 15 years and live together in the home Susan purchased 20 years ago. Before meeting Susan, Linda bought a small house, which she now maintains as a rental property. Susan and Linda have always been active. They enjoy traveling and socializing with friends. They are open about their relationship with most friends and family. However, they have not talked about their relationship with their medical care providers or other business contacts.

Recently, Susan was diagnosed with early-stage Alzheimer's disease. Linda feels that their relationship has changed completely because of Susan's new limitations. Susan is no longer able to travel for extended periods of time. Her confusion about everyday matters is increasing. Linda speaks of moving back to her house with comments such as, "I have to keep my options open." Linda has not talked with Susan about these thoughts. Neither woman is knowledgeable about services in their local community to help them maintain stability in their lives.

Frequently, when relationships begin, lesbians do not talk about their long-term future in concrete, real-life terms. Often, no plans are made for long-term care or for dealing with potential changes in health or financial status. Because there is no legal recognition of lesbian relationships in most jurisdictions, partners must discuss future plans so that both parties have a measure of security in their later years, particularly because traditional, government-sponsored solutions are often not available to them.

Although literature about aging within the LGBT communities is scant, even less is known about race and class diversity within these communities. Much of the available research has been conducted using random samples, which reflect the racial and ethnic diversity within the communities only to a limited degree. Although theories can be proposed regarding the possible similarities and differences in aging experiences between white and nonwhite LGBT individuals, or between persons who are members of different nonwhite groups, these cannot currently be substantiated with solid research data. In addition to their mistrust of the research process, many LGBT people of color have also experienced discrimination within the general LGBT community. As a result, they may be reluctant to participate in surveys and studies conducted under traditional research protocols. This is particularly unfortunate, as some research (MetLife, 2006) has found that African American and Hispanic LGBT elders may be more likely than their white/European American peers to find their LGBT identity beneficial as they approach midlife and old age. Further research that includes nonwhite older lesbians, and other nonwhite LGBT elders, will be a necessary aspect of understanding resilience among older adults, as well as a needed service on behalf of LGBT older persons and communities of color.

More research has been conducted on behalf of lesbians and gay men who are African American than on behalf of those who are members of other racial and ethnic groups, such as Latinos and Latinas, Asian Americans, Pacific Islanders, and Native Americans. However, that research has been limited and has included participants of all ages, without much discussion of differences between age cohorts (Cahill et al., 2000). Few data are available regarding the experience of elderly sexual or gender-minority-identified individuals in any racial group (Cahill et al., 2000; Harel, McKinney, & Williams, 1990; Mays, Chatters, Cochran, & Mackness, 1998), although some studies have included respondents with a variety of racial identities (MetLife 2006, 2010) that have used statistical weighting to more closely approximate the racial makeup of the United States in their analyses. There is a significant need to learn more about the aging experiences of members of these populations through focusing on community-based, culturally sensitive research and consumer evaluation of currently available programs and services.

Across demographic groups, several general studies on aging have identified two major themes that concern women as they age. First is their desire to maintain good health, a factor they view as essential to continue to function independently (Hooyman & Kiyak, 2010; Kaufman, 1994). The second emergent theme is the concern regarding their ability to stay in their own homes for as long as possible (Hamburger, 1997; Hooyman & Kiyak, 2010). These are major factors for successful aging both for the general population and for lesbian and gay populations (Jones & Nystrom, 2002; Kimmel, 1995).

Richard Friend's (1990) study of successful aging among lesbians and gay men found that those who successfully maintain independence are those who have a social structure of friends and family that is closely identified with, or supportive of, the lesbian and gay experience. *This connectedness to others who are like oneself offers an environment that does not need to be defended, explained, or justified and helps to ease the transitional stresses associated with the aging process, which are frequently compounded by outside forces such as worry about income and health* (Friend, 1990). The concept of having a connectedness through commonalities is hypothesized to be essential to healthy and successful aging. Establishing and strengthening the sense of community, or belonging, enables those who are aging to have access to resources needed to maintain a network of support (Amadio, 2005; Anetzberger, Ishler, Mostade, & Blair, 2004). The greater importance of supportive friends and "chosen family" for LGBT older adults, especially lesbians and gay men, has been a consistent finding over time and is reflected in recent studies (MetLife 2006, 2010) and policy documents and reviews (IOM, 2011).

Connections and support are vital to most lesbians. Research indicates that lesbians tend to face growing older with a greater sense of freedom than they experienced in their younger years (Cahill et al., 2000; Jones & Nystrom, 2002). Lesbians often report a strong sense of fulfillment in old age. This is built on a broad foundation of diverse circles of friends and families (Jones & Nystrom, 2002). Research indicates that lesbians tend to build these friendship bases more readily than gay men (Cahill et al., 2000), although both lesbians and gay men place great importance on friendships as they age (MetLife, 2010). In one recent survey (MetLife, 2010) of LGBT adults born during the baby boom years (1946–1964), lesbians were more likely than gay men, or men and women who identified as bisexual or transgender, to be open about their sexual orientation ("completely" or "mostly" out), to report that their families were "completely" or "very" accepting of their identity, and to characterize their LGBT identity as "strongly" or "somewhat" important to how they think of themselves. These findings support the belief that older lesbians, as a group, are making the connections that they need for healthy aging. However, little research has addressed the conditions, status, and adjustment difficulties old lesbians may face if they do not experience this sense of community or a network of support.

BIOLOGICAL, PSYCHOLOGICAL, AND SOCIAL CONCERNS FOR AGING LESBIANS

Lesbians often have more in common with heterosexual women, biologically, psychologically, and socially, than they do with gay-identified men (Gabbay & Wahler, 2002). In other words, lesbians may have a political identification with the civil rights quest based on sexual orientation but may indeed more closely identify with their heterosexual and bisexual female peers in society, reflecting that the commonality based on gender is stronger than the political connection based on sexual orientation (Clunis, Fredriksen-Goldsen, Freeman, & Nystrom, 2005; Gabbay & Wahler, 2002). Although this statement may seem disconcerting, particularly for those who seek to build political coalitions, it simply means that gender can be a greater factor than sexual orientation when examining many important issues that affect older women and all women (Gabbay & Wahler, 2002).

For aging and old lesbians, these perceptions are likely a direct result of the ageism manifest within American society, as well as within the LGBT communities (Healy, 1994). Mainstream American culture focuses on youth, emphasizing staying young—appearing young and physically fit regardless of age. The prevailing view of older persons is stereotypic and usually negative. Within the LGBT communities, this focus on youth is replicated, with most efforts and activities focused on events that will attract younger members of these communities. Aging and old lesbians often report that they are not included in most activities and social events within the larger lesbian community (Cahill et al., 2000; Jones & Nystrom, 2002). The closer ties between old lesbians and their heterosexual and bisexual women peers, whose experience of aging is similar in many ways, may be an unintended consequence of ageism and exclusion by the larger communities, both the general society and the greater community of LGBT people.

BIOLOGICAL ASPECTS OF AGING

Aging lesbians generally report having a good overall sense of well-being, with their priorities centering on their ability to maintain their independence, their health, and their sense of "place" (Gabbay & Wahler, 2002; Jones & Nystrom, 2002). The qualitative study of aging and old lesbians conducted by Clunis et al. (2005) addressed demographic factors and current social, physical, emotional, and financial concerns. Participants were recruited through mailings to organizations, articles in lesbian and gay community newspapers, and snowball sampling, which entails asking current research participants for names of others who might fit the study criteria. Qualitative methods were employed because these techniques were in concert with the research team's underlying philosophy. The women's life stories were paramount. Therefore, research methods emphasized participants' perspectives and allowed those perspectives to emerge within the context of interactions between interviewer and participant (Seidman, 1991). Team members conducted tape-recorded, semistructured interviews with 62 older lesbians living in three western states. Questions to which the women responded included:

1. What do the words "coming out" mean to you?
2. When I say "your family," what does that mean to you?
3. What are your anticipations about getting older?
4. Compared to others, how do you rate your physical health?

The findings of Clunis et al. (2005) were consistent with previous research. Most lesbians reported that they have strong social networks and friendship circles, that their identity is strong, and that their main concerns are primarily centered on the potential loss of physical ability, the loss of independence, the lack of money to survive old age, and the potential loss of mental faculties (Almvig, 1982; Bradford & Ryan, 1991; Claes & Moore, 2000; Jones & Nystrom, 2002; Kehoe, 1986b; MetLife, 2006, 2010).

In another study conducted in 2002 by the advocacy organization Old Lesbians Organizing for Change (OLOC), elder lesbians were asked about their perceptions of growing older and the current status of their health. The 62 participants were all older than age 60 years. These women were asked how they perceived their overall physical health on a scale of 1 to 4, with 1 representing excellent and 4 representing poor. Of the 62 respondents, 88.5% ($n=54$) reported their physical health as good or excellent. Only 7 of the women reported their health as fair.

None of the respondents indicated that they were in poor health. When asked about their perceptions of their mental health status, using the same Likert scale of 1 to 4, 95% ($n = 58$) of the respondents indicated that their overall mental health was good or excellent. Only 3 of the women indicated that their mental health was fair. None of the respondents reported their mental health status as poor. Although aging and old lesbians who are in poor health are the least likely to become participants in research studies, the OLOC findings support the belief that many healthy and vibrant older lesbians are living in the community, although they may not form a highly visible political or demographic group.

Later years are usually a time of emerging physical illnesses, regardless of the gender or identity of the individual. Health problems that confront many aging women, including old lesbians, include hypertension, heart disease, arthritis, osteoporosis, cancer, and other illnesses associated with aging (IOM, 2011). These and other health difficulties generally require medical care. In addition, a variety of programs and services such as Seattle's Lesbian Cancer Project and the National Black Women's Health Project (www.nationalblackwomenshealthproject .org) have been developed to help women maintain better health and access support from other women facing similar life and health concerns (O'Hanlan, Dibble, Hagan, & Davids, 2004).

HEALTH RISKS AND OLD LESBIANS

Neither identifying as a lesbian nor living as a lesbian *causes* the development of any known illness or disability. Rather, younger women who have sex exclusively, or nearly exclusively, with women experience the health benefits of much lower rates of unwanted pregnancy, HIV and other sexually transmissible infections, relative to their heterosexually active women peers. The beneficial consequences of these earlier life experiences also positively influence the health of aging and old lesbians. However, older lesbians may face risks to their health because of other lifestyle-related physiologic factors (O'Hanlan et al., 2004) and of lack of preparation for managing lesbian health concerns on the part of medical and nursing professionals (IOM, 2011).

Lesbians are less likely than their heterosexually identified peers to be underweight and are more likely to be overweight or obese (Conron, Mimiaga, & Landers, 2010). Although this finding probably reflects a relative immunity to media and other societal messages, which exaggerate the value of bodily thinness, and are damaging to women's self-esteem, being overweight has been associated with a higher risk, in the middle and older years, of developing type 2 diabetes, hypertension, coronary artery disease, arthritis, and certain cancers—and a lower risk of developing osteoporosis (Case et al., 2004; O'Hanlan et al., 2004).

Although many lesbians are mothers, lesbians as a group are less likely to have borne children, or to have used oral contraceptives, than their heterosexually identified peers. Because pregnancy and oral contraceptive use lower the relative risk of developing malignancies of the ovary and endometrium (uterine lining), lesbians as a group experience a higher risk of developing these cancers, although old lesbians who have borne children or used oral contraceptives earlier in their lives do not (Case et al., 2004; O'Hanlan et al., 2004). However, data are somewhat conflicting; the IOM report (2011, p. 6-24) notes that "it appears that rates of hysterectomy, oral contraceptive use, and hormone replacement therapy may be similar for lesbians, bisexual women, and heterosexual women."

Lesbians are also more likely to smoke than are heterosexually identified women (Conron et al., 2010; IOM, 2011). Therefore, illnesses that are caused or worsened by smoking, such as lung cancer, emphysema, hypertension, and coronary artery disease, may be more common among older lesbians than among their heterosexually identified peers. However, many old lesbians have never smoked or have quit smoking in the distant past and therefore do not experience high rates of lung disease (Case et al., 2004; O'Hanlan et al., 2004). Heart disease is common among older persons in all demographic groups but is more common among smokers. The IOM report (2011, p. 6-24) recognizes the need for more data, stating that "data on whether lesbians have a higher risk for cardiovascular disease are conflicting."

Lesbians are also more likely to overuse alcohol than are heterosexually identified women (Conron et al., 2010; IOM, 2011), perhaps because of the combination of discrimination and stigma-related emotional stress and the use of bars as a means of meeting potential partners. As with the aforementioned illnesses, alcohol-related risks should be assessed individually, rather than using lesbian identity as a proxy for any particular health risk or disease state (Case et al., 2004; O'Hanlan et al., 2004).

O'Hanlan et al. (2004) also report that misperceptions about the lives of lesbians by physicians and other health care professionals may lead to diagnostic delays and treatment complications. For example, cervical cancer is most often caused by cellular damage from certain strains of the human papillomavirus (HPV), which are usually acquired sexually (American College of Obstetrics and Gynecology, www.acog.org). Male-to-female transmission occurs much more frequently than female-to-female. Therefore, women who have never had sexual intercourse with a male partner are at lower risk for this disease, although transmission can occur in lesbian sex, particularly if sex toys are shared. Also, many young women—and some who are not young—have sex with male partners before coming out as lesbians, or possibly after coming out, and may acquire HPV infection in these sexual relationships.

Rates of cervical cancer have fallen dramatically since the introduction of the Papanicolou (Pap) test, a relatively painless sampling of cervical cells, which are then examined microscopically for signs of precancerous change. However, lesbians sometimes receive Pap testing less frequently than heterosexual women because health care providers may mistakenly believe that their lesbian patients have never had sex with men and are therefore not at risk (Bonvicini & Perlin, 2002; Marrazzo, 2004; O'Hanlan et al., 2004), or because they seek care less frequently because of discomfort with health care settings or lack of medical insurance. Also, Pap testing is recommended during prenatal care and medical visits for contraception—health services some lesbian women may not need. This can lead to lack of preventive treatment (i.e., following patients with HPV-related cellular changes closely to be sure that the cervical tissue normalizes and ablating the surface cells if they do not) and diagnostic delay in cases in which cervical cancer develops (Bonvicini & Perlin, 2002; Marrazzo, 2004; O'Hanlan et al., 2004).

Cervical cancer is most commonly diagnosed between ages 40 and 59 years but can occur at any adult age (American Cancer Society, 2007). Older lesbians may become exposed to HPV when they begin new sexual relationships involving exposure of the cervix to partner bodily fluids, particularly semen, and should receive cervical cancer screening based on individual risk assessment and gynecologic history.

Some improvement in cervical cancer screening in the lesbian population may be occurring. In aggregated data from the 2001–2008 Massachusetts Behavioral Risk Factor Surveillance surveys ($n = 67,359$), Conron et al. (2010) found no difference in likelihood of having received Pap testing within the last 3 years among lesbian, bisexual, and heterosexually identified women aged 40 and older, though in a previous analysis using pooled data from seven studies conducted in 1987–1996 ($n = 11,896$, approx.), lesbian and bisexual women (data combined for these groups) had been less likely than national norms to have had a pelvic examination within the last 5 years (Cochran et al., 2001). However, Cochran et al. noted that this difference may have been partially explained by lower rates of insurance coverage.

Rates of cervical cancer are expected to further decrease in coming decades, as vaccination against the strains of HPV that most frequently cause cervical cancer becomes more widespread. In the United States, vaccination is currently recommended for adolescent girls, and has been found to be effective for females and males aged 9–26 years (www.cdc.gov/vaccines). Young women who identify early as lesbians should receive vaccination against these strains of HPV, even if they do not plan to have sex with men. It is to be hoped that cervical cancer eventually will be eliminated through vaccination; however, the current cohort of older women did not have the benefit of vaccination and must rely on early detection of cervical dysplasia through Pap testing to prevent cervical cancer.

Older lesbians can also experience difficulty in obtaining adequate health care services because of social and interpersonal factors. These include a lack of access to medical professionals who are openly welcoming of LGBT patients, fear of receiving discriminatory health services, uncertainty regarding whether to reveal their sexual orientation, and difficulty developing trust in medical and nursing providers and the available health care systems, in light of past negative experiences (Gabbay and Wahler, 2002; O'Hanlan et al., 2004). The IOM report (2011, p. 5-38) notes that "very little research has been done on health outcomes resulting from LGBT people's lack of access to and utilization of health care services . . . [and on] the quality of care experienced by sexual and gender minorities." Additional health services research, "particularly related to identity disclosure and interactions with providers" is recommended (p. 5-39).

Research indicates that lesbians often do not seek health care services or do not disclose their sexual orientation during visits to medical professionals because they fear discrimination (Boehmer & Case, 2004). Reasons for these findings include fear of homophobia, being single (and therefore without partner support), and the belief that sexual orientation is a private matter and not relevant to the health concern that prompted the medical visit (Boehmer & Case, 2004). Lesbians who have partners often prefer to bring their partners with them to medical visits in cases of serious illness. Having a partner present can make the decision to reveal one's sexual orientation much easier. The importance of this lesbian family structure is a significant factor in lesbians' reports about their feelings about medical care and disclosure. Despite the importance of these relationships, many health professionals do not acknowledge the partner's role in their patient's recovery and well-being (Bonvicini & Perlin, 2002). New federal regulations, however, require hospitals that receive funds through the Medicare and Medicaid programs to prohibit discrimination in visitation based on sexual orientation. These regulations have been in effect only since January 2011 and have likely not yet had much influence on older lesbians' experiences in health care settings (www.hrc.org/resources/entry/map-of-state-laws-policies).

Because health care professionals often do not ask about sexual orientation and may have received little education regarding lesbian health concerns, lesbian patients must decide whether to make their sexual orientation known and how to obtain the best care (Bonvicini & Perlin, 2002). Although research shows that the incidence of overt homophobia in health care settings is now low, many lesbians report receiving neutral responses from their doctors regarding the disclosure of their sexual orientation. These neutral responses are perceived as more negative than affirming (Boehmer & Case, 2004). Considering the emotional investment required to disclose one's sexual orientation, most older lesbians would appreciate receiving a more definitely welcoming response from their health professionals. Interestingly, when asked about the strengths and challenges of being LGBT identified, 17% of lesbian respondents in one major study (MetLife, 2010) named feeling vulnerable with health care providers as a "difficulty," as did 19% of gay men, 18% of bisexual men and women, and 36% of transgender respondents (p. 27). Although no older adult should have to feel vulnerable when seeking physical or mental health care, these results suggest a relatively high degree of self-confidence on the part of these older lesbians and other LGBT adults.

SOCIAL AND PSYCHOLOGICAL ASPECTS OF AGING

Older lesbians, as a group, report a positive sense of well-being and good health, including good mental health (Clunis et al., 2005; Horwitz, Weis, & Laflin, 2003; IOM, 2011; Jones & Nystrom, 2002). Nonetheless, aging and old lesbians may experience greater emotional stress than their female heterosexual counterparts. Being female, lesbian, and old presents opportunities and challenges. Stigma and discrimination faced by old lesbians are stressors that can have negative effects on these women's psychological well-being (Adelman, 1990; Herek & Garnets, 2007; Meyer, 2003), and the memory of more virulent oppression from earlier in their lives can continue to affect current quality of life.

Being lesbian in contemporary culture brings difficulties that each lesbian woman must address. Regardless of the age or period of life during which sexual orientation is acknowledged, coming out can often lead to emotional distress. Being "out" and making decisions about when to "pass" (as a presumed heterosexual) can add stress to daily living. Fear of rejection, particularly by friends and family, is often experienced. When difficulties arise, useful social services may be absent or difficult to locate, particularly in smaller communities (Adelman, 1990; Donahue & McDonald, 2005; Grossman, D'Augelli, & Hershberger, 2000; Jones & Nystrom, 2002). The conclusion that their heterosexual loved ones, including friends and family, can never fully understand the realities of lesbian life and identity adds to the potential for depression, isolation, or anger that lesbians sometimes experience (O'Hanlan et al., 2004).

Research indicates that those who are able to come to terms with the stigma associated with being lesbian or gay during their younger years often report a stronger ability to manage the challenges of aging later on (Adelman, 1990; Woolf, 2002). Resilience is often linked to the presence of social networks and a strong sense of self and self-identification, all of which contribute to a positive aging experience (Adelman, 1990; Friend, 1990; MetLife, 2010). Recent research has indicated that several specific themes contribute to a successful aging experience for lesbians (Jones & Nystrom, 2002). Feeling the freedom to come out to friends and family; having a sense of pride and accomplishment, primarily at work; creating supportive social networks; having a strong sense of self; and having satisfying family and relationship experiences are major indicators of successful aging for lesbians (Jones & Nystrom, 2002).

The era in which they grew up (e.g., the 1940s vs. the 1960s), and the social events in which they participated, affected when and how older lesbians were able to manage the coming out process (Clunis et al., 2005; Jones & Nystrom, 2002). Older lesbians who came out early in life, at least to themselves, often indicate that, over time, they have resolved many of the effects of the stigmatization and alienation related to their sexual orientation. Consequently, by the time they reach old age, these lesbians have developed skills that enable them to weather the stigmas associated with aging and with identity stress (Adelman, 1990; Berger, 1982; MetLife, 2010). Learning to cope with these difficulties at an early age offers opportunities to develop resilience and lesbian social networks, which may prove useful in later years.

Vignette 2: Coming Out

Diane is 72 years old. She works for the county government in the small, rural town where she lives. She knew she was different than most girls when she was about 10 years of age but did not "figure it all out" until her last year of high school. It was then that she realized that she did not understand dating and boyfriends in the same way that her girlfriends did. Even so, she continued dating and looking for the "right guy." After high school, Diane met and fell in love with another woman and immediately realized that she was a lesbian. This relationship did not last long. Because the thought of being lesbian frightened her, she redoubled her efforts, over the next few years, to succeed in the world of heterosexual relationships.

Soon after graduating from college, Diane married a longtime acquaintance from her town. She had three children, but she knew throughout her marriage that she was not happy. She began drinking and became addicted to alcohol. After 12 years of marriage, her internal conflicts began to take their toll. Her husband threatened to divorce her. After a long series of conversations, she finally told her husband that she believed she was a lesbian. For the sake of their children, the two of them decided to stay together and make the best of the situation. However, the increased tension in their relationship further worsened her alcoholism. When the children were grown, Diane and her husband divorced. Diane was finally able to live more openly as a lesbian. With this new life, Diane entered an addiction recovery program, got a full-time job, and began dating other women. She feels now that she is much healthier—and much more empowered—than in her earlier years.

Repressing or denying one's sexual orientation and giving in to traditional societal pressures was a common occurrence for many lesbians who are now old. The keys to successful aging are support and the confidence to be true to oneself and to live a genuine life.

Lesbians who report pride in their accomplishments at work and in community involvements have often developed a strong sense of self-esteem that contributes to successful aging (Clunis et al., 2005; Jones & Nystrom, 2002). This fosters confidence in their personal decision making and in their development of social support networks that may include lesbian and straight friends, family members, and work colleagues (Jones & Nystrom, 2002).

Developing strong social support networks is important to the well-being of all aging adults, but it is particularly valued by aging lesbians. Many lesbians who have participated in research studies indicate that their connection to social and friendship groups is especially important to them. These groups provide stable social environments, a sense of belonging, the opportunity to participate in group activities, and potential sources of mutual aid (Clunis et al., 2005; IOM, 2011; Jacobs, Rasmussen, & Hohman, 1999; Jones & Nystrom, 2002; MetLife, 2010; Woolf, 2002).

The definition of family among older lesbians is an important area of study. In the Jones and Nystrom (2002) study of old lesbians, all but one participant indicated that their definition of family is broader than that of the general society, which is primarily based on biological relationships (Clunis et al., 2005; Jones & Nystrom, 2002). Most reported that their family includes the partner, friends, social contacts, and biological family members. Although children were often primary, equal weight was often given to significant relationships with partners and supportive friends. This inclusive definition of family gave these women a sense of belonging and trust, built over time by developing these critical social networks (Jones & Nystrom, 2002).

This sense of belonging, which Friend (1991) has termed *connectedness*, has emerged as a factor in successful aging among lesbians. Many aging lesbians do not exclusively depend on biological family members for support. Instead, they garner emotional warmth and practical assistance from friendship networks (Jones & Nystrom, 2002; Woolf, 2002). This may be a primary factor in successful aging, as these "families of choice" are tailored to the particular needs of the individual (Friend, 1991). The strength and cohesion of these networks reflect the definition of family usually described by older lesbians (Clunis et al., 2005; Jones & Nystrom, 2002).

Most research regarding the lives of aging lesbians has focused on women who are visible members of a lesbian community and who are generally open about their lesbian lives. Lesbians who are more secretive about their sexual orientation, who have not stayed involved in an identifiable community, who have "returned to the closet," or blended into the mainstream culture are generally not represented in existing literature. There is currently a strong need for research behalf of lesbians who are not members of stable social networks, who may be uncomfortable with their sexual orientation, or who lack self-esteem or personal effectiveness, which are necessary for taking a visible role in society (Cruikshank, 1991; Faderman, 1996).

Much of the research of the 1980s and 1990s focused on identity adjustment and mental health, from the perspective of identifying emotional pathology (Adelman, 1990; Berger, 1986; Dorfman et al., 1995; Fredriksen-Goldsen & Muraco, 2010). This research illuminated the consequences of experiencing chronic stress brought about by overt legal and social discrimination, as well as the consequences of the absence of the protective factors described above. These include an increased risk of depression and an increased prevalence of substance abuse and alcohol dependence. In some studies, as many as one-fourth of aging and old lesbian participants have indicated that they were in recovery from alcoholism or other substance use disorders (Jones & Nystrom, 2002). Although depression, anxiety, and substance abuse remain significant concerns in lesbian (and LGBT) health, recent work has also focused on the psychological resiliency of lesbians and other sexual and gender minority persons (Fredriksen-Goldsen & Muraco, 2010; IOM, 2011; MetLife, 2010).

Vignette 3: Substance Abuse and Recovery

Mary has been in recovery for six years after a long history of alcoholism. She is now 62 and feels that she must start taking care of herself to stay healthy in her later years. Because her recovery is important to her, she maintains strict personal guidelines. All of the people in her social support system and her friendship circle support her recovery. Although she has found a solid support network, she feels that she cannot participate in most lesbian social activities because of the emphasis on alcohol, especially because most social activities are located in what she terms "the gay ghetto" (i.e., the bars).

Mary has formed a group of lesbians 50 years of age and older, most of whom are also in recovery. They participate in healthier activities such as camping trips, book club meetings at the local community center, potluck dinners, and trips to plays and other events. The women in the group frequently express their gratitude for the support and friendship they share and for the alcohol-free environment critical to their recovery.

Creating support systems to meet individual needs is important for the physical and emotional well-being of older people. Aging and old lesbians often emphasize these networks more than do members of other demographic groups. Chosen and biological family, friends, and informal or organized lesbian support groups can be the foundation for meaningful primary support systems.

Lesbians who come out later in life often find this process somewhat more difficult than younger lesbians usually do. Building systems that will give them balance and support requires a significant investment of personal energy. Managing the specific stresses of aging also requires ongoing effort. For aging lesbians who are experiencing both of these demands simultaneously, achieving success in the aging process can be challenging. However, despite these difficulties, and with strong support systems in place, lesbians may indeed be more resilient than many other demographic groups.

Many older lesbians did not acknowledge their lesbian sexual orientation until fairly late in life, often after children were raised or after retirement (Clunis et al., 2005; Jones & Nystrom, 2002). Social norms and restrictions of the times dictated that women marry and raise children, particularly those who reached young adulthood during the 1950s (Kochman, 1997). More than half of lesbians in the Jones and Nystrom (2002) study indicated that they did not identify as lesbians, even privately, until after their children reached adulthood. As society became less restrictive with regard to sexual and social behavior, these women felt free to live more authentically, even if it meant extensive changes in many aspects of their lives (Clunis et al., 2005; Jones & Nystrom, 2002).

Women who acknowledged their sexual orientation during the 1950s and 1960s often experienced the additional stressors of societal discrimination and police harassment. Although they may have experienced a greater sense of personal freedom, their lesbian social contacts were limited to tightly woven social circles, often referred to as *friendship circles* (Kochman, 1997). Today's older lesbians have reported the historical experiences of losing custody of children, being fired from jobs, being rejected by biological families, being declared deviant or mentally ill, being involuntarily hospitalized or medicated, and even being threatened with lobotomy surgery (Clunis et al., 2005; Nystrom, 1997).

Until 1973, the mental health professions reinforced these fears by diagnosing gay men and lesbians as deviant or mentally ill, thereby providing a "psychological" or "medical" basis for social repression. In 1973, the Assembly of the American Psychiatric Association voted to remove homosexuality from the list of mental disorders codified in its *Diagnostic and Statistical Manual of Mental Disorders*, which set the stage for the appropriate treatment of lesbian, gay, and bisexual persons who were suffering from bona fide emotional difficulties. Although subsequent change in mental health practice has been gradual, many younger lesbians and gay men who suffer from depression and anxiety now report satisfactory treatment with mental health professionals, and their experiences in older age may improve as a result. However, for contemporary aging and old lesbians, trusting mental health professionals is often difficult.

Most women who are currently in late middle age or among the "young old" grew up during the 1940s and 1950s, when attempts to "cure" lesbians and gay men through psychoanalysis or hospitalization were customary (Kochman, 1997). Many have reported that, when they were younger, their families sent them to psychologists, psychiatrists, or hospitals to be "cured" of their lesbianism. The candor of these women in reporting these traumatic experiences has made it possible to record the lesbian history of events that took place before the modern lesbian rights movement.

Despite the challenges older lesbians have faced, most report an overall sense of good mental health. However, these positive findings do not negate the need for appropriate mental health and supportive services that older lesbians can turn to when needed (Boxer, 1997). There is currently a paucity of such services available to most aging lesbians (Boxer, 1997; Claes & Moore, 2000; IOM, 2011;

O'Hanlan et al., 2004). Examples of services that could be created or made available are grief and loss support groups; counseling, financial, and legal assistance; and coming-out groups for older lesbians.

Most physical and mental health service systems also do not adequately address the concerns of lesbians or members of other sexual and gender minorities, even when appropriate interventions would be straightforward and inexpensive (Cahill et al., 2000). Simple solutions include adding sexual orientation as a checkbox choice when asking for relationship information, posting information relevant to lesbians on bulletin boards, and encouraging allied health providers to contact lesbian organizations about their ability to offer advice regarding service provision (Cahill et al., 2000).

SOCIOECONOMIC CONCERNS OF AGING AND OLD LESBIANS

A common stereotype regarding gay men and lesbians is that they are financially well off or wealthy. This myth has been perpetuated both by those who oppose granting civil rights to lesbian- and gay-identified persons, and those within lesbian and gay communities who seek to profit from merchandizing within these groups (Cahill et al., 2000). Those who support the continued marginalization of lesbian and gay people use the image of an active and wealthy lesbian and gay community to perpetuate the belief among the general society that these individuals are not discriminated against and, therefore, do not need protection from bigotry. Often, these political groups obtain their information from advertisements aimed at lesbians and gay men. Companies that publish commercial magazines, offer travel opportunities, or seek to sell lesbian- and gay-identified persons specific goods and services all promote an image focused on leisure, travel, and wealth. These marketing strategies are also employed in the heterosexual marketplace, in which retired persons are often portrayed as wealthy and at leisure (Cahill et al., 2000).

For aging lesbians, the consequences of these misperceptions are severe, especially when the general society does not respond to existing data about the higher rates of poverty experienced by women as they age. Because of the scarcity of research focusing on aging and old lesbians, most data are extrapolated from small samples or from mathematical averages gleaned from general population data. Most data regarding older lesbians indicate annual incomes similar to those of aging women in general. The poverty rate of the older American female population is 13%. The poverty rate for aging and old lesbian women is likely similar. Yet with the image of a well-off community, the reality of lesbians experiencing financial difficulties is often unrecognized (Cahill et al., 2000; Jones & Nystrom, 2002).

The American Association of Retired Persons reports that 40% of all those older than age 65 years live on annual incomes less than 200% of the poverty level (Cahill et al., 2000; Hooyman & Kiyak, 2004). The National Gay and Lesbian Task Force Policy Institute reports that the poverty rates for aging and older gay men are likely higher than for heterosexual men. However, this comparative relationship does not seem to exist between old lesbians and their female heterosexual counterparts, most likely because of the older women's generally higher poverty rate (Cahill et al., 2000). This higher level of poverty can be attributed to several factors; the most prevalent is lower wages earned by women relative to men. Other factors include more breaks in work history due to raising children, fewer available higher-level job positions for women, and lower educational opportunities and attainment. For lesbians, additional factors include exclusion from receiving their partners' Social Security and pension benefits and a greater likelihood of lesbians living alone when older (Kohn, 1999; Liu, 1999). Since 2006, the federal Pension Protection Act (http://aging.senate.gov/crs/pension9 .pdf) has provided some assistance in accessing partner pension survivor benefits to same gender couples. Social Security benefits, however, remain inaccessible to surviving same gender partners. If enacted, the Respect for Marriage Act would make federal benefits, such as spousal Social Security benefits, available to same-sex couples who are legally married, but its future remains uncertain.

A major factor in preventing the fall into poverty is maintaining good health and adequate health care covered by medical insurance. Lack of health insurance is a major societal problem that affects the aging and old lesbian community as well as members of other demographic groups. The National Lesbian Health Care Survey reports that 27% of lesbians between ages 40 and 60 years have no health insurance (Bradford & Ryan, 1991), and many are still uninsured or underinsured, particularly with regard to long-term care (MetLife, 2010). This survey also found that 16% of lesbian respondents indicated that they could not afford any health care (Bradford & Ryan, 1991). As is true for women and men in general, lack of affordable health care directly contributes to an increase in poverty levels. As the percentage of all Americans without health insurance increases, a further increase in poverty rates among aging and old lesbians is likely (Bradford & Ryan, 1991). Although health finance reform efforts are under way at the time of this writing, the success of these policies, and their impact on older adults, remains to be determined.

Older lesbians may be more likely to live alone than older gay men or heterosexual women (Cahill et al., 2000). In a study conducted by Senior Aging in a Gay Environment (SAGE) in New York City, lesbians older than age 65 years were twice as likely as their gay male peers to live alone (42% vs. 21%). The primary contributing factor is women's longer life spans. In the SAGE study, fewer than 20% of the lesbian and gay elders living in the city had partners. By comparison, in the Jones and Nystrom (2002) study, 39% ($n = 24$) of lesbians studied lived alone, while 51% ($n = 31$) lived with a partner.

Vignette 4: Living Arrangements

Vera is 83 years old and has lived alone since her last long-term relationship ended more than 20 years ago. She has been active in the civil rights and lesbian rights movements for many years. She has two grown children and several grandchildren, all of whom have good relationships with her. She is independent and believes that this is what keeps her healthy. Living alone feels good to her, as it gives her personal freedom and allows her to travel and to socialize as she wants to.

Long ago, she had an attorney document her decisions regarding her care, should she be unable to communicate her wishes to care providers in later life. She has a long-term care plan in place and has insurance to cover her costs. She believes that having taken care of these things in her middle age was the best thing to do because she does not have to worry about these things now. There are times when she feels frustrated by the lack of social supports within her local community, but she appreciates her strong support network of caring friends and family.

Community-based supports for older lesbians, such as social and educational groups and health and financial services, can be valuable resources. However, personal health and well-being can be enhanced through developing strong personal support systems, making and documenting decisions regarding end-of-life care, and maintaining control over important life decisions.

Despite high numbers of lesbians living alone, most consistently report having an active life and a healthy adjustment to old age. Overall, studies indicate that most older lesbians report a high level of satisfaction with their lives, whether they live alone or with a partner. These reports are consistent with their descriptions of having strong social networks. Many research participants have reported that they associate primarily with other lesbians, some to the virtual exclusion of gay and straight men. Participation in nongay community groups, such as churches and Twelve Step programs, has also been frequently mentioned as a source of social support and connection (Clunis et al., 2005; Jones & Nystrom, 2002).

Although many older lesbians participate in lesbian and gay community events, most report that the LGBT civil rights movement has positively affected the lives of younger lesbians and gay men but only had minimal impact on their own lives. Despite this, they continue to be active in the LGBT community, staying informed on issues, attending rallies and workshops, and volunteering for local lesbian and gay organizations (Clunis et al., 2005; Jones & Nystrom, 2002).

AGEISM, DISCRIMINATION, AND LEGAL CONSIDERATIONS

Discrimination against the LGBT communities is well documented and affects LGBT people throughout the nation. Discrimination occurs in housing, health care, employment, service delivery, pension exclusions, credit applications, and law enforcement response, as well as many other important areas of life. Although several states and municipal governments have adopted antidiscrimination policies (www.hrc.org/about_us/state_laws.asp), these changes are not uniform. Most were enacted to create at least some equality in the workplace or in housing. However, without more comprehensive antidiscrimination policies, many serious problems facing members of sexual and gender minorities remain unresolved (van der Meide, 2000).

Discrimination regarding legal recognition of partnered relationships often deeply affects lesbians as they grow older, particularly when one partner becomes ill or dies. When treating persons with serious or terminal illness, health care providers often defer to biological relatives—the "next of kin"—instead of the partner, as the partner may have no legal standing in that environment. New federal regulations were enacted in January 2011 that prohibit hospitals participating in Medicare and Medicaid programs from discrimination in visitation based on sexual orientation and gender identity, but many other aspects of equality in illness and terminal care remain unaddressed. If the ill member of the relationship has verbalized her wishes about end-of-life care only to her partner, medical providers may not honor those plans, because of significant liability concerns.

When an old lesbian dies, the partner may be prohibited from participating in decision making regarding funeral or memorial services or the disposition of the estate. Without formal recognition of the relationship, the partner is left without any legal standing. This can particularly affect disposition of property holdings that, even if bought with shared resources, will not revert to the surviving partner unless advance legal documentation has been obtained (van der Meide, 2000).

All aging and old lesbians must prepare legal documentation to prevent these forms of exclusion. Currently, many old lesbians report that they have powers of attorney and wills in place to ensure that their partners are protected and that their estates are handled according to their wishes, but some do not (Jones & Nystrom, 2002; O'Hanlan et al., 2004).

Societal refusal to legally recognize lesbian partnerships often denies these women equal access to their partners' retirement benefits, such as pensions and Social Security—access that is routinely granted to married heterosexual couples (Human Rights Campaign, 2006; van der Meide, 2000). Legal relationship status and provision for partner benefits would ease the financial burden experienced by aging and old lesbians at their most vulnerable time in life. The federal Pension Protection Act of 2006 provides some ability for lesbians and gay men to leave their retirement savings to their partners, who can then inherit as "nonspouse beneficiaries," an important first step on the road to financial equality, although many more steps are needed. The ability to participate in a partner's health insurance plan would also reduce financial distress created by high costs of health care, including prescription medications, which consume a significant portion of elderly persons' incomes and which are expected to rise (Cahill et al., 2000). Six states and the District of Columbia currently (in 2011) allow same-gender couples to marry, and an additional ten states offer lesser forms of relationship recognition, or legal recognition of same gender marriages entered into in other states, and two have passed statutes that will go into effect in 2012. Marriages recognized at the state level, however, do not allow same gender couples access to marriage benefits of federal programs, such as Social Security and veterans' family services.

Discrimination in employment is common and has been documented repeatedly. Although many discriminatory acts are perceived as occurring on the basis of gender rather than sexual orientation, study participants also report discrimination perpetrated because they were lesbian (Cahill et al., 2000; Jones & Nystrom, 2002; van der Meide, 2000). Discrimination and oppression outside of the workplace have frequently been reported, particularly when lesbians seek employment or at employer-sponsored social events. For example, when employers sponsor holiday parties to which families are invited, lesbian employees may be made to feel uncomfortable about bringing their partners. They may also choose not to attend the event for fear of ostracism by co-workers.

In addition to these heterosexist practices, old lesbians are also affected by ageism within the LGBT communities. *Ageism* is defined as the systemic exclusion of or discrimination against people because of their age. Within the LGBT communities, ageism is prevalent, a problem that aging and old lesbians perceive as affecting them, although their younger peers often do not recognize it. OLOC, SAGE, and other advocacy groups have been confronting ageism within the LGBT communities since the late 1980s. Over the years, the founders of OLOC have helped to bring about greater visibility for older lesbians and have improved understanding of the extent of ageism within the LGBT communities. OLOC members attend community conferences, organize old lesbians, and lobby national LGBT groups to draw attention to ageism and to address its practical consequences (Cahill et al., 2000).

Ageism within LGBT communities is demonstrated by the exclusion of older people from community planning and decision making, lack of outreach to older individuals, and a failure to acknowledge contributions of older members of these communities (Healy, 1993). Few organizations sponsor events that attract older persons, particularly aging and old lesbians. While the general society has begun to reach out to elderly persons through the creation of specific events, senior discounts, and product development, the LGBT communities have yet to recognize the potential for growth through including more elderly members (Cahill et al., 2000).

Lesbians recognize that the focus on youth within the LGBT community alienates older women, sometimes overtly, such as through negative humor or ridicule of the old perpetrated by younger members (Healy, 1993). The use of negative stereotypes of older women as weak, feeble, asexual, demented, or frail is common. As OLOC illustrates in their workshops, even such simple things as birthday card messages exploit ageism as humorous, which most shoppers do not think about when they buy them (Healy, 1994; Warren, 2000).

In response to ageism and exclusion, lesbians are creating their own networks and activities. Aging women, especially lesbian women, are forming housing communities, social groups, camping groups, and athletic events specifically tailored to their skills, talents, and interests (Jones & Nystrom, 2002).

RECOMMENDATIONS

The most common concerns among aging and old lesbians include maintaining their housing and financial security, becoming seriously ill, losing the support of partners and friends through death, and ensuring that they and their partners continue to control their own lives (Orel, 2004). Considering the anticipated growth in the population of older adults in the United States, within the next decade, the need for affordable and safe housing is urgent. Affordability is the key for old lesbians to be able to maintain their own homes and their independence. A variety of forms of communal and shared housing are being planned and developed around the country, by and for aging and old lesbians. For these and other lesbian housing initiatives to be successful, attention must be paid to the costs for each woman over time, the accessibility of lesbian-appropriate services, and the authority of residents to determine who will be allowed to join the cooperative housing arrangement (Nystrom, 1997).

Misperceptions about the lives of lesbians, and assumptions of heterosexuality, contribute to the lack of development and delivery of appropriate medical and social services. The limited amount of available research that has focused on these issues has come to similar conclusions: (1) current services are inadequate for addressing the concerns of aging lesbians; and (2) lesbians are aware of the potential for experiencing discrimination in health services and, therefore, may choose not to seek physical and mental health care. Changes in many aspects of the medical and social service systems are critical to the long-term health and well-being of old lesbians. A simple starting point would be to include "Partnered" on intake and information forms that request relationship status. This small change would begin the process of recognizing the existence and legitimacy of lesbian relationships and promoting the inclusion of partners in medical and social service decisions and treatment. Education regarding the LGBT community and its older members, for health professionals such as physicians, nurses, psychologists, social workers, and home care assistants, would be a crucial step in improving these professional relationships.

The creation and maintenance of supportive social networks is important to lesbians as they age. Stable social support networks help older lesbians maintain control of their lives. Studies indicate that many lesbians are interested in living in communities with other older lesbians in which support networks can be developed and sustained (Jones & Nystrom, 2002). These networks can be enhanced in all communities through the development of informal support groups, age-specific lesbian gathering places, information about service providers who welcome lesbians in their practices, free or low-cost legal information centers, and organizations focused on the concerns of aging and old lesbians.

In October 2009, the U.S. Department of Health and Human Services and the Administration on Aging announced plans to fund a resource center to address the needs of LGBT older adults (SAGE, 2011). The National Resource Center on LGBT Aging (lgbtagingcenter.org) is a partnership of service and research organizations and represents progress in governmental awareness of the needs of old lesbians and other older LGBT persons, as well as a potential means for locating services in different parts of the country.

Many aging and old lesbians have had success in their careers and in planning for their retirement. However, poverty among old lesbians is common, especially as they grow into the "oldest of the old" category (Cahill et al., 2000; Hooyman & Kiyak, 2010). Legal recognition of partnerships and the right of inheritance are critically needed to ensure that women who build a life together are not deprived of the benefits of that partnership. Policy changes that would fully include partners in pension and Social Security benefits are also required to ensure a minimum income for all lesbians and members of other sexual and gender minorities, as is currently the case for married heterosexual couples.

Many older lesbians have made provisions to protect the right of inheritance of their partners through wills and living trusts. However, legal costs can be prohibitive, and lesbian partners are usually not eligible for the discounted attorney's fees offered to married couples who are conducting estate planning. Despite these costs, it is imperative for aging and old lesbians to work with qualified estate attorneys to ensure that their property and other assets will be distributed as they intend.

Combating ageism in LGBT and broader communities is a major undertaking. Changing long-ingrained attitudes about older persons will take the concerted efforts of individuals and organizations from a wide spectrum of society, but change in this arena is clearly possible. The first step within the LGBT community is for aging and old lesbians to engage in dialogue about the realities and the impact of ageism and about their own internalization of ageist attitudes. Lesbians must develop a full understanding of the issues related to ageism and use their combined power to demand changes in how the larger LGBT community responds to them. With greater visibility and stronger voices, older lesbians can focus attention on the ways in which ageism damages the LGBT community and society at large.

CONCLUSION

Aging and old lesbians, on the whole, are a highly self-sufficient group of women who have achieved personal and professional success despite numerous obstacles, including discrimination based on gender, sexual orientation, and age. Many convey their belief that hardships and adversity have made them stronger. Through marriages, raising children, attending school, and working, these women made critical decisions, reflecting the social and political times in which they grew up, about whether to reveal their sexual orientation at different times of life.

Although some women live in relatively small social circles, most old lesbians are actively involved in networks that include partners, family, friends, community groups, and religious affiliations. These women express their ardent desire to remain independent and healthy and to continue to maintain their own housing as they age. The possibility of living in lesbian communities appeals to many older lesbians.

Additional research on behalf of aging and old lesbians is strongly needed. Despite the contributions of the existing body of literature, little is known about this population, relative to other older persons. In addition to basic demographic information, further investigation of support structures, stressors, health status, aging processes, and practical needs is critical to understanding the lives of these women and to creating or enhancing appropriate service systems.

Service development is needed, both within the lesbian community and in general society, to meet the requirements of older lesbians. This will require the full inclusion of older lesbians in defining assets and needs, planning, and implementation. All aspects of these processes must be conducted with respect for these women's lives and choices.

Finally, new research and service efforts must focus on aging and old lesbians as viable groups unto themselves. The lesbian and gay community has often been regarded as more homogeneous than it really is. Research and service programs have been designed for members of the communities as a whole. Lesbians, gay men, bisexual women and men, and persons who identify as transgender or intersex share many goals with regard to advocacy and legal and political struggles. However, the perspectives and needs of older members of these groups are often different than those of their younger peers. Also, the needs of older women and older men are usually similar in some ways and not in others. Research and service projects concerning older lesbians should reflect this diversity and be tailored to their specific strengths, needs, and histories. Recognizing the life struggles and triumphs of aging and old lesbians will also enrich the human experience of the LGBTI communities and of contemporary culture as a whole.

REFERENCES

Adelman, M. (1990). Stigma, gay lifestyles, and adjustment to aging: A study of later-life gay men and lesbians. *Journal of Homosexuality*, 20(3/4), 7–32.

Almvig, C. (1982). *The invisible minority: Aging and lesbianism.* (Unpublished master's thesis). Utica College of Syracuse, Syracuse, NY.

Amadio, D. (2005). Internalized heterosexism, alcohol use, and alcohol-related problems among lesbians and gay men. *Addictive Behaviors.* Retrieved from www
.sciencedirect.com.offcampus.lib.washington.edu/science

American Cancer Society. (2007). *Cancer facts and figures 2007.* Retrieved from www
.cancer.org/downloads/STT/CAFF2007PWSecured.pdf

Anetzberger, G. J., Ishler, K., Mostade, J., & Blair, M. (2004). Gray and gay: A community dialogue on the issues and concerns of older gays and lesbians. *Journal of Gay and Lesbian Social Services,* 17(1), 23–41.

Berger, R. M. (1982). The unseen minority: Older gays and lesbians. *Social Work,* 27(3), 236–242.

Berger, R. M. (1984). Realities of gay and lesbian aging. *Social Work,* 29(1), 57–62.

Berger, R. M. (1986). Working with homosexuals of the older population. *Social Casework,* 67(4), 203–210.

Boehmer, U., & Case, P. (2004). Physicians don't ask, sometimes patients tell. *Cancer,* 101(8), 1882–1889.

Bonvicini, K. A., & Perlin, M. J. (2002). The same but different: Clinician-patient communication with gay and lesbian patients. *Patient Education and Counseling,* 51, 115–122.

Boxer, A. M. (1997). Gay, lesbian, and bisexual aging into the twenty-first century: An overview and introduction. *Journal of Gay, Lesbian, and Bisexual Identity,* 1(2), 187–197.

Bradford, J., & Ryan, C. (1991). Who we are: Health concerns of middle aged lesbians. In B. Sang, J. Warshow, & A. Smith (Eds.), *Lesbians at midlife.* San Francisco: Spinsters Book.

Cahill, S., South, K., & Spade, J. (2000). *Outing Age: Public policy issues affecting gay, lesbian, bisexual, transgender elders.* Washington, DC: National Gay and Lesbian Task Force Policy Institute.

Case, P., Austin, S. B., Hunter, D., Manson, J. E., Malspeis, S., Willett, W. C., & Spiegelman, D. (2004). Sexual orientation, health risk factors, and physical functioning in the Nurses' Health Study II. *Journal of Women's Health,* 13(9), 1033–1447.

Claes, J. A., & Moore, W. (2000). Issues confronting lesbian and gay elders: The challenge for health and human service providers. *Journal of Health and Human Services Administration,* 23(2), 181.

Clunis, D. M., Fredriksen-Goldsen, K., Freeman, P., & Nystrom, N. (2005). *Lives of lesbian elders.* New York: Haworth Press.

Cochran, S. D., Mays, V. M., Bowen, D., Gage, S., Bybee, D., Roberts, S. J., . . . White, J. (2001). Cancer-related risk indicators and preventive screening behaviors among lesbians and bisexual women. *American Journal of Public Health,* 91(4), 591–597.

Conron, K. J., Mimiaga, M. J., & Landers, S. J. (2010). A population-based study of sexual orientation identity and gender differences in adult health. *American Journal of Public Health,* 100(10), 1953–1960.

Cruikshank, M. (1991). Lavender and gray: A brief survey of lesbian and gay aging studies. In J. A. Lee (Ed.), *Gay midlife and maturity* (pp. 77–87). New York: Haworth Press.

Donahue, P., & McDonald, L. (2005). Gay and lesbian aging: Current perspectives and future directions for social work practice and research. *Families in Society,* 86(3), 359–366.

Dorfman, R., Walters, K., Burke, P., & Hardin, L. (1995). Old, sad, and alone: The myth of homosexual aging. *Journal of Gerontological Social Work,* 24(1/2), 29–44.

Faderman, L. (1996). Out of sight: Lesbian lifestyles. *The Advocate,* 7(23), 72.

Fassinger, R. E. (1991). The hidden minority: Issues and challenges in working with lesbian women and gay men. *Counseling Psychologist,* 19(2), 157–176.

Fredriksen-Goldsen, K. I., & Muraco, A. (2010). Aging and sexual orientation: A 25-year review of the literature. *Research on Aging,* 32(3), 372–413.

Friend, R. A. (1990). Older lesbian and gay people: A theory of successful aging. *Journal of Homosexuality,* 20(3/4), 99–118.

Gabbay, S., & Wahler, J. (2002). Lesbian aging: Review of a growing literature. *Journal of Gay and Lesbian Social Services,* 14(3), 1–21.

Gartrell, N., Banks, A., Hamilton, J., Reed, N., Bishop, H., & Rodas, C. (1999). The National Lesbian Family Study II: Interviews with mothers of toddlers. *American Journal of Orthopsychiatry,* 69(3), 362–369.

Grossman, A. H., D'Augelli, A. R., & Hershberger, S. L. (2000). Social support networks of lesbian, gay, and bisexual adults 60 years of age and older. *Journal of Gerontology, Series B, Psychological Sciences and Social Sciences,* 55B(3), 171–179.

Gwenwald, M. (1983). The SAGE model for serving older lesbians and gay men. *Homosexuality and Social Work,* 2(2/3), 53–61.

Hamburger, L. J. (1997). The wisdom of non-heterosexually based senior housing and related services. *Journal of Gay and Lesbian Social Services,* 6(1), 11–25.

Hare, J. (1994). Concerns and issues faced by families headed by a lesbian couple. *Families in Society,* 75(1), 27–35.

Harel, Z., McKinney, E. A., & Williams, M. (Eds). (1990). *Black aged: Understanding diversity and service needs.* Newbury Park, CA: Sage.

Healey, S. (1993). Confronting ageism: A must for mental health. *Faces of Women and Aging,* 41–54.

Healey, S. (1994). Diversity with a difference: On being old and lesbian. *Journal of Gay and Lesbian Social Services,* 1(1), 107–117.

Hequembourg, A. L., & Farrell, M. P. (1999). Lesbian motherhood: Negotiating marginal mainstream identities. *Gender and Society,* 13(4), 540–557.

Herdt, G., Beeler, J., & Rawls, T. W. (1997). Life course diversity among older lesbians and gay men: A study in Chicago. *Journal of Gay, Lesbian, and Bisexual Identity,* 2(3/4), 231–246.

Herek, G., & Berill, K. (1992). *Hate crimes: Confronting violence against lesbians and gay men.* Newbury Park, CA: Sage.

Herek, G. M., & Garnets, L. D. (2007). Sexual orientation and mental health. *Annual Review of Clinical Psychology, 3*, 353–375.

Hooyman, N., & Kiyak, A. (2010). *Social gerontology* (9th ed.). Needham Heights, MA: Allyn & Bacon.

Horwitz, S. M., Weis, D. L., & Laflin, M. T. (2003). Bisexuality, quality of life, life-style, and health indicators. *Journal of Bisexuality, 3*, 5–28.

Human Rights Campaign. (2006). *Pension law includes important protections for same-sex couples under federal law.* Retrieved from www.hrc.org/resources/entry/maps-of-state-laws-policies

Hutchinson, E. D. (1999). *Dimensions of human behavior: Person and environment.* Thousand Oaks, CA: Pine Forge Press.

Institute of Medicine. (2011). *The health of lesbian, gay, bisexual, and transgender people: Building a foundation for better understanding* [Prepublication e-copy, uncorrected proofs] (pp. 6–24). Washington, DC: National Academies Press. www.nap.edu/catalog/13128.html

Jacobs, R., Rasmussen, L., & Hohman, M. (1999). The social support needs of older lesbians, gay men, and bisexuals. *Journal of Gay and Lesbian Social Services, 9*(1), 1–30.

Jones, T., & Nystrom, N. (2002). Looking back . . . looking forward: Addressing the lives of lesbians 55 and older. *Journal of Women and Aging, 14*(3/4), 59–76.

Kaufman, S. R. (1994). The social construction of frailty: An anthropological perspective. *Journal of Aging Studies, 8*(1), 45–58.

Kehoe, M. (1986a). Lesbians over 65: A triply invisible minority. *Journal of Homosexuality, 12*(3/4), 139–152.

Kehoe, M. (1986b). A portrait of the older lesbian. *Journal of Homosexuality, 12*(3/4), 157–161.

Kehoe, M. (1988). Lesbians over 60 speak for themselves. *Journal of Homosexuality, 16*(3/4), 3–111.

Kimmel, D. C. (1978). Adult development and aging: A gay perspective. *Journal of Social Issues, 34*(3), 113–130.

Kimmel, D. C. (1992). The families of older gay men and lesbians. *Generations, 16*(3), 37–38.

Kimmel, D. C. (1995). Lesbians and gay men grow old. In L. A. Bond, S. J. Cutler, & A. Grams (Eds.), *Promoting successful and productive aging* (pp. 289–303). Thousand Oaks, CA: Sage.

Kochman, A. (1997). Gay and lesbian elderly: Historical overview and implications for social work practice. *Journal of Gay and Lesbian Social Services, 6*(1), 11–10.

Kohn, S. (1999). *Domestic partnership organizing manual.* New York: Policy Institute of the National Gay and Lesbian Task Force.

Liu, G. (1999). Social Security and the treatment of marriage: Spousal benefits, earnings sharing and the challenge of reform. *Wisconsin Law Review, 1*, 1–64.

Lott-Whitehead, L., & Tully, C. T. (1993). The family lives of lesbian mothers. *Smith College Studies in Social Work, 63*(3), 265–280.

Marrazzo, J. M. (2004). Barriers to infectious disease care among lesbians. *Emerging Infectious Diseases, 10*(11), 1974–1978.

Mays, V. M., Chatters, L. M., Cochran, S. D., & Mackness, J. (1998). African American families in diversity: Gay men and lesbians as participants in family networks. *Journal of Comparative Family Studies, 29*(1), 73–87.

McDougall, G. J. (1993). Therapeutic issues with gay and lesbian elders. *Clinical Gerontologist, 14*(1), 45–57.

MetLife. (2006). *Out and aging: The MetLife Study of Lesbian and Gay Baby Boomers.* Westport, CT: MetLife Mature Market Institute. www.metlife.com/assets/cao/mmi/publications/studies/mmi-out-aging-lesbian-gay-retirment.pdf

MetLife. (2010). *Still out, still aging: The MetLife Study of Lesbian, Gay, Bisexual, and Transgender Baby Boomers.* Westport, CT: MetLife Mature Market Institute. www.metlife.com/assets/cao/mmi/publications/studies/2010/mmi-still-out-still-aging.pdf

Meyer, I. H. (2003). Prejudice, social stress, and mental health in lesbian, gay, and bisexual populations: Conceptual issues and research evidence. *Psychological Bulletin, 129*(5), 674–697.

Muzio, C. (1993). Lesbian co-parenting: On being/being with the invisible (m)other. *Smith College Studies in Social Work, 63*(3), 215–229.

Nystrom, N. (1997). *Oppression by mental health providers: A report by gay men and lesbians about their treatment.* Ann Arbor, MI: UMI Dissertation Services.

O'Hanlan, K. A., Dibble, S. L., Hagan, H. J. J., & Davids, R. (2004). Advocacy for women's health should include lesbian health. *Journal of Women's Health, 13*(2), 227–234.

Orel, N. A. (2004). Gay, lesbian, and bisexual elders: Expressed needs and concerns across focus groups. *Journal of Gerontological Social Work, 43*(2/3), 57–77.

Orel, N. A. (2006). Community needs assessment: Documenting the need for affirmative services for LGB older adults. In D. Kimmel, T. Rose, & S. David (Eds.), *Lesbian, gay, bisexual, and transgender aging: Research and clinical perspectives* (pp. 175–194). New York: Columbia University Press.

Parks, C. A. (1999). Lesbian identity development: An examination of differences across generations. *American Journal of Orthopsychiatry, 69*(3), 347–361.

Potter, S. J., & Darty, T. E. (1981). Social work and the invisible minority: An exploration of lesbianism. *Social Work, 26*(3), 187–192.

Rothblum, E. D. (1990). Depression among lesbians: An invisible and unresearched phenomena. *Journal of Gay and Lesbian Psychotherapy, 1*(3), 67–87.

Seidman, I. E. (1991). *Interviewing as qualitative research.* New York: Teachers College Press.

Services and Advocacy for GLBT Elders (SAGE). (2011, Spring). History in the making: How SAGE built the country's first National Resource Center on LGBT Aging. *Sage Matters: The Magazine of Services & Advocacy for GLBT Elders,* pp. 3–5. sageusa.org

Slusher, M. P., Mayer, C. J., & Dunkle, R. E. (1996). Gay and lesbians old and wiser (GLOW): A support group for old gay people. *Gerontologist, 36,* 118–123.

Trippet, S. E. (1994). Lesbians' mental health concerns. *Health Care for Women International, 15,* 317–323.

Tully, C. T. (1989). Caregiving: What do mid-life lesbians view as important? *Journal of Gay and Lesbian Psychotherapy, 1*(7), 87–103.

van der Meide, W. (2000). *Legislating equality: A review of laws affecting gay, lesbian, bisexual, and transgendered people in the United States.* New York: Policy Institute of the National Gay and Lesbian Task Force.

Warren, P. N. (2000). Elephant graveyards, gay aging and gay ageism in the year 2000. *Outword Magazine.* American Society on Aging, San Francisco. Retrieved from www.gaywired.com/wildcat/wildedt10.htm#graveyards

West, D. J. (1983). Homosexuality and lesbianism. *British Journal of Psychiatry, 143,* 221–226.

Woolf, L. M. (2002). *Gay and lesbian aging.* Siecus Report No. 17.

CHAPTER FIVE

Aging in the Bisexual Community

PAULA C. RODRÍGUEZ RUST, PH.D.

What experience, event, or circumstance caused you to realize that you might not be heterosexual?

> My first sexual activity was with men, but I was so sexually ignorant when I entered the Army I naively and innocently answered "no" to the queries about homosexual activity. It had just felt good—I didn't know it was sex.
>
> *—A 67-year-old man who first had sex with a man at age 17, came out as "homosexual" at age 35, and as "bisexual" at age 45*

> I have concluded, following the death of my husband, . . . [that] my sexual needs are more likely to be met at my age by [an] intimate relationship [with] a woman . . . [I knew that] there were less available men near my age as I reached 60 . . . [and my a]wareness [that] I needed sexual outlet and sharing, still at my age, caused me to give more thought to how and with whom.
>
> *—A 69-year-old woman who came out for the first time as "bisexual" at age 62*

Bisexual elders are a diverse population (Boxer, 1997). Some older bisexual men and women have been out for decades, living as visible members of sexual minority communities through significant historical events and changes in political climate. Others have come out more recently, adopting bisexual identities at a later stage of life, often after lengthy heterosexual marriages and child rearing. Issues facing bisexual persons as they age are similarly diverse. The goal of this chapter is to explore these issues by examining the many different life journeys that lead to bisexual elderhood.

DIVERSITY AMONG ELDERLY BISEXUALS

Diversity among bisexual elders reflects diversity among older persons in general. The bisexual elderly population includes individuals of different racial, ethnic, and religious backgrounds; persons of different genders, including transgender; able-bodied people and people living with disabilities; and individuals with different marriage, partnership, and parental histories. Age is also a significant factor. Although one's 50th birthday is a current cultural marker for the beginning of "older age," in an era in which many people will live into their 80s, the age of 50 is only slightly more than halfway through life. The needs of 50-year-olds are often different from the needs of people in their 60s, 70s, 80s, or 90s.

The population of bisexual elders is also diverse in ways unique to sexual minority communities. The historical time period in which an individual came out, and the age at which she or he did so, are factors that have profound and lasting effects on that person's needs and experiences. For example, a person who first identified as bisexual before the Stonewall Rebellion in 1969 experienced a very different world as a sexual minority person than did someone who came out in the 1970s during the gay macho and lesbian feminist era or in the 1980s during the HIV/AIDS crisis. Furthermore, during each historical time period, individuals who came out as teenagers were affected differently than those who came out as young adults—perhaps in the context of marriage and child rearing—and differently than those who came out during older age.

Therefore, sexual minority individuals belong to three different *cohorts*, or age-related groups. Like other elderly persons, they belong to a generational cohort based on chronological age. As members of a sexual minority, they belong to a cohort of individuals who came out within a given historical time period and also to a cohort of individuals who came out at a certain age, or stage, in their own life courses (Rodríguez Rust, 2004; see also Keppel & Firestein, 2006;*

* My appreciation to Bobbi Keppel and Beth Firestein, who provided me with a prepublication copy of their chapter "Bisexual Inclusion in Addressing Issues of LGBT Aging: Therapy with

Ritter & Terndrup, 2002). These three age-related groupings form a *temporal trilogy*: one's age at coming out plus the number of years one has been out equals one's current age. Although correlated with one another, each factor in the temporal trilogy exerts an independent influence on the individual experience of minority status and therefore on personal needs and concerns during the aging process.

HISTORICAL EVENTS AND THE IMPACT OF CHRONOLOGICAL AGE AND YEAR OF COMING OUT

During the past century, occidental society has experienced dramatic changes in attitudes toward sexuality, in the context of important historical events. The challenges faced by bisexual elders depend in part on whether they identified and lived as heterosexuals, as bisexuals, or as lesbians or gay men during each historical period experienced by their generation.

During the lives of the current cohort of elderly persons, several major social changes occurred that affected all members of society, including World War I, the more open sexuality of the 1920s, Prohibition, the Great Depression, World War II, the postwar baby boom with its emphasis on domestic conformity, the sexual revolution of the 1960s, the black civil rights movement, the feminist movement, and advances in electronic communication during the latter twentieth century.

Many of these events affected sexual minority persons differently than their heterosexual peers. For example, during World War II, the gender segregation that occurred as men were drafted into the military and as women entered the industrial workplace to support the war economically gave many individuals the opportunity to discover and explore same-sex desires of which they were not previously aware (Keppel & Firestein, 2006). During McCarthyism in the 1950s, homosexuals were targeted for particular persecution. Many gay men and lesbians participated in the black civil rights movement because they understood the importance of social justice but were not yet in a position to fight for their own civil rights. The sexual revolution of the 1960s was primarily a heterosexual revolution, but it made sexual activity motivated only by sexual desire—and not by a desire to procreate—more acceptable, which paved the way for the acknowledgment of same-sex desire. The feminist movement taught women to value one another in new ways; lesbianism was both a threat to early feminists' social

---

Older Bisexuals," later published in Firestein's *Becoming Visible: Counseling Bisexuals across the Lifespan* (Columbia University Press).

respectability and a natural outcome of women working together against male dominance. In the cultural lesbian feminist branch of the feminist movement, bisexual women were regarded as "traitors" to the lesbian feminist cause. Advances in electronic information technology now allow members of hidden minorities to communicate anonymously with persons outside their local area, leading to new forms of social support for individuals who had previously struggled in lonely silence.

Other historical milestones of the twentieth century affected sexual minority persons even more directly. These include the Kinsey studies of 1948 and 1953; the Stonewall Rebellion; the homophile, gay, and queer rights movements; the removal of "homosexuality" as a diagnostic category in the *Diagnostic and Statistical Manual of Mental Disorders* (*DSM*) of the American Psychiatric Association; the "bisexual chic" of the 1970s; the HIV epidemic; and the bisexual political movement. The Kinsey studies shocked a generation with their estimates of same-sex sexual experience among both men and women. To heterosexuals, this was the first suggestion that homosexual behavior, long regarded as a rare perversion of "normal" sexual expression, might be more common than previously thought. To isolated homosexuals, it meant they might be able to find others like themselves (Gagnon, 1990; Pomeroy, 1972; Voeller, 1990). The Stonewall Rebellion reflected the growing unwillingness of gay men and lesbians to tolerate police harassment and public bigotry, symbolizing the transformation of the homophile movement into the gay and lesbian civil rights movement. The HIV epidemic focused public attention on gay men. Although this attention was decidedly negative, it gave gay men and lesbians a visibility that could eventually be used toward positive ends. The existence of bisexuality was also negatively recognized during the HIV epidemic, first by public health officials and then by the general public, because of fears that bisexuals would transmit HIV from gay men into the "general population." The contemporary bisexual movement, whose roots date back to the 1950s, became increasingly vocal and visible in response to gay and lesbian rejection of bisexuals as traitors and heterosexual characterizations of bisexuals as HIV carriers.

The effect of each of these historical events on an elderly bisexual person depended in part on whether he or she had already come out and, if so, whether he or she had come out as gay or lesbian identified or as bisexual identified. For example, a 55-year-old woman who is currently bisexual-identified and was in college during the early 1970s may have experienced the feminist movement differently if she were heterosexual identified at the time than if she had already come out as lesbian or bisexual. If she were living a heterosexual life at the time, she would have found her life choices complicated by her increasing understanding of patriarchal social structures. If she identified as a lesbian, initially she may have been told to stay closeted in the interest of feminist public respectability, but a few years later, she might have found herself regarded as the embodiment of feminist ideals. If she called herself bisexual, she probably would have experienced greater rejection than either her lesbian or her heterosexual peers during this ideological evolution, because her bisexuality would have been considered an embarrassment by both. If, however, this 55-year-old did not go to college but was a young wife and mother during the 1970s, without any personal involvement in the feminist movement, and later came out as bisexual at age 50, she might have been surprised to find that some of her lesbian age-mates still carried an antipathy toward bisexual women that she did not even know existed. Unfamiliar with the sexual identity politics of this subculture of her own generation, she might feel at a loss in her struggle to find acceptance and support.

Chronological age differences further complicate these distinctions. Compared with college women and young mothers in the 1970s, the experiences of women who were in their 40s at that time were quite different. For a middle-aged, heterosexually married woman, the feminist movement of the 1970s may have presented her with difficult choices regarding her relationship to her husband, her role in their marriage, and her career choices—or lack of them. If she were a butch or femme lesbian, instead of finding support from the lesbian feminists of that era, she might have found herself rejected as an outdated imitator of heterosexual masculine or feminine roles.

WHAT IS BISEXUALITY?

Although bisexual visibility has increased in recent decades, contemporary culture is still deeply imbued with a belief that there are two fundamental forms of sexuality—heterosexuality and homosexuality—and that bisexuality does not exist as a "true" sexual orientation. A brief history of the development of modern concepts of sexual orientation illuminates the roots of this "nonexistence belief." Once this has been identified as a cultural product rather than as a reflection of scientific or social reality, the question of what bisexuality *is* can be addressed.

The Nonexistence Belief

Many social scientists have discussed the history of the evolution of the concepts of heterosexuality and homosexuality, and of the "heterosexual person" and "homosexual person." Contemporary concepts of sexual orientation, which classify people according to their sexual desires for males or females, date to the late nineteenth century (Katz, 1995; cf. Boswell, 1990; Trumbach, 1977). Before that period, men and women were defined primarily by their roles as husbands and wives, mothers and fathers. Marriage was necessary for economic stability and procreation; it was not primarily a route for expressing personal sexual desire (Smith-Rosenberg, 1975). Sexual passion was considered antithetical to marriage, because it was too short lived to sustain lifelong marriage. Over the course of the late 19th and early 20th centuries, increased economic prosperity allowed greater attention to the fulfillment of personal desires and needs, including sexual ones, and the pursuit of one's own desires became more socially acceptable. Before that time, some individuals had same-sex desires that were sometimes satisfied outside of marriage, but it was not until the late 19th century that individuals came to be defined as *types of persons*, depending on the gender to which they were more sexually attracted, that is, as homosexuals and heterosexuals. Heterosexuals enjoyed a birthright of legal and social privilege, and the resulting homosexual, gay, and lesbian rights movements further cemented the distinction between heterosexuals and homosexuals and created gay, lesbian, and heterosexual *identities*, communities, and politics.

The ironic consequences of this development regarding the concept of bisexuality are described by Rodríguez Rust (2002):

> The late 19th century development of the concepts of *homosexuality* and *heterosexuality* as forms of sexuality characterized by sexual impulses directed toward members of either one's own gender or the opposite gender made it possible to conceptualize the combination of both such impulses (i.e., *bi*-sexuality). Paradoxically, however, the same historical developments—the conceptualization of heterosexuality and homosexuality as distinct forms of sexuality, predicated upon concepts of men and women as opposite genders—also made it difficult for contemporary lay people . . . to believe that such a combination could exist within a single individual. (pp. 181–182)

Before the division of the social world into populations of heterosexuals and homosexuals, there was no need, nor any basis, for creating the concept of bisexuality. One cannot theorize a *combination* of two things that are not distinguished from each other, and there would be no need for such a concept. But the cultural construction of heterosexuality and homosexuality simultaneously made their combination both *possible* and *inconceivable*. Men and women are culturally constructed as opposites, and if men and women are opposites, how can attractions toward both genders coexist in a single individual? Whatever one is attracted to in men would not exist in women, and vice versa, so how could one be attracted to both? This cultural belief in "opposing genders," therefore, is at the root of the misperception that bisexuality *cannot* exist. It is also the root of many contemporary stereotypes regarding bisexual persons. For example, bisexuals are stereotyped as promiscuous, incapable of monogamy, or experiencing internal conflict between their "heterosexual and homosexual sides." Bisexuals are also often believed to be lesbians and gay men who lack self-awareness, are afraid to embrace their homosexuality, or have not yet finished coming out.

As the gay and lesbian civil rights movements gained momentum in the mid- to late twentieth century, the lack of conceptual "space" for bisexuality grew into a lack of social and political space as well. Bisexual men and women were regarded as disingenuous homosexuals who would not come out to join the lesbian and gay community and political struggle and who wanted the "best of both worlds" without sharing the burdens of minority status. To lesbians and gay men, continued heterosexual desires and behavior implied a lack of commitment to the struggle for gay and lesbian equality; bisexual persons were often labeled as traitors or told to "finish" coming out as lesbian or gay.

There are many logical flaws in the argument that attractions to men and women are opposing drives that cannot coexist in one person. First, men and women are not *opposites*. Men and women are different in some ways and similar in many others. Bem (1974) and numerous others have demonstrated that our cultural concepts of masculinity and femininity overlap substantially and that women and men display more similarity than do our cultural stereotypes. Personality traits, social skills, economic and educational levels, music and activity preferences, age, and ethnicity are characteristics shared across genders, by all adults. Among people of all sexual orientations, these nongendered characteristics influence sexual desire by determining which males or which females will appear most attractive. Second, attraction to a particular man, or woman, is not necessarily an attraction to the aspects of the individual that distinguish men from women, such as genitalia, secondary sex characteristics, and gendered social markers. It could be an attraction to nongendered characteristics, such as intelligence, personality, hobbies, or hair color.

Because heterosexuals, gay men, and lesbians tend to be attracted only to people with particular sex and gender characteristics, it can be difficult for them to imagine that other people might be attracted to other people primarily on the basis of nongendered aspects of personhood, regardless of which genitalia or how much body hair they have. The difference between lesbians, gay men, and heterosexuals—collectively known as *monosexuals* because they are attracted to only one sex or gender—and bisexuals is whether an individual's sex or gender is a necessary criterion for sexual attraction. It is easy for monosexuals to discount the existence of bisexuality, because they experience sexual attraction as conflated with an attraction to sex characteristics. But for bisexual women and men, it often is not. Some bisexual persons are attracted to both male and female sexual anatomy and gendered social markers, and some find the male-female distinction irrelevant because they are primarily attracted to other—nongendered—characteristics that men and women share. For example, a 73-year-old bisexual woman respondent in the International Bisexual Identity, Community, Ideology, and Politics (IBICIP) study (a study of more than 900 bisexual men and women conducted by the author) wrote, "I am drawn to certain characteristics in a person . . . more and more those traits that attract me happen to be in women."*

The Spectrum of Bisexuality

Bisexuality is a culturally marginalized concept, without a clear and universal definition. Bisexuality means different things to different people, and there are many ways to be bisexual. The different ways of being bisexual are a source of diversity among bisexual persons, especially bisexual elders whose sexual self-perceptions were shaped during decades when the existence of bisexuality was most strongly denied.

Most individuals who identify themselves as bisexual use the term to indicate that they are attracted to both men and women. Their attractions may be stronger for one gender or the other, and they may or may not have sexual or romantic experience with members of both genders (Rust, 2001). Some individuals call themselves bisexual because they have had sex with both men and women, or because they could picture themselves in a long-term or lifetime committed relationship with either a man or a woman. Others who identify as bisexual do so because they consider gender a relatively unimportant characteristic; that is, they are attracted to *people*, not to "men and women." There are also individuals who self-identify as heterosexual, gay, or lesbian and who have exactly the same patterns of attraction to both genders or histories of sexual behavior with both men

---

* Questions and quotes are from respondents in the author's International Bisexual Identity, Community, Ideology and Politics Study (IBICIP), a survey of more than 900 individuals who either identify as bisexual, have ever felt attractions for men and women, or who have lifetime sexual histories that include sexual activity with at least one man and at least one woman. Methodological details can be found in Rust (2001) or Rodríguez Rust (2006).

and women that can be found among self-identified bisexuals. For medical and mental health practitioners, whether a given individual *is* bisexual in some essentially "true" sense is not a useful question. Rather, it is important to understand the various forms that bisexuality can take and the medical and mental health implications of this cultural concept.

The multiple dimensions of sexuality, including sexual identity, sexual behavior, sexual fantasies, sexual attractions, and romantic attractions, can be used to characterize various forms of bisexuality (Kinsey, Pomeroy, & Martin, 1948; Klein, 1978, 1990; Klein, Sepekoff, & Wolf, 1985; Weinberg, Williams, & Pryor, 1994). These dimensions vary independently of one another. If a person can be regarded as bisexual on one or more of these dimensions (i.e., if she or he self-identifies as bisexual, has engaged in both same- and other-sex sexual activity, or has romantic, sexual, or fantasized attractions to both men and women), then his or her concerns during the aging process fall within the scope of this chapter. The term *bisexual* will be used to refer to this diverse population. This is not meant to imply that these individuals are in any essential way "truly" bisexual, nor that they should self-identify as bisexual.

The independent variability of the multiple dimensions of sexuality produces an enormous variety of possible combinations of sexual identity, behavior, fantasies, and attractions. However, certain patterns occur more frequently than others. Many researchers have outlined common forms of bisexuality, often developing descriptive typologies (e.g., Klein, 1978, 1993; Ross, 1991). Types of bisexuality found in the United States include sequential, historical or lifetime, concurrent, polyfidelitous, Latin, situational, and transitional or experimental.

Sequential bisexuality consists of relationships or sexual activity with both men and women over time. The individual may be involved with only one partner at a time, but when one coupled relationship ends, the next partner may be either a man or a woman. The result is a pattern of bisexual behavior that can only be recognized over time.

Historical, or *lifetime,* bisexuality is a term that can be applied to anyone whose entire life sexual history includes activity with both men and women. Some researchers and theorists include only adult, or postpubertal, sexual experiences in this definition. For purposes such as public health research, attention may be focused on recent experiences with both men and women.

Concurrent bisexuality involves simultaneous relationships with a man or men and a woman or women. There are many different forms of concurrent bisexuality (Rust, 1996b; Weinberg et al., 1994). A common pattern consists of a primary relationship with an individual of one gender and concurrent secondary relationships with one or more individuals of the other gender. The primary relationship may be an open relationship in which the partner is aware and accepting of the secondary relationships. For example, a 55-year-old man in the IBICIP study wrote that he is still deeply in love with his wife of 32 years. She accepts that, during the course of their relationship, he has also been involved with more than 30 men, 5 or 6 at any given time, including a 23-year relationship with another man. A 73-year-old woman, married to a man for six years, reported that she had recently begun a relationship with a woman who lives in another city. She does not think that this would surprise her husband, because they both had same-sex experiences earlier in their lives. Sometimes, both members of a primary relationship are involved in concurrent secondary relationships; if this is done as a couple, it is sometimes colloquially referred to as *swinging*. Some individuals have two primary relationships, one with a man and one with a woman. Bisexual persons who are not in committed relationships may date or form sexual friendships with individuals of both genders. These patterns are also forms of concurrent bisexuality. Multiple concurrent sexual relationships are probably less common among elderly persons than among the young, but nonsexual romantic relationships in the pursuit of companionship can be just as complicated.

Polyfidelity refers to sexual fidelity among more than two people. In such relationships, each person may be involved with all of the other individuals, or only certain pairs of individuals may be sexually involved. In either case, all participants confine their sexual contacts to other members of the polyfidelitous group.

Latin bisexuality refers to Latino conceptions of sexuality in which a man— who may be married or primarily attracted to women—is considered heterosexual as long as he plays only the insertive (*activo*) role in sex with men. In European-American constructions of sexuality, this would be considered bisexual behavior because of the genders of the sex partners (Carrier, 1991, 1995; Magaña & Almaguer, 1993).

Situational bisexuality (also called situational homosexuality) involves sexual activity with members of one's less preferred sex because of situational constraints. Examples include sex between individuals in single-sex environments, such as prisons or boarding schools, same-sex activity among female prostitutes who find it difficult to form satisfying romantic relationships with men, and same-sex prostitution among men whose sexual desire is toward women but who "trick" for economic reasons (Burkhart, 1973/1996; Giallombardo, 1966; James, 1976; Wooden & Parker, 1982).

Bisexuality can be referred to as *transitional*, or *experimental*, if it occurs during a period of coming out or of personal sexual experimentation, such as during adolescence, during college, or following a divorce. These terms have been used in the past to discredit bisexuality as a "true" sexual orientation by implying that any past sexual activity with an individual's currently nonpreferred sex must have been just a "phase" or "not really serious." These terms, therefore, should be used with care because they are offensive to bisexual-identified persons who have repeatedly faced censure or devaluation of their sexuality. The fact that some people choose to interpret their *own* previous sexual experiences in this way should also be respected.

Bisexual diversity interacts with the aging process in some important ways. The percentage of persons with bisexual experience increases with age. This does not mean that older generations contain more bisexual individuals but, rather, that the elderly have had more years in which to have a greater variety of experiences. People with any inclination toward both same-sex and other-sex activity become more and more likely to have engaged in these behaviors as they age, simply because they have had more years in which to encounter opportunities. However, partnered relationships tend to be more transient among the young. As individuals age, they often settle down into more stable life patterns, whether these are monogamous, polyfidelitous, or celibate. Therefore, among the elderly, lifetime bisexuality is more common relative to younger cohorts, whereas concurrent and situational bisexuality are probably less common.

STEREOTYPES OF BISEXUALS AND THE ELDERLY

Elderly bisexual individuals must contend with sexual stereotypes pertaining to both old age and bisexuality. In large part, these are conflicting: The elderly are characterized as sexless, whereas bisexuals are perceived as overly sexual. Of course, neither of these stereotypes is accurate. All aging individuals, not only bisexual older adults, must contend with the societal belief that sexual desire and activity decrease with age. Some older persons find that their personal experience is consistent with this image. Others find that when they are no longer worried about pregnancy or have fulfilled their social obligation to marry and procreate, older age brings the freedom to express formerly suppressed social and sexual desires.

Conversely, all bisexual persons, not only elderly bisexuals, face stereotypes that they are oversexed, nonmonogamous, and sexually indiscriminate. Many of these beliefs derive from the cultural conception of bisexuality as an unstable and inherently conflict-laden combination of heterosexuality and homosexuality. This faulty reasoning maintains that a heterosexual's partner must be other sex and a lesbian's or gay man's partner must be same sex. Therefore, a bisexual's "heterosexual side" must have an other-sex partner, whereas his or her "homosexual side" must have a same-sex partner, resulting in a need for partners of both sexes. However, the defining characteristic for most bisexual individuals is an openness to partners of either sex, not a need for both. Nor do bisexual persons necessarily have twice the opportunity for sexual activity as heterosexuals, lesbians, or gay men. Some experience fewer possibilities, because social prejudices and fears (e.g., of HIV) make some monosexual persons reluctant to become involved with bisexual partners.

The combination of these conflicting stereotypes presents unique psychological and social challenges for elderly bisexuals. They are perceived as overly sexual at a time in their lives when younger adults would prefer that they not be sexual at all. As elders, they are not "supposed" to have sexual desires, and yet they desire not only one sex but both. Bisexual elderly persons who express sexual interest risk others perceiving them as "dirty old men and women" to an even greater degree than their sexually active monosexual peers. Heterosexuals can reach old age, perhaps still in a lifetime marriage or having found a new partner after the death of a spouse, and others will comfortably approve of the fact that they have companionship in their later years, although it will be presumed to be platonic or minimally sexual. In contrast, if elders assert a bisexual self-identity, this may be perceived as a statement of active sexual desire or behavior, which, for older adults, is unexpected at best and taboo at worst.

There are many different patterns of sexual activity among bisexual elderly persons. Some people experience a decrease in sexual activity with age because of physical difficulties or social circumstances. Some individuals who have spent their youth with a number of different sexual partners eventually find one person with whom they want to spend the remainder of their lives and settle into monogamous relationships. Decreasing energy or physical capacity may also limit the older person's ability to maintain multiple partnered relationships or to travel to spend time with a partner, and these factors can result in de facto monogamy or celibacy. For example, an 86-year-old man in the IBICIP study reported that he has an "ongoing committed emotional and sexual relationship with a man 55 years old—but we seldom see each other."

Non-bisexuals may believe that a bisexual elder whose sexual path has led into a monogamous relationship has "become" heterosexual, lesbian, or gay, or that he or she has finally "matured" into his or her true identity and lifestyle. These perceptions are used to support cultural beliefs regarding the nonexistence of bisexuality. The tendency for many aging individuals to "settle down" in two-person relationships should not be interpreted as "settling down into one sexuality or the other" with age, nor as proof that bisexuality is an immature sexuality. Monogamous or celibate elderly bisexual men and women are no less bisexual than their younger peers.

For other bisexual elderly persons, the social freedom attached to old age brings opportunity to express new or previously suppressed sexual desires. A 67-year-old woman in the IBICIP study wrote that she had been married for 20 years, but following her divorce, she spent several years in relationships with women, followed by relationships with both men and women during the past 10 years. A male study participant of the same age reported that he "realiz[ed] I could be truly attracted to both sexes" after divorcing his first wife. The 60-year-old woman quoted at the beginning of this chapter found that she still wanted companionship after her husband's death. Knowing that women live longer than men, on average, she realized that her chances of finding a woman companion were greater than her chances of finding a man companion. She did not write about a suppressed same-sex desire that she was "freed" to express by the death of her husband; rather, she was *open* to the possibility of a female partner, and changing circumstances provided her with different opportunities at different times in her life. The result in her case was—given the cultural penchant for labeling people according to the genders of their sexual partners—serial bisexuality.

LIFE COURSE DYNAMICS AND PEER SUPPORT
AMONG BISEXUAL OLDER ADULTS

Each stage of life is associated with characteristic life course events. By the time they reach older age, most persons have experienced the loss of their parents, children leaving home, the birth of grandchildren, the loss of a partner or spouse, retirement, changing economic circumstances, new physical ailments and limitations, and changing medical needs.

As significant events are experienced over the life course, individuals find support and solace in their friendships. Social networks in American mainstream culture are age graded; individuals socialize with friends of similar ages, and members of friendship groups tend to experience life course events contemporaneously. For example, a young woman giving birth to her first child will share her joy with her friends, particularly those who have already given birth and understand what she is experiencing. When that child leaves for college, her friends' children are also leaving their homes, and she can share her "empty nest" feelings with other mothers who have been her friends for years. With increasing age, however, more of one's long-term friends die or become mentally disabled. Those who survive meet one another through various social networks—a common residence in a retirement community or shared activities at a senior center—and become new friends. Elderly persons find support among their new companions who are facing similar challenges as they age, and who have often experienced similar life events in the past, although they did not know one another at the time.

Bisexual elders face many of the same life course events as other older persons regardless of sexual orientation, but they also have experiences unique to sexual minority individuals. People whose lives have followed atypical paths have greater difficulty finding the support of new companions as they age. As their long-term friends die, it can be difficult for them to meet others who share similar histories. For example, sexual minority individuals share the important experience of "coming out"—a momentous event in the lives of lesbian, gay, bisexual, and transgendered people. For most, the coming out process changed their understanding of self, expectations for romance and lifestyle, and relationships with friends and family. Those who came out in young adulthood may have been rejected by their parents. Those who came out later in life may have been married, perhaps with children, at the time. They had to decide whether and how to tell their spouses and children. Some lost custody of their children because, as sexual minority persons, they were considered unfit parents. Those who retained custody or visitation rights sometimes had to curtail or conceal their romantic lives because some courts imposed restrictions on same-sex relationships as a condition of these parenting rights. A heterosexual woman who lost a husband can walk into any senior center and find dozens of other women who share her experience; elderly lesbians, gay men, and bisexuals cannot expect to find many other individuals who have shared their coming out experiences.

COMING OUT

The process of coming out is different for bisexual persons than for lesbians and gay men (Diamond & Savin-Williams, 2000; Rust, 1996a; Weinberg et al., 1994). In traditional models of lesbian and gay identity development, the coming out process begins with an assumed heterosexual identity, the gradual recognition and acknowledgment of same-sex desires, the adoption of a lesbian or gay identity—perhaps after a period of bisexual identification—and, finally, acceptance of and pride in one's lesbian or gay self. In this model, the individual "comes out" only once; after the "true" sexuality has been acknowledged and accepted, the process is complete, and there is no reason for further identity change. Many lesbians and gay men experience their coming out times in this way and, looking back, perceive any periods during which they identified as bisexual as "transitional," periods that served as stepping-stones toward their true lesbian or gay identity.

Some individuals do not follow this "linear" model of the coming out process; for example, some individuals change sexual identities several times over the life course (Diamond, 1998, 2000; Rodríguez Rust, 2009; Rust, 1993). Evidence suggests that individuals who identify as bisexual at any given time have, in the past, reexamined their sexual identities more times than their peers who identify as lesbian or gay (Rodríguez Rust, 2009; Rust, 1993). Although this finding may be interpreted as evidence of bisexual "instability," it likely reflects cultural reluctance to acknowledge the validity of the bisexual identity. Bisexual persons often adopt either a homosexual or a heterosexual identification during some portions of the life course, perhaps because maintaining a bisexual identity in the face of others' invalidation or censure can be difficult. Many bisexual adults come out at least twice, first, as lesbian or gay and, second, as bisexual. Whereas older lesbians and gay men often have difficulty meeting companions who understand the coming out experience, it can be even harder for bisexual elders to find true peers, that is, other older persons who acknowledge both their same- and other-sex attractions and who have struggled to be acknowledged as bisexual in both heterosexual society and lesbian or gay culture.

Coming out is unusual among life course events, in that it can occur at any time during adolescence or adulthood. Most life course events occur at typical ages. Marriage, childbearing, retirement, and loss of a partner to death generally occur at specific times during adulthood and in a particular order. Individuals who experience these events at atypical ages tend to experience them somewhat differently than their peers. For example, widowhood usually occurs at older ages. A woman who loses her husband at an early age—for example, in a motor vehicle accident at age 25, two years after the birth of their child—experiences this event differently than a woman who loses her husband at the more typical age of 75 to a heart attack or chronic illness. In contrast, coming out can normally occur at any time of life. This is particularly true in the current cohort of elderly persons, who reached adulthood during more sexually repressive times.

Many sexual minority individuals in the current elderly population were at least somewhat aware of their same-sex attractions early in life but married and remained closeted for decades because of social pressure. The experience of the 67-year-old military veteran quoted at the beginning of this chapter—who had enjoyed contact with other men but "didn't know it was sex"—is not unusual.

Another man in the IBICIP study, who was consciously aware of his same-sex attractions in 1934 at age 15, wrote that he married in part because he wanted children. He and his wife had talked about his same-gender sexual attraction before they married, but he reported that they "thought that once in a hetero-sexual relationship" his orientation would change. At age 61, when a male friend came out to him as bisexual, he realized that this trusted person was describing his own orientation as well. When his wife passed away after 40 years of marriage, he became involved with the friend. Like these two men, many sexual minority individuals who were unable to come out earlier in life do so in old age because of increasing social tolerance in the contemporary social world and decreasing pressure to fulfill heterosexual expectations and obligations in their own lives.

Coming out as a member of a sexual minority parallels many of the processes that occur during normal adolescence, for example, the search for identity and acceptance and the struggle to find one's niche in the world. When coming out occurs during adolescence—as it does for many of today's youth—it becomes part of the age-appropriate struggle to grow into adulthood. When it occurs at older ages, the process of coming out can be dissonant with other life course events and challenges (Keppel & Firestein, 2006; Ritter & Terndrup, 2002). An individual who has already reached social and psychological maturity can find herself, or himself, again facing the struggles of youth—but now, at a much later stage of life and in the more complex contexts of established career and family, instead of during high school, college, or single young adulthood.

The timing of coming out, relative to the life stage of the individual, significantly influences the needs and challenges facing bisexual elderly persons. Those who came out early in life have experienced many relevant historical events with their lesbian, gay, and bisexual peer group. Their sexual-minority-identity status is long-standing and is often comfortable and well integrated with other aspects of their psyches and social lives. Unlike those who have recently come out, they may have little need to relay the latest story of interaction with an intolerant person or to tell and retell their coming out stories. They have "been there and done that." They are no longer actively working on their social and psychological identities as sexual minority individuals; they are now engaged in the business of *being* who they are.

Elderly persons who have recently come out, or are in the process of coming out, are still engaged in an "adolescent" developmental experience. They may need to discuss their sexual minority status with supportive peers and to tell their coming out stories. They are still learning what it means to be a bisexual person in this culture and time. The dissonance of facing these issues at a time in life when others are comfortably enjoying the fruits of bygone struggles can be a challenge for all sexual minority persons who come out late in life. These "late-comers" may have difficulty finding support among peers who consolidated this aspect of personal identity long ago, and who did so in more repressive times. These peers are also less likely to share their histories of heterosexual marriage and child rearing, and may have some lingering resentment toward—and there-fore less available emotional support for—persons who spent their younger adult-hoods enjoying the legal and social privileges of heterosexuality that they were denied (see also Barón & Cramer, 2000; Keppel & Firestein, 2006).

For those who come out during their older years, however, one advantage is the fact that increasing age brings increasing likelihood of coming out as bisex-ual rather than as lesbian or gay (Rust, 2004). Individuals who have been hetero-sexually married and raised children are often unwilling to negate this important part of their lives by coming out as lesbian or gay and so come out as bisexual to acknowledge both their newly recognized same-sex feelings and their heterosex-ual histories. Therefore, a support group for older people who are questioning their sexual identities or in the process of coming out is likely to yield support for elderly bisexual persons.

WIDOWHOOD AND WIDOWERHOOD

Another life course event unique to sexual minority individuals is the death of a long-term *same-sex* partner. Although sexual minority and heterosexual individu-als share the common experience of partner loss, the death of a same-sex partner is different because of the lack of social support and legal validation for same-sex relationships. The survivor of a same-sex relationship may have been denied the right to make medical decisions for or to be at the deathbed of a dying partner. She or he may have lost the shared home following the death because of the lack of legal protections afforded the deceased's estate. The relationship was not afforded full social recognition or legal protection during life. Same-sex couples, especially among generations who are now elderly, did not have weddings sanc-tioned by religious bodies and publicized by congratulatory friends and family. In the recent past, after decades of secrecy and censure, some older couples have obtained civil unions or state-recognized legal marriages, but such recognition remains unavailable to same-sex couples in most of the United States.

At death, the surviving partner may not have received any expressions of sym-pathy from friends and co-workers. They may not even have known that the widow or widower was partnered, much less that the partner had just passed away. Family leave or equivalent benefits for same-sex couples are rare. Sexual minority individuals who lose partners sometimes encounter attitudes from heterosexuals such as "I feel sorry for you, but it's not as if it was a marriage or anything." In this regard, bisexual elders who lose same-sex partners are not different from lesbians and gay men. However, a bisexual individual who has both other-sex and same-sex partners is likely to receive very little comfort from non-bisexuals following the death of a same-sex partner. Such a relationship is not merely less valued than a heterosexual partnership but is still sometimes considered illegitimate and better ended.

The death of a spouse or a partner results in both loss of companionship and a psychological challenge to one's personal identity as a member of that partnership or marriage. For sexual minority individuals, one's identity as a partner in a couple bears a complex relationship to one's sexual orientation identity. After the death of a spouse, heterosexuals are still perceived as heterosexual; heterosexuality is assumed, even in the absence of an other-sex spouse. Regardless of whether they are sexually active, their heterosexual identities remain unchallenged. Sexual minority persons, however, face a loss of perceived sexual orientation identity as well as the loss of identifying as part of a couple. In the absence of a same-sex partner, it can be difficult for others to recognize the survivor as a sexual minority individual and to understand the continued importance of the survivor's sexual minority identity.

Sexual orientation is usually a more salient aspect of identity for sexual minority individuals—lesbians, gay men, and bisexual persons—than for heterosexually identified persons. A heterosexual identity is assumed. It does not have to be achieved, discovered, or fought for. One does not have to come out as heterosexual, either to oneself or to others. Heterosexual elders have not spent their lifetimes correcting the assumption underlying the question, "And what does your wife [or husband] do?" each time they meet a new person. Sexual minority individuals have faced these challenges. Their identities are often hard won and may be continually problematic in a society that still assumes, and favors, heterosexuality. For elderly sexual minority individuals, the heterosexual assumption resurfaces each time a new acquaintance, seeking to build a friendship based on shared past experiences, asks, "And when did you lose your husband [or wife]?"

THE ROLE OF FAMILY SUPPORT AMONG
ELDERLY BISEXUAL PERSONS

In addition to the support of their age peers, many elderly persons receive assistance from their adult children and grandchildren. Some elderly lesbians and gay men do not have children and therefore lack this important source of emotional, physical, and financial support in their old age. Bisexual elders—whether they came out early or late in life—are more likely to have had children. However, if the children are intolerant of the parent's sexual orientation, these potentially helpful relationships will be compromised. One recent study (MetLife, 2010, p. 18) found that bisexual older adults were less likely than their gay and lesbian peers to report that family members were accepting of their lives as sexual minority people. See also Goldberg (2007) and Grossman et al. (2000) for further discussion of family and social support.

The relationships between elderly individuals and their children depend on many factors. Those who came out early in life may have had full knowledge of their own bisexuality when they married and as they raised their children, but they may not have shared this information with their spouse and children. Children may have experienced significant strife, depending on how this information was handled within the family and whether it resulted in extramarital affairs or in the separation or divorce of their parents. Some children may have found out in early childhood, some during their own turbulent adolescent years, and some after they reached adulthood. In some cases, children of bisexual elders prevent them from having relationships with their grandchildren. When family support is lacking, establishing relationships between elderly and young sexual minority persons, such as teenagers or young adults from a community Pride center, high school Gay-Straight Alliance (GSA), or college LGBTIAQQ group, can provide intergenerational assistance not only for the older individuals but also for youth who lack approval from their own parents and grandparents.

LEGAL AND MEDICAL ISSUES AMONG THE BISEXUAL ELDERLY

Legal issues for the bisexual elderly are similar to those all sexual minority persons face. The inability to marry a same-sex partner means that the surviving partner cannot collect Social Security payments as a surviving spouse and may be denied other financial, legal, and medical rights before and following the partner's death. These legal issues become more problematic with age, because individuals become more likely to require the financial and legal benefits of recognized marriage as they age such as the right to control assets left in an estate and the right to make medical decisions for a partner who becomes incapacitated.

Many of the medical needs of bisexual older persons are similar to the needs of other elderly individuals. However, research has shown that sexual minority individuals underutilize medical resources (Institute of Medicine, 2011) for a number of reasons, including negative past experiences with intolerant medical practitioners, lack of health coverage due to lack of marriage rights, and a lower frequency of events, such as pregnancy, which often motivate heterosexual individuals to seek medical care (e.g., Diamant et al., 2000; Smith, Johnson, & Guenther, 1985). There is also some evidence of higher rates of smoking and alcohol use among some populations of sexual minority individuals than among their heterosexual peers (e.g., Diamant et al., 2000; Drabble, Midanik, & Trocki, 2005; Institute of Medicine, 2011; cf. Horowitz, Weis, & Laflin, 2001). This may be a result of the stress of social repression or because gay life was centered in the "bar scene" before the 1970s. Elderly bisexual persons may therefore experience both a greater morbidity from common conditions and a stronger reluctance to seek medical attention.

One specific area in which the needs of elderly sexual minority persons differ from the needs of elderly heterosexuals is sexual health. Elderly people often do not receive adequate sexual health care because health care providers assume that older persons are sexually inactive. Medical practitioners must avoid assuming that elderly patients are not sexually active and avoid assuming that any sexual activity among elderly patients is heterosexual. Older adults, who grew up during times when sexuality was not as openly discussed as it is currently, may be unwilling to discuss sexual issues with medical practitioners (Keppel & Firestein, 2006).

During medical examinations, older patients should be asked many of the same questions regarding sexual activity that younger patients are asked. Introductory questions could include, "Are you sexually active with any other person?" or "How long ago was your last sexual contact with another person?" An affirmative answer should be followed up with a question to elicit—without prejudice—information about both same- and other-sex activities, for example, "Are you sexually active with men, women, or both?" A patient who is married to someone of the other sex should not be assumed to be exclusively heterosexual. He or she may be bisexually identified and may be bisexually active. Conversely, a patient with a same-sex partner should be asked questions that would elicit information about any other-sex contacts and relationships. Bisexually active individuals may identify as heterosexual, lesbian, or gay. Therefore, a patient's stated sexual identity should not be interpreted to indicate his or her sexual behavior. Seemingly heterosexual patients and self-labeled lesbian and gay patients should be asked for information regarding both same- and other-sex contacts if they are sexually active. Many of the books and online resources listed at the end of this chapter can be used by medical practitioners to increase their knowledge, understanding, and comfort with bisexuality and with the needs of elderly bisexual patients.

All sexually active individuals, regardless of the gender of their partner, or partners, should receive accurate information about sexually transmitted infections, including HIV. Rates of HIV infection are increasing among elderly people, probably because the assumption that older persons are not sexually active and therefore not at risk has led to a lack of education about HIV in this population group (Ginty, 2004; Institute of Medicine, 2011). Elderly individuals who spent much of their adult lives in long-term partnerships and are now seeking new relationships—either because of partner death or a change in their own sexual identity—need to learn new sexual negotiation skills, including how to discuss safer sex. Elderly persons are less likely to use condoms for many reasons: postmenopausal women are not at risk for pregnancy, older adults often do not perceive that they are at risk for infection, HIV-prevention efforts do not target senior environments for HIV education and condom distribution, and decreased mobility can prevent seniors from discretely acquiring condoms. Medical service providers can help elderly bisexual patients and clients develop safer sex attitudes and practices, primarily by maintaining an awareness that they may be at risk for infection.

RESOURCES FOR ELDERLY BISEXUALS
AND FOR SERVICE PROVIDERS

Bisexual organizations and support groups exist in many areas of the United States. The Bisexual Resource Center (BRC) in Boston, Massachusetts, publishes a list of bisexual and bi-inclusive organizations around the world (www .biresource.org). LGBT community organizations can provide additional contact information for bisexual groups or for elderly LBGT groups, such as SAGE USA (Services and Advocacy for LGBT Elders, formerly Senior Action in a Gay Environment, sageusa.net). Universities and colleges also often have LGBT organizations or GSAs (Gay-Straight Alliances). Although the members of these organizations will be young adults, elderly individuals who lack relationships with their own grandchildren and young adults seeking support from an older generation may benefit from pursuing intergenerational friendships. The BRC website also offers downloadable pamphlets and information about bisexuality for both service providers working with bisexual clients and bisexual individuals. Elderly individuals able to travel may be interested in attending conferences on bisexuality. Information about upcoming conferences can be found through the BRC.

The internet provides a wealth of information and access to sources of support. Many isolated individuals, especially those belonging to small minorities, have been able to use the internet to find others like themselves for the first time.

The online bisexual community includes chat rooms, electronic mailing lists, and websites. The BRC website serves as a gateway to many resources. This website also features a bibliography, including books on bisexual health, audio books, fiction with bisexual characters or written by bisexual authors, and nonfiction, including anthologies "by and for" bisexual people.

Keppel and Firestein (2006) recommend the following books for bisexual elders: *Still Doing It: Men and Women over Sixty Write about Their Sexuality* by Joani Blank, *Getting Bi: Voices of Bisexuals around the World* by Robyn Ochs and Sarah E. Rowley, and *Growing Old Disgracefully* and *Disgracefully Yours* by the Hen Co-op. Other online resources for bisexual persons include BiNet USA at www.binetusa.org, the Bisexual Foundation at www.bissexual.org, and Gay & Gender Research at www.gaygenderresearch.org. Online resources for information about STD/HIV safety and other health issues include the San Francisco Department of Public Health at www.sfdph.org, Fenway Community Health at www.fenwayhealth.org, and HIV > 50 at www.hivoverfifty.org. Magazines and newsletters such as *BiNetUSA* are a source of up-to-date information about conferences, events, news, and people of interest to bisexual persons.

Professionals with bisexual clients currently have access to many resources. Most professional organizations in the social and psychological sciences have divisions, committees, or interest groups devoted to enhancing professional awareness of sexual minority needs. These include Division 44 of the American Psychological Association; the Caucus of Lesbian, Gay and Bisexual Psychiatrists of the American Psychiatric Association; the Lesbian, Gay, Bisexual, and Transgender Caucus of the American Sociological Association; and the Gay and Lesbian Medical Association at www.glma.org. Many books about bisexuality are directed toward professional audiences. For example, resources for psychotherapists include Beth Firestein's books *Bisexuality: The Psychology and Politics of an Invisible Minority* and *Becoming Visible: Counseling Bisexuals across the Lifespan* and Esther D. Rothblum and Lynne A. Bond's *Preventing Heterosexism and Homophobia*. To serve the elderly bisexual population well requires both information about the needs and concerns of bisexual elderly persons and comfort with—and an understanding of—this aspect of human sexuality.

REFERENCES

Almaguer, T. (1993). Chicano men: A cartography of homosexual identity and behavior. In H. Abelove, M. A. Barale, & D. M. Halperin (Eds.), *The lesbian and gay studies reader* (pp. 255–273). New York: Routledge.

Barón, A., & Cramer, D. W. (2000). Potential counseling concerns of aging lesbian, gay, and bisexual clients. In R. M. Perez, K. A. DeBoard, & K. J. Bieschke (Eds.), *Handbook of counseling and psychotherapy with lesbian, gay and bisexual clients* (pp. 207–223). Washington, DC: American Psychological Association.

Bem, S. L. (1974). The measurement of psychological androgyny. *Journal of Consulting and Clinical Psychology, 42*(2), 155–162.

Boswell, J. (1990). Sexual and ethical categories in premodern Europe. In D. P. McWhirter, S. A. Sanders, & J. M. Reinisch (Eds.), *Homosexuality/heterosexuality: Concepts of sexual orientation* (pp. 15–31). New York: Oxford University Press.

Boxer, A. M. (1997). Gay, lesbian, and bisexual aging into the twenty-first century: An overview and introduction. Coming of age: Gays, lesbians and bisexuals in the second half of life. *International Journal of Sexuality and Gender Studies, 2*(3/4), 187–197.

Burkhart, K. W. (1996). *Women in prison: Inside the concrete womb.* Boston: Northeastern University Press. (Original work published 1973)

Carrier, J. M. (1995). *De los otros: Intimacy and homosexuality among Mexican men.* New York: Columbia University Press.

Diamant, A. L., Wold, C., Spritzer, K., & Gelberg, L. (2000). Health behaviors, health status, and access to and use of health care: A population-based study of lesbian, bisexual, and heterosexual women. *Archives of Family Medicine, 9,* 1043–1051.

Diamond, L. M. (1998). Development of sexual orientation among adolescent and young adult women. *Developmental Psychology, 34,* 1085–1095.

Diamond, L. M. (2000). Sexual identity, attractions, and behavior among young sexual-minority women over a 2-year period. *Developmental Psychology, 36,* 241–250.

Diamond, L. M., & Savin-Williams, R. (2000). Explaining diversity in the development of same-sex sexuality among young women. *Journal of Social Issues, 56,* 297–313.

Drabble, L., Midanik, L. T., & Trocki, K. (2005). Reports of alcohol consumption and alcohol-related problems among homosexual, bisexual, and heterosexual respondents: Results from the 2000 National Alcohol Survey. *Journal of Studies on Alcohol, 66,* 111–120.

Firestein, B. A. (Ed.). (1996). *Bisexuality: The psychology and politics of an invisible minority.* Thousand Oaks, CA: Sage.

Firestein, B. A. (Ed.). (2007). *Becoming visible: Counseling bisexuals across the lifespan* (pp. 164–185). New York: Columbia University Press.

Gagnon, John H. (1990). Gender preference in erotic relations: The Kinsey scale and sexual scripts. In D. P. McWhirter, S. A. Sanders, & J. M. Reinisch (Eds.), *Homosexuality/heterosexuality: Concepts of sexual orientation* (pp. 177–207). New York: Oxford University Press.

Giallombardo, R. (1966). *Society of women: A study of a women's prison.* New York: Wiley.

Ginty, M. M. (2004). HIV/AIDS cases still rising among older women. *The Call* [Internet edition]. Kansas City, MO. Retrieved from www.kccall.com/News/2004/0326/Community/082.html

Goldberg, A. E. (2007). Talking about family: Disclosure practices of adults raised by lesbian, gay, and bisexual parents. *Journal of Family Issues, 28,* 100–131.

Horowitz, S. M., Weis, D. L., & Laflin, M. T. (2001). Differences between sexual orientation behavior groups and social background, quality of life, and health behaviors. *Journal of Sex Research, 38,* 205–218.

Institute of Medicine (IOM). (2011). *The health of lesbian, gay, bisexual, and transgender people: Building a foundation for better understanding* [Prepublication e-copy, uncorrected proofs]. Washington, DC: National Academies Press. Retrieved from www.nap.edu/catalog/13128.html

James, J. (1976). Motivations for entrance into prostitution. In L. Crites (Ed.), *The female offender* (pp. 177–198). Lexington, MA: D. C. Heath & Co.

Katz, J. N. (1995). *The invention of heterosexuality.* New York: Dutton.

Keppel, B., & Firestein, B. (2007). Bisexual inclusion in issues of LGBT aging: Therapy with older bisexuals. In B. Firestein (Ed.), *Becoming visible: Counseling bisexuals across the lifespan* (pp. 164–185). New York: Columbia University Press.

Kinsey, A. C., Pomeroy, W. B., & Martin, C. E. (1948). *Sexual behavior in the human male.* Philadelphia: W. B. Saunders.

Kinsey, A. C., Pomeroy, W. B., Martin, C. E., & Gebhard, P. H. (1953). *Sexual behavior in the human female.* Philadelphia: W. B. Saunders.

Klein, F. (1978). *The bisexual option: A concept of one-hundred percent intimacy.* New York: Arbor House.

Klein, F. (1990). The need to view sexual orientation as a multivariable dynamic process: A theoretical perspective. In D. P. McWhirter, S. A. Sanders, & J. M. Reinisch (Eds.), *Homosexuality/heterosexuality: Concepts of sexual orientation* (pp. 277–282). New York: Oxford University Press.

Klein, F., Sepekoff, B., & Wolf, T. J. (1985). Sexual orientation: A multivariable dynamic process. *Journal of Homosexuality, 11*(1/2), 35–49.

Magaña, J. R., & Carrier, J. M. (1991). Mexican and Mexican American male sexual behavior and spread of AIDS in California. *Journal of Sex Research, 28*(3), 425–441.

MetLife. (2010). *Still out, still aging: The MetLife study of lesbian, gay, bisexual, and transgender baby boomers.* Westport, CT: MetLife Mature Market Institute.

Pomeroy, W. B. (1972). *Dr. Kinsey and the Institute for Sex Research.* New York: Harper and Row.

Ritter, K. Y., & Terndrup, A. I. (2002). *Handbook of affirmative psychotherapy with lesbians and gay men.* New York: Guilford Press.

Rodríguez Rust, P. C. (2002). Bisexuality: The state of the union. *Annual Review of Sex Research, 13,* 180–240.

Rodríguez Rust, P. C. (2004, July). *Eye of the storm: Young adults creating sexual identity in a world of shifting sexual meanings.* Paper presented at the 31st annual meeting of the International Academy of Sex Research, Ottawa, Canada.

Rodríguez Rust, P. C. (2009). Bisexuality in a house of mirrors: Multiple reflections, multiple identities. In P. L. Hammack & B. J. Cohler (Eds.), *The story of sexual identity* (pp. 107–129). New York: Oxford University.

Ross, M. W. (1991). A taxonomy of global behavior. In R. Tielman, M. Carballo, & A. Hendriks (Eds.), *Bisexuality and HIV/AIDS: A global perspective* (pp. 21–26). Buffalo, NY: Prometheus Books.

Rothblum, E. D., & Bond, L. A. (Eds.). (1996). *Preventing heterosexism and homophobia* (pp. 87–123). Thousand Oaks, CA: Sage.

Rust, P. C. (1993). "Coming out" in the age of social constructionism: Sexual identity formation among lesbian and bisexual women. *Gender and Society, 7*(1), 50–77.

Rust, P. C. (1996a). Finding a sexual identity and community: Therapeutic implications and cultural assumptions in scientific models of coming out. In E. D. Rothblum & L. A. Bond (Eds.), *Preventing heterosexism and homophobia* (pp. 87–123). Thousand Oaks, CA: Sage.

Rust, P. C. (1996b). Monogamy and polyamory: Relationship issues for bisexuals. In B. Firestein (Ed.), *Bisexuality: The psychology and politics of an invisible minority* (pp. 127–148). Thousand Oaks, CA: Sage.

Rust, P. C. (2001). Two many and not enough: The meanings of bisexual identities. *Journal of Bisexuality, 1*(1), 31–68.

Smith, E. M., Johnson, S. R., & Guenther, S. M. (1985). Health care attitudes and experiences during gynecologic care among lesbians and bisexuals. *American Journal of Public Health, 75,* 1085–1087.

Smith-Rosenberg, C. (1975). The female world of love and ritual: Relations between women in nineteenth-century America. *Signs, 1*(1), 1–29.

Trumbach, R. (1977). London's sodomites: Homosexual behavior and Western culture in the 18th century. *Journal of Social History, 2,* 1–33.

Voeller, B. (1990). Some uses and abuses of the Kinsey scale. In D. P. McWhirter, S. A. Sanders, & J. M. Reinisch (Eds.), *Homosexuality/heterosexuality: Concepts of sexual orientation* (pp. 32–38). New York: Oxford University Press.

Weinberg, M. S., Williams, C. J., & Pryor, D. W. (1994). *Dual attraction: Understanding bisexuality.* New York: Oxford University Press.

Wooden, W. S., & Parker, J. (1982). *Men behind bars: Sexual exploitation in prison.* New York: Plenum Press.

CHAPTER SIX

Transgender and Aging

Beings and Becomings

TARYNN M. WITTEN, PH.D., L.C.S.W.,
AND A. EVAN EYLER, M.D., M.P.H.

The process of aging can be more complex for transgender and other gender minority persons than for members of normatively identified non-transgender populations (Witten, 2002a, 2002b, 2002c, 2003). There are also often significant differences between the concerns of transgender older adults and those of their lesbian, gay, and bisexual (LGB) peers because of the medical realities of physical gender transition and the associated difficulties that can occur in dependent care settings. During recent years, a number of works have been published that include transgender aging (Currah & Minter, 2000; Feldman & Bockting, 2003; Harcourt, 2006; Kimmel, Rose, & David, 2006; Institute of Medicine, 2011; Meezan & Martin, 2003; MetLife, 2010; National Gay and Lesbian Task Force, 2005; Shankle, 2006; Wallace, Cochran, Durazo, & Ford, 2011) though this remains an evolving and often poorly understood field. This chapter discusses the experiences and concerns of aging transgender and gender nonconforming persons, from midlife through old age and death.

Important principles gleaned from the available information about transgender and gender nonconforming older adults include the following:

- Transgender older adults are a heterogeneous group and are less likely to be "out" regarding the transgender history than their younger peers.
- Many transgender older adults have experienced discrimination or victimization both on the basis of gender (being identifiable as transgender or as women) and sexual orientation (being perceived as lesbians or gay men either before or after gender transition).
- Older adults who have transitioned gender are more likely than their LGB peers to be identifiable in medical settings because of the visible effects of surgery or having not had genital surgical transition.
- The need for ongoing hormonal support creates a medical and financial requirement throughout life that many fear will not be met in older age.
- Many older adults who have transitioned gender are fearful of being mistreated in care settings on the basis of the transgender presentation (including "anatomical mismatch"), some to the point of considering "de-transition" (resuming presentation in the birth-assigned gender), regardless of how dysphoric this may be, or suicide.
- Age at the time of transition significantly affects the life experience of transgender older adults.
- Transgender and gender-atypical older adults are becoming more visible and are facing these challenges with an emerging strength and voice.

In contemporary North American society, persons who identify as female-to-male (FTM) transgender, or transmen, often come out during their teens, 20s, or 30s, sometimes following a period of lesbian identification (Bockting & Coleman, 2007; Lev, 2004; Witten & Eyler, 1999). Individuals who identify as male-to-female (MTF) transgender, or transwomen, have more often attempted to conceal their gender variance for years or decades, sometimes delaying publicly coming out and sometimes suppressing the awareness of difference to themselves (Cole, Dallas, Eyler, & Samons, 2000). They may seek medical assistance for the physical aspects of gender transition during midlife or older age. Some transmen follow this pattern as well, particularly those attracted to males who manage to "pass" as heterosexual women for years (Bockting & Coleman, 2007). This is changing; greater numbers of adolescents, both FTM and MTF, are presenting for transgender-specific therapies and services (Zucker, 2004, 2005, 2007). However, the current cohort of transgender older adults has arrived in older age after either having transitioned gender during the younger adult years, which was fairly uncommon, or having transitioned during the more recent past. Some seek medical and mental health services related to gender transition in the final stages of life. They may not have previously done so or may have been dissuaded by other competing responsibilities. In some non-Western cultures, expression of gender variance can occur in a variety of ways and at a variety of times of life, and sometimes, though not always, integrates into the cultural structure in a positive and supportive way.

TRANSGENDER IDENTITIES AND NOMENCLATURE

It is beyond the scope of this book to present an exhaustive discussion of the concepts and construction of sex, gender, sexuality, and the body as they affect the production of transgender identities. Witten (2006a) reviews current literature in that regard (see also Roughgarten, 2005, and the *Standards of Care* of the World Professional Association for Transgender Health [WPATH, 2011], pp. 4–9).

The terminology of the transgender-identified population is culturally dynamic; meanings vary for personal and political reasons (Witten, 2003). Unpublished data from the TranScience Longitudinal Aging Research Survey study (TLAR, 1999) include more than 50 different terms respondents used to describe their gender, gender identity, or gender presentation. When the large number of non-Western, cross-gender identities is included, this number exceeds 200 worldwide (Witten, 2003). This diversity of gender referents is supported by the more recent results of an international survey (Witten, 2011). This chapter uses commonly understood Western terms and is not meant to exclude or to render invisible the experience of persons who describe their experience—or themselves—differently. Although this discussion will focus on the needs, experiences, and struggles of older persons who identify as transsexual or transgender, members of other gender minority population groups will be briefly discussed. As these terms do not have precise, fixed meanings, we begin by defining some of the terminology used in this chapter (see also Steckley, 2009; WPATH, 2011), recognizing that other authors or transgender older adults may define them somewhat differently.

Transsexual-identified persons experience variance between their natal sex (genital sex, birth body, "origin identity") and their psychological gender ("target identity"; Witten, 2005, 2006a; Witten & Eyler, 1999). Often, but not always, they seek medical sex reassignment ("realignment") services, including hormonal treatments, genital sex reassignment surgery (also called gender confirmation surgery, or gender affirmation surgery), and sometimes other procedures (such as female breast augmentation or male chest reconstruction, facial cosmetic surgery, and electrolysis), usually accompanied by a change in gender presentation or role (WPATH, 2011, p. 97).

Transgender is a general term with an evolving meaning. Kaufman (2008) notes that "transgender people are individuals who transgress societally constructed gender norms in one manner or another" and includes persons such as full-time cross-dressers, drag queens, drag kings, gender-blended people, and gender queers, as well as myriad other members of the "gender community" (Sims, 2007). Transgender persons often identify strongly with the "other" sex and adopt a lifestyle and appearance consistent with the psychological gender self-perception. This may be supported by hormonal medications without genital sex reassignment surgery. Some transgender-identified individuals eventually seek genital surgery; gender self-perception can have an element of fluidity over the life span. Some transgender persons present as members of their natal sex in certain situations for practical reasons, such as to avoid premature termination of employment or precipitating a family crisis.

The Harry Benjamin International Gender Dysphoria Association (Meyer et al., 2001, p. 4) notes:

> Between the publication of the DSM-III and DSM-IV, the term "transgender" began to be used in various ways. Some employed it to refer to those with unusual gender identities in a value-free manner—that is, without a connotation of psychopathology. Some people informally used the term to refer to any person with any type of gender identity issues. Transgender is not a formal diagnosis, but many professionals and members of the public found it easier to use informally than GID NOS [Gender Identity Disorder, Not Otherwise Specified] which is a formal diagnosis. (Meyer et al. 2001)

Given the lengthy history of assigning pathology to variation in sexual behavior or gender identity in the mental health and other health care professions, this broad definition, with its acknowledgment of the scope and import of gender variance, was significant. The most recent version of the *Standards of Care* (WPATH, 2011, 7th version) is even more straightforward, simply defining *transgender* as an "adjective to describe a diverse group of individuals who cross or transcend culturally defined categories of gender. The gender identity of transgender people differs to varying degrees from the sex they were assigned at birth" (Bockting, 1999; WPATH, 2011, p. 97).

People who *cross-dress*, or *cross-dressers*, usually cultivate the appearance of the other gender, particularly with regard to clothing and makeup. Cross-dressing may be undertaken part time or recreationally, such as at clubs and social events, and may or may not have erotic significance. Women who prefer men's clothing for comfort or practicality, but self-identify as fully female, are not usually considered cross-dressers (Witten & Eyler, 1999) nor are individuals who cross-dress only for erotic satisfaction, without other gender concerns. It is interesting to consider whether drag queens who take hormones to enhance their appearance for work and performance purposes, but regard themselves as members of their birth-assigned gender, are "expert cross-dressers" or are somewhat transgender. Similar discussions have been raised with regard to child and adolescent cross-gender dressing (Olson, Forbes, & Belzer, 2011) and in different cultural contexts (Nichols, 2010).

Clearly, the lines can be blurry at times, sometimes reflecting individual flexibility and sometimes further complicating practical matters in which identification can be important, such as hate crime prosecution.

The term *transvestite* derives from the diagnosis of psychopathology with functional impairment ("Transvestic Fetishism," American Psychiatric Association, 2000, pp. 574–575). It is generally considered pejorative, though some older adults who cross-dress use it more neutrally, and despite its negative connotations, some people who cross-dress have reclaimed it, much as many LGBT-identified persons have reclaimed the word *queer*. For example, British comedian Eddie Izzard has referred to himself as an "executive," or "action," transvestite, and candidly describes his sexuality: "I'm a straight transvestite or male lesbian. It seems we are beyond the idea that I am gay and hiding it. If I had to describe how I feel in my head, I'd say I'm a complete boy plus half a girl" ("Eddie Izzard," 2004). He has remarked in his shows, "Women wear what they want, and so do I." *Tranny*, short for "transsexual" or "transgender," is also being reclaimed in the United Kingdom but is still often considered insulting in the United States. A more thorough discussion of trans-identities in the United Kingdom is found in Monro (2003).

Specific terminologies have cultural impact. For example, in the Army Medical Services *Standards of Medical Fitness* (2002), the U.S. Army lumps transsexualism (which is increasingly considered a normal, human variation rather than a form of mental illness) with sexual paraphilias. The *United States Army Standards of Medical Fitness* (2002) states, in chapter 2-30 on "Psychosexual Conditions," that "the causes for rejection for appointment, enlistment, and induction are transsexualism, exhibitionism, transvestitism, voyeurism, and other paraphilias" (p. 13). Individuals who decide to transition gender or come out regarding their transgender identity while in the U.S. military service can be prosecuted under military law. Identified case law illustrates the military's use of LGB-based case law surrounding "cross-dressing" as the pathway to prosecute transsexual servicemen and servicewomen. Principal cases are *U.S. v. Guerrero* and *U.S. v. Modesto*. (See also Witten, 2007b, for an extensive discussion of gender identity and the U.S. Armed Forces.) This restriction is not shared worldwide; for example, in the Thai and Israeli armed services, transsexual military personnel are allowed to serve and are treated as members of their posttransition gender (Witten, 2007b).

On June 9, 2011, the Department of Veterans Affairs released VHA Directive 2011-024, "Providing Health Care for Transgender and Intersex Veterans," which mandates the delivery of respectful, confidential medical care for U.S. military veterans who are transgender identified or intersex, including mental health and general medical services needed for gender transition, except for sex reassignment surgical procedures. This directive applies to military veterans rather than currently enlisted military personnel, though its promulgation may signal the potential for active servicemen and servicewomen who are transgender to serve openly in the future. The 2011 repeal of the "Don't Ask, Don't Tell" policy for the United States uniformed services (in process at the time of this writing; Servicemembers Legal Defense Network, 2011) may provide indirect support for active service by transgender enlisted personnel, though it does not address gender identity directly.

Gender variance is sometimes conceptualized on a continuum (Eyler & Wright, 1997) or spectrum. Cross-dressing is often considered a form of gender variance, as are other social "gender transgressions," such as the evident male femininity and female masculinity sometimes seen among persons who do not identify as transgender. Bullough and Bullough (1993) noted, "The major area in which people depart from societal expectations is in sexual orientation . . . The second most common area of cross-gender behavior is in the area of the symbolic expression of gender through clothing (including jewelry, tattoos, and other adornments). A smaller group of cross-gendered people seek a complete and permanent identity as a member of the . . . [other] sex" (Bullough & Bullough, 1993, p. 313; see also Brown et al., 1996). Others consider gender as a multidimensional construct that is not captured by a binary (male/female, woman/man), a spectrum, or a representative act or action. Gender can be temporally dynamic, across the life span and in daily living, and can be understood as composed of several interacting facets, such as self-perception, self-presentation, or representation in society and response to that presentation (Witten, 2001).

The terms that describe gender identity evolve and change, reflecting the social and political emergence of persons whose gender self-perception is not adequately described by existing terminology and the evolving dialogue regarding gender identity in social and social science contexts. Some people feel they are not defined by usual understandings of man and woman, masculine and femi-nine, but are psychologically a blend of the two or are in some sense apart from both groups. This has been described as gender blended (e.g., Devor, 1989) and, more recently, as gender queer, particularly among adolescents and young adults (Welle, Fuller, Mauk, & Clatts, 2006). Whittle also notes that "many in the [transgender] community would see themselves as existing outside of gender, of being oppressed by it, but using its icons and signifiers to say who they are" (Whittle, 1996, p. 212). Indeed, some people who choose to live publicly in the gender usually associated with their natal sex, but who do not feel that this ad-equately captures the blended or "none of the above" nature of their gender self-perception, use this as a "flag of convenience" in superficial social and regulatory contexts.

The difference between self-understanding and public perception with regard to gender can also be significant, as described in the WPATH SOC (2011, p. 9):

> Other individuals affirm their unique gender identity and no longer consider themselves either male or female (Bornstein, 1994; Kimberly, 1997; Stone, 1991; Warren, 1993). Instead, they may describe their gender identity in specific terms such as transgender, bigender, or genderqueer, affirming their unique experi-ence that may transcend a male/female binary understanding of gender (Bock-ting, 2008; Ekins & King, 2006; Nestle, Wilchins, & Howell, 2002). They may not experience their process of identity affirmation as a "transition," because they never fully embraced the gender role they were assigned at birth or be-cause they actualize their gender identity, role, and expression in a way that does not involve a change from one gender role to another. For example, some youth identifying as genderqueer have always experienced their gender identity and role as such (genderqueer). Greater public visibility and awareness of gender diversity (Feinberg, 1996) has further expanded options for people with gender dysphoria to actualize an identity and find a gender role and expression that is comfortable for them.

Transgender is often used as a general term, meant to encompass everyone with a minority gender identity or gender self-perception, including persons who are transsexual or who have had sex reassignment surgery, as well as those who cross-dress or transgress gender norms in other significant ways. From a Western viewpoint, persons with cultural gender identities that are outside the dyadic female-feminine/male-masculine structure, such as the Hijra of India and Pakistan (discussed subsequently), may also be considered transgender.

THE (TRANS)GENDER COMMUNITY

The literature regarding gender minority persons and gender transition often refers to the *gender community*, referring either to all gender-variant persons, such as in a particular geographic area, or to persons who are identifiable—out—as transsexual, transgender, cross-dressing, or gender variant in some other way. This conceptualization is open to question, as many MTF and FTM individuals who have transitioned gender are not open about this aspect of personal history, wishing only to live fully in the true, or chosen, gender, without reminders of the pretransition gender. Their position in the cultural milieu may be similar to men and women who have had same-sex sexual experiences but are fully closeted and never identifiable as gay, lesbian, or bisexual. However, same-sex sexual expression does not require any alteration of the body, whereas gender transition usually does. In addition, medical treatments, although improving in quality, often leave detectable signs of the natal sex, such that a closeted transsexual person may be outed at any time, particularly in older age, as the need for medical services becomes more frequent and less predictable. *Gender community* can therefore be conceptualized as referring either to the self-identified gender minority population—the T people of LGBT—or to the larger population of gender-variant persons, including those who are posttransition and currently closeted or "living stealth."

As sexual diversity and gender variance become less stigmatized in the larger society, the number and proportion of gender minority persons is increasing. Thus, all terminology and conceptualizations regarding this population of people must be considered dynamic and evolving, as has been the case for lesbians and gay men. In reporting on gay male American culture in the early 1990s, Frank Browning described his work as "an inquiry into the faiths, practice, structure, and meanings of gay life in America, an exploration of the unwinding and reformulation of gender, the dissolution and reconstruction of family, the impulse toward community, the passage of generations, and an emerging reconciliation with death . . . inspired by scores of private lives that, intentionally or not, became the stuff of a social movement" (Browning, 1993, p. 1).

Transgender studies, the culture of transgender and the experience of gender variance in contemporary Western culture, are following a similar path, as the need to remain secretive about a universal aspect of the human psyche—gender identity and, therefore, gender variance—is dissipating somewhat. It is to be hoped that greater openness about gender identity and gendered experience will be increasingly available to gender minority persons in the years ahead. Unfortunately, this has not often been the experience of the current cohort of older adults, many of whom are still living stealth, despite the difficulties that this can cause in receiving medical, nursing, and other services.

GENDER IDENTITY IN A MULTICULTURAL CONTEXT

Population estimates for sexual and gender minority groups are difficult to obtain and verify primarily because of the currently stigmatized nature of homosexual, bisexual, transgender, and gender-variant identifications and behavior, as well as the lack of available resources for sexual or gender minority persons in many geographic regions. This often leads to private solutions such as passing as a member of the other sex without medical or mental health services and, consequently, to epidemiological invisibility. This occurs in a variety of forms and in many parts of the world (Witten et al., 2003) and is sometimes a result of data collection decisions by policy makers. Worldwide, large government-sponsored surveys regarding older adults almost never include options for gender identity other than female or male. For example, recent attempts by Brown, Brennan, and Witten (personal communication, 2011) to add gender and sexuality questions to the Health and Retirement Study (HRS), a longitudinal study sponsored by the National Institute of Aging (hrsonline.isr.umich.edu), were unsuccessful, though these items may be added in the future.

This discussion centers on Western views of gender and sexuality and the evolving LGBT aspects of contemporary culture. However, cultural dynamics can alter the expressions and interpretations of gender, gender identity, and sexuality. It is worth examining these cultural variations in light of parallel cultural views on aging and when working with patients or clients whose gender self-perception is rooted in a cultural framework that defines gender differently from majority Western culture. The current professional literature regarding gender variance is largely based on the experience of transgender persons, and the professionals who interact with them, in Western nations. Winter (2006b) points out that between 1992 and 2002 approximately 89% of the published articles concerning psychology and transgender were based on European and North American populations. Although progress in representing other cultures within the transgender literature has been made, this primacy is still present. There are many reasons for this besides the prominence of European and North American researchers, including cultural precepts concerning personal privacy, and fear of disclosure and its negative consequences, in many parts of the world (Witten, 2011).

The traditional Western view of gender is dichotomous (i.e., including only women and men). However, some other cultures, such as some Native American, Pan Asian, African, and South Pacific population groups, include alternate genders in their social organizations (Blackwood & Wieringa, 1999; Davis & Whitten, 1987; Elkins & King, 1996; Godlewski, 1988; Hoenig & Kenna, 1974; Kockett & Fahrner, 1988; Kröhn, Bertermann, Wand, & Wille, 1981; Langevin, 1983; Satterfeld, 1988; Sigusch, 1991; Tsoi, 1988; van Kesteren, Gooren, & Megens, 1996; Walinder, 1971, 1972; Weitze & Osburg, 1996; Witten et al., 2003). Therefore, the study of gender variance must be expanded to include persons whose gender self-perception is other than woman or man within a cultural context that includes more than these two gender groups. Recognition of the specific cultural populations present within the location in which one practices clinically can be an important aspect of cultural competence for transgender care and service provision. The following is a brief summary of some of the cultures that include alternate genders.

The Americas

Many indigenous peoples recognize gender groups other than women and men (Jacobs, Thomas, & Lang, 1997; Lang, 1990; Prince-Hughes, 1999). Some of the First Nations tribes historically identified many forms of gender identity (Blackwood, 1984; Fulton & Anderson, 1992; Murray, 1994). For example, traditional North American Tewa culture recognizes three genders: women, men, and *kwidó*. Kwidó persons have certain spiritual talents and are usually identifiable to adults in their lives by age 4 or 5 years (Jacobs & Cromwell, 1992). Other examples include the Chukchi people of the Artic regions (Balzer, 1996), who traditionally recognized seven genders in addition to women and men, and the MTF transgender *Berdache* of a number of tribal groups (Fulton & Anderson, 1992). (*Berdache* was a European term, based on intercultural confusion and is often considered pejorative. See Epple [1998] for a discussion of *alternate genders* and other terminology used instead of berdache.)

In South America, the cross-gendered priests of the Araucanian people are found in Chile, and the *travesti* (persons who are MTF transgender or cross-dressing) are found in many parts of Latin America (Kulick, 1998a, 1998b; Lancaster, 1998).

Southern Asia and the Middle East

In India (Gupta, Singh, & Rastogi, 1988; Jaffrey, 1997; Mahalingam, 2003), the *Hijra* define themselves as a third gender. Hijra (Agrawal, 1997; Bakshi, 2004; Baqi, Shah, Baig, Mujeeb, & Memon, 1999; Baskaran, 2004; Basu, 2001; Lal, 1999; Nanda, 1990, 1997, 2000) individuals are physical males or intersexed persons that identify as the "third sex" of India, Bangladesh, and Pakistan. They describe themselves as neither man nor woman, although they use the female pronoun and are referred to as female. In Hindu contexts, they belong to a special caste devoted to the mother goddess Bahuchara Mata. They are also known as the Tritiya-Prakriti (Wilhelm, 2004). The Indian government has recently protected the Hijra by granting them legal status as members of a third gender.

Cross-gender behavior in Turkey is somewhat less stigmatized than in some other parts of the Muslim world and is discussed in Atamer (2005); Yueksel, Kulaksizouglu, Tuerksoy, and Sahin (2000); and Yueksel, Yuecel, Tuekel, and Motavalli (1992).

Iranian LGBT persons, particularly natal males, are subject to severe persecution. For example, two Iranian gay teens reportedly were executed by hanging because of their homosexual identification ("Iran Executes Two Gay Teens in Public Hanging," 2005). However, medical sex reassignment is commonly practiced as a means of changing homosexuals to heterosexuals. As Ellison (2008) reported in his description of Tenaz Eshagian's 2008 documentary film *Be Like Others*: "Explaining the apparent paradox, one Muslim cleric says that while homosexuality is explicitly outlawed in the Qur'an, sex-change operations are not. They are no more an affront to God's will than, for example, turning wheat into flour and flour into bread. So while homosexuality is punishable by death, sex-change operations are presented as an acceptable alternative—as a way to live within a set of strict gender binaries, as a way to, well, live like others." This creates a complex situation in which some Iranian natal males seek gender transition medical services because they are MTF transgender, whereas others may be gay men who feel that sex reassignment is their only option for living without fear in their own country. An Iranian woman and her transman fiancé, who had been a close female friend for years prior to gender transition, petitioned for the legal right to marry in 2009. (See also Hines, 2006; Kurtz, 2000; Tait, 2009, for similar examples, including outside Iran.)

Pan Asia and Oceania

Sexual and gender diversity are widespread and sometimes relatively well-accepted in many Southeast and East Asian countries, including the Philippines, Malaysia, Cambodia, China, Japan, Indonesia, Singapore, Myanmar (Burma), Thailand, and in New Zealand, and the Pacific Islands (Johnson, Jackson, & Herdt, 2000; Transgender Asia, 2006).

Japanese culture contains a number of "folk categories" considered to be transgender, "such as *okama, gei bli, bur^bli* and *ny^h#fu*" (Lunsing, 2003; McLelland, 2004). Fans of Japanese anime state that the most powerful characters in anime are the cross-gender characters. Cross-gender behavior in Japan is discussed in Higashi, Nomiya, and Morino (2000); Kameya and Norita (2000); Leupp (1995); Mackie (2002); Nakamura and Matsuo (2003); Stringer (2000); and Sugihara and Katsurada (1999). The dynamics of cross-gender behavior in China are complex and are discussed in Chong (1990, 1991); Cui, Ren, Fang, and Xia (1998); Emerton (2004a, 2003b, 2006); Furth (1993); Li (2003); Ma (1997, 1999); Mackie (2002); Ng et al. (1989); Ruan (1991); and Ruan, Bullough, and Tsai (1989).

The transgender culture of Oman is discussed in Wikan (1977, 1991). Transgender Singapore is discussed in Kok (1993); Tsoi (1993); Tsoi, Kok, and Long (1977); and Tsoi, Kok, Yeo, and Ratnam (1995), and the transgender culture of Cambodia is discussed in Earth (2006). Myanmar (Burmese) cross-gender behavior is described in Coleman, Cogan, and Gooren (1992). In Malaysia, the *mak nyahs* are MTF transgender (Teh, 1998, 2001), and the *pak nyah* are FTM transgender, also known as *abang* (Teh, 2002). Indonesian cross-gender culture is discussed in Anderson (1996), and Beyrer (1998), Boellstaff (2001), and Filipino transgender identities are considered in Johnson (1997, 1998) and Tolentino (2000). Thai transpersons, *kathoey*, or "lady boys," are discussed in Costa and Matzner (2006), Ford and Kittisuksathit (1994), Humes (1996), Jackson (1995a, 1995b, 1997, 1998, 1999), Morris (1997), Sinnott (2000, 2004), ten Brummelhuis (1999), Totman (2003), and Winter (2005, 2006a, 2006b). The terminology for Thai transgender persons contains nearly 15 different descriptors.

Hawaii's *Mahu* are MTF transgender and still play an important role in traditional society (Matzner, 2001a, 2001b; Tengan, 2002). Alternate gender identities exist in the *Maori*, an indigenous New Zealand people, along with the *Mahu* (Ellison-Loschmann & Pearce, 2006; Williams, Labonte & O'Brien, 2003).

The traditional cultures of Tonga and Samoa identify the MTF *Fa'afafine* and FTM *Fa'afatama* as additional genders (Poasa & Blanchard, 2004; Schmidt, 2003; Zucker & Blanchard, 2003). Fa'afafine means "in the manner of a woman";

members of this alternate gender are usually interested in activities associated with women and are often sexually attracted to men. Although biologically male, most gender-identify either as fa'afafine or as women (Vasey & Bartlett, 2007). Although this is a heterogeneous group, many fa'afafine do not experience discomfort with their male sexual anatomy because, "in cultures like Samoa, where having a penis is not seen as incompatible with living socially 'in the manner of a woman,' many fa'afafine may 'feel like girls or women' but experience no discomfort with their sexed bodies" (Vasey & Bartlett, 2007).

Africa

More than 25 different cross-gender or minority gender identity groups have been identified in Africa, including the *Sango, Nkontana, Sekrata, Ndongo-l-echi-la*, and *Mudoko dako* (Murray & Roscoe, 1998). Little is known about African transgender elders, but some extremely concerning reports of antitransgender human rights abuses have surfaced in recent years.

> In Africa, transgender people are seriously punished for being who they are. While still with my parents, I was always beaten by my father for "behaving" like a boy. In school, the same story. While peeing one day my neighbour's daughter found me peeing while squatting and she screamed like she had seen a monster. I became the laughing stock of the village and I expelled myself because of the humiliation. I could speak the whole day about the discomforts I have suffered in life more because I am a transgender person. (Mukasa, 2006)

Mukasa documents a wide variety of abuses against transgender persons in Africa, including severe emotional harm, sexual and other physical acts of violence; discrimination; and persecution in school, in church, in other aspects of village life, and by police and government agencies. The status of transgender persons in many parts of Africa requires investigation and inclusion in the agendas of human rights organizations. This has not historically been an area of concern by the relevant agencies, though some progress is being made. On June 17, 2011, the United Nations Human Rights Council passed a resolution endorsing the rights of lesbian, gay, bisexual, and transgender persons, the first such achievement in the history of the United Nations ("UN Rights Body Hits Out against Violence Based On Sexual Orientation," 2011).

Understanding the dynamics of gender and culture will have potentially important effects on how gender-variant older persons are able to live and thrive, not only within their countries of origin but also cross-culturally, as they move from one part of the world to another (Davis & Whitten, 1987; Puar, 2001). In many parts of the world, certain groups of transgender older adults are at particularly high risk for poor health and social outcomes. For example, elder transgender-identified persons who are disabled (Hines, 2007; Morgan, Mancl, Kaffar, & Ferreira, 2011), HIV positive (Clements-Nolle, Marx, Guzman, & Katz, 2001), members of disadvantaged racial and ethnic groups (Nemoto, Operario, Keatley, Han, & Soma, 2004a; Nemoto, Operario, Keatley, Nguyen, & Sugano, 2005; Nemoto, Operario, Keatley, & Villegas, 2004b), working in the sex industry (Clements-Nolle et al., 2001), incarcerated (Alexander & Meshelemia, 2010; Brown & McDuffie, 2009; Jenness, 2010; Linder, Enders, Craig, Richardson, & Meyers, 2002; Philips et al., 2010; Rickard & Rosenberg, 2007), or military veterans (Witten, 2007b) face additional obstacles to peaceful and successful aging and deserve additional study and practical assistance.

GENDER IDENTITY, POPULATION COHORTS, AND AGING

Little research-based information is available regarding the life course concerns faced by transgender individuals in mid- to late life (Witten, 2004), as this group has been particularly "epidemiologically invisible" (Shankle, Maxwell, Katzman, & Landers, 2003; Witten & Eyler, 1999; see also Institute of Medicine, 2011, and WPATH, 2011, pp. 4–9), with many older adults who have transitioned gender preferring to conceal this history (i.e., by "going stealth"; Witten, 2003). Recent studies (Whittle, 2007) are beginning to shed light on the lives of people in this demographic group. Most out (i.e., publicly identified), transgender, or gender-nonconforming persons are young and middle adults, many of whom have chosen to be politically active on behalf of the transgender community or involved in other LGBT causes. In contrast, many older adults who have transitioned gender no longer consider themselves trans-identified and therefore do not participate in research studies of the transgender or LGBT communities, as exemplified in these quotations from Witten (2011):

> I almost didn't take your survey. I do not identify as trans. I am a woman who was born a man. I've taken care of the problem and now I am a woman.

> Please stop using the umbrella term transgender. There has always been but [sic] a growing group of people will not take this survey (I almost didn't) because of the blanket use of the term transgender. It erases an entire group of people.

My worst fear? . . . that this soup I've bee[n] coopted into will erase my being seen for what I am. A straight heterosexual woman and my fear is the social backlash will revoke my leagal [*sic*] rights and cast me as some wanker in a dress and my husband as gay.

The current cohort of older gender minority persons has arrived in the elder years through several life course paths. These include

- growing up in a culture that acknowledges transgender or minority gender identities as at least marginally acceptable, and growing old in that culture;
- transitioning in young or middle adulthood and growing old in the true gender, either "out" or as a "stealth" transgender-identified person;
- coming out or transitioning gender later in life and therefore experiencing a shorter period of time in the true gender or gender of choice; and
- remaining unaware of the true gender (not out even to oneself) until later in life, sometimes followed by transition in the older adult years or at least by some private true-gender expression.

These different possibilities play an important role in the aging experience of transgender-identified persons. The influence of the historical cohort is also crucial. For example, individuals who came out or transitioned in the 1990s had very different experiences than those who did so during the 1950s. The impact of these life paths on the present quality of life of older transgender persons remains to be well addressed in clinical and social science research. Nonetheless, in an era in which forecasting the health status of elderly populations and recognizing disparity among different subpopulations of older persons are increasingly important (Anderson, Bulatao, & Cohen, 2004; Manton, Singer, & Suzman, 1993), preliminary discussions regarding the life experience and concerns of older gender minority persons should be undertaken (Witten, 2003, 2004), even as additional studies are planned. As one respondent in Witten (2011) stated:

Aging and end of life issues are extremely important for people. Many must draw final emotional and spiritual conclusions about our lives and how we experience those final days. For all of us who have outlived our partners and friends we need others in the LGBTIQ community who accept us to be the family we have outlived, and creating alternative formal relationships to supplant the ones society denies us is all important. Old age is a time of extreme vulnerability to the same degree that infancy is, but the elderly lives are devalued in comparison. We need to change this, along with far more cultural competency demands and trainings for health care and mental health providers for the services we cannot provide in the LGBTIQ community. We need more trans-research. Thank you for doing this survey.

Much of the currently available information consists of case reports and discussions of clinical experience, although larger studies are in progress. One of the challenges of more extensive survey research projects is that they are usually aimed at the LGBTQ populations rather than the transgender communities exclusively, so questions and their wording may not accurately capture the responses of the transgender and gender atypical respondents. Conversely, trans-specific surveys often have relatively low response rates, for reasons discussed earlier in this chapter.

Gerontological research has demonstrated the importance of life course events on the aging process. For example, factors such as socioeconomic status, severity of past abuse and victimization, experiences of prejudice and discrimination, and the presence of depression have been demonstrated to mediate later life mortality, morbidity, and quality of life. Data from the gerontological literature contain a well-documented fact base, supporting the argument that social conditions (Kubzansky, Berkman, & Seeman, 2000), social network support (Everard, Lach, Fisher, & Baum, 2000; Pinquart & Sorenson, 2000), socioeconomic status (Rautio, Heikkinen, & Heikkinen, 2001), and even social role (Krause & Shaw, 2000) can have significant positive or negative impact on mortality, morbidity, health status, depression prevalence, overall psychological well-being (Zhang & Hayward, 2001), successful aging, and numerous other life course outcomes of current importance in public health policy, such as are reflected in the objectives of *Healthy People 2020* (U.S. Department of Health and Human Services, 2010).

Results of these studies can be summarized as follows: The lower the income, the less social support (e.g., friends, spiritual activity, supporting organizations, neighbors one can depend on), the less habitable the social conditions (e.g., isolation, poor environment), the lesser the educational attainment, then the higher the risk for psychological dysfunction, long-term poor quality of life, poor health status, increased morbidity and mortality, and the less likely the person is to become "a successful ager" in the sense of the MacArthur Foundation's Successful Aging Project.

Central themes in the lives of gender minority persons include fear of violence and discrimination, and fear of inappropriate or abusive care in mental health, medical, and nursing care settings. This is usually based on personal experience or that of friends (Witten, 2004, 2011). This is particularly significant for transgender older adults, who have often been recipients of stigmatization or abuse related to gender identity or gender presentation at multiple times of life. The current cohort of older persons also came of age during eras when gender transition was not an option for most people and when gender variance was regarded both as evidence of mental illness and as an acceptable excuse for hate crime violence (Kidd & Witten, 2007b; National Coalition of Anti-Violence Programs, 2009). Many identified as gay or lesbian, either before or after transition, and therefore experienced discrimination and sometimes violence on that basis as well. In addition, physical evidence of gender transition is often readily apparent in care settings, further enhancing the vulnerability of trans older adults who have been living stealth:

> My worst fear is how I may be treated as a result of my half male / half female anatomy and how my spouse might be treated as a result of this. I worry that I may be denied care or treated roughly or neglected if I am unable to self-advocate. I worry about the lack of knowledge of the effects of long-term hormone treatments on transsexuals [sic] bodies and brains. I worry that my spouse will decide she needs to return to being a visible lesbian and leave me. I worry that I will never be able to afford GRS [gender/genital reassignment surgery] and when/if I am able to afford it, that I will be too old or unhealthy to get it done anyway . . . Mostly, I worry about leaving my family without means to survive after I am dead.

> I'm angry about conditions for aging in general as well as specifically for GLBTQ people in nursing homes, hospitals and assisted living facilities.

> I feel that as a disabled trans person I will be treated disrespectfully at best . . . I shudder to think whats [sic] going to happen when im [sic] less able to self advocate.

The next section contains basic information regarding antitransgender violence and abuse and a brief discussion of its ramifications for older persons.

ANTITRANSGENDER MISTREATMENT, ABUSE, AND THREAT

Members of any stigmatized group are at higher risk for victimization than those who do not bear the burden of stigmatization, prejudice, or hatred. Global, gender-based violence and abuse is well-documented (World Health Organization, 2007).

Kidd and Witten (2007a) argue that, from a global perspective, violence against transgender and gender nonconforming people can be seen as a form of genocide in need of intervention on a multinational scale. Although gender minority persons may be respected and valued in some indigenous cultures, violence and abuse against transgender persons, including transgender older adults, is a substantial problem in the United States, many Western nations, and many other parts of the world (Witten, 2011; Witten & Whittle, 2004).

Persons who are transgender or who do not conform to expected gender roles often experience stigmatization and abuse, sometimes beginning early in life, when gender nonconformity becomes evident. (See Perrin, 2002, pp. 5–22, 49–69, for a cogent discussion of the "different child" as applied to children with gender atypical characteristics, many of whom become gay or lesbian adults or, less commonly, transgender adults.) These experiences can subsequently influence self-perception and development of minority identification, as well as quality of life over the life span, including increased morbidity and mortality in later life. In his doctoral dissertation, Valentine (2000) points out that a principal "common binding" of the identifiable transgender community is the experience of violence and abuse (see also Witten, 2004). Although the extent of this problem remains to be fully determined, existing evidence suggests that it is widespread (Kidd & Witten, 2007a, 2007b; Lombardi, Wilchins, Priestling, & Malouf, 2001; Witten & Eyler, 1999; Xavier & Simmons, 2000). The large and growing literature on violence based on actual or perceived sexual orientation, or "queerness," supports this view (see Bowles, 1995; Dittman, 2003; Dunbar, 2006; Herek, 1989, 2009; Herek, Cogan, & Gillis, 2002; Herek, Gillis, Cogan, & Glunt, 1997; Jenness, 2003; Los Angeles County Commission on Human Relations, 2006; Mansey, 2006; Mason, 2005; McPhail, 2002; McPhail & DeNitto, 2005; Moran & Sharpe, 2004; Nolan, Akiyama, & Berhanu, 2002; Otis, 2007; Patton, 2006; Rubenstein, 2004; Schrank, 2007; Seelau & Seelau, 2005; Sisk, 2006a; Tomsen & Mason, 2001).

Black's Law Dictionary (Garner, 1999) defines *hate crime* as "a crime motivated by the victim's race, color, ethnicity, religion or national origin." In recent decades, some states and jurisdictions within the United States have expanded hate crimes statutes to include gender, gender identity, and other personal attributes (Transgender Law and Policy Institute, 2006). Hate crimes based on the (actual or perceived) sexual orientation or gender identity of the victim have historically not been well addressed in federal law. However, on October 28, 2009, President Obama signed into law Public Law No. 111-84 (United States Government Printing Office, 2009), the Matthew Shepard and James Byrd, Jr.

Hate Crimes Prevention Act. This statute expanded the demographic groups covered by hate crime legislation in the United States. On this basis, the U.S. Department of Justice currently has the power to investigate and prosecute violent crimes based on the victim's actual or perceived race, color, national origin, religion, gender, gender identity, sexual orientation, or disability, and to pursue investigations not undertaken by local authorities. Statistics about hate crimes based on these characteristics are kept by the FBI.

Unfortunately, despite the apparent legal clarity regarding hate crimes, Perry (2005–2006) points out that academicians, politicians, the media, and the public do not always use the word *hate* in a conceptually uniform way. Recently, critics of hate crimes laws have adopted an emotive, individualized conceptualization of "hate," maintaining that to prosecute a hate crime is to criminalize "thought" and "belief" (Rosebury, 2003, p. 37). This reductionist interpretation inappropriately broadens the phrase "hate crime" to describe any crime motivated by dislike of another person. Perry points out that hate crimes are not based simply on emotive responses but are a manifestation of power and assertion of one's own identity over the identity of another. She also demonstrates that reducing a hate crime to an emotional dislike of another person narrowly pathologizes the perpetrator as an unstable individual acting out irrationally when, in reality, "racist or gendered violence, for example, is not aberrant. It is not un-usual or ab-normal in cultures like ours, that is, in cultures which are permeated by bigotry and prejudice" (Rosebury, 2003, p. 125). Therefore, a hate crime is more accurately depicted as "rational, at least within the world view of the perpetrator" (p. 125). This sociological and cultural rather than individualist or even psychodynamic conceptualization of "hate" is the basis of the legal distinction between hate crimes and other types of violent crime. Public Law No. 111-84 reflects the sociological conceptualization of hate crimes, that is, crimes in which the victim is selected as a member of a group.

The following examples of antitransgender hate crime illustrate the difference between violent acting out based on dislike of another person and criminal behavior based on the decision of the perpetrator (usually a heterosexually identified male) to intimidate, to brutalize, or to murder the victim, either to punish the person for his or her "difference" or to psychologically eliminate or "erase" the minority identity. Some crimes also illustrate the perpetrator dynamic of combining hatred of the transgender identity of the victim and the sense of betrayal and disgust when the victim's genital anatomy (a fundamental aspect of the transgender experience) is revealed.

— *August 12, 2002:* Two MTF transgender teens were shot 10 times as they sat in the front seat of their vehicle in a Washington, D.C., neighborhood. This was the third antitransgender shooting in Washington, D.C., that week. (Fahrenthold, 2002)

— *October 4, 2002:* A 15-year-old young transwoman named Gwen Araujo, was beaten, tied up, and strangled by four men in Newark, California, after her male sexual anatomy was revealed. Two of the convicted perpetrators had had sex with Araujo during the summer of 2002. (Locke, 2006)

— *Summer 2005:* Three transgender people were sexually assaulted at gunpoint in San Diego, California. The Associated Press (2006) reported that prosecutors felt that the perpetrator preyed on people who were less likely to report crimes and threatened to kill them.

— *April 2011:* A 22-year-old transgender woman was beaten in the restroom at a McDonald's restaurant in Rosedale, Maryland. The assault was captured on video and uploaded onto the internet, despite her pleas to stop both the attack and the filming. She reported that her experience would have been even worse, but an older female customer came to her aid. ("Chrissy Lee Polis, Victim in Maryland McDonald's Attack, Alleges Hate Crime," 2011)

Additional examples and expanded explanatory material can be found on the Remembering Our Dead website (rememberingourdead.org). Remembrance events, honoring the lives of trans-identified persons who had been killed because of their transgender identity or presentation, were sponsored by Gender Education and Advocacy from the late 1990s through 2007 (Gender Education and Advocacy, 2011).

One aspect of antitransgender acts of violence that supports their inclusion as hate crimes is the extreme intensity of brutality that is sometimes used, such as strangulation, mutilation, and group or multiple rape. This can reflect the desire to deface and mutilate the bodies of transgender people because they challenge the normative worldview of the perpetrator with respect to gender, including the perpetrator's self-construct of his own gender identity and sexuality. Some perpetrators also express a profound visceral disgust with the gender expression, in combination with the genital anatomy, of their victims. The desire to remove from society the group of people that provokes such disgust motivates some assailants to acts of shocking brutality. This is not dissimilar to feelings expressed by some perpetrators of hate crime violence based on the sexual orientation of the victim, particularly against gay men, and of some perpetrators of sexual brutalization and murder of non-transgender women, most of whom are also heterosexually identified men.

The pervasive psychological burden of prejudice and the potential for hate crime victimization on transgender persons is evident. For example, one 50-year-old transwoman reported (in Wave 1 of the TranScience Longitudinal Aging Research Survey, or TLARS) that "every time I leave the house I leave with three strikes against me. I can be raped for being a woman. I can be raped and murdered because I am perceived as 'gay' (a drag queen) or I can be violently murdered because I am read as trans." Individuals who responded to the TLAR survey questions as having suffered some sort of violence were asked a series of clarifying items that addressed whether respondents believed that any of these acts of violence constituted "hate crimes," and approximately 70% reported that they believed that this was the case. Other research findings are similar. The National Coalition of Anti-Violence Programs (2009) found that 12% of anti-LGBT bias crimes tracked by that organization in 2008 had transgender victims.

The results of the Washington Transgender Needs Assessment Survey (Xavier & Simmons, 2000) are equally disturbing, particularly regarding difficulties that respondents reported encountering when they sought help from appropriate authorities following experiences of victimization; about two-thirds of respondents who had been criminally victimized reported dissatisfaction with the actions taken in their case or cases. In approximately 13% of crimes included in the 2009 study of the National Coalition of Anti-Violence Programs, the victim contacted police, who refused to take a report. In the Wave 1 TLARS, many respondents who had been victimized reported that they did not take any action because they believed that they would not be listened to or taken seriously. Because many crimes against gender and sexual minority persons go unreported, in part because of fears of further mistreatment by law enforcement, health care, and social services personnel, high-profile crimes, such as murders, must be regarded as the "tip of the iceberg" with regard to victimization of transgender persons. Public Law No. 111-84 will likely improve the response to victims of hate crimes over time, but at present, much room for improvement remains.

Although (MTF) transwomen are almost certainly victimized more frequently during adulthood than (FTM) transmen, Kidd and Witten (2007a, 2009) documented that transmen (and boys) also suffer abuse based on transgender personal attributes. The following examples are taken from their research and from the TLAR project (spelling and grammar preserved as written by the respondent):

When I was about 14, a boy (stranger) asked me if I were a boy or a girl. When I didn't answer, he threatened to shove his hand in my pants, "to see if there is a hole there." I punched him and ran. (Kidd & Witten, 2007a, p. 39)

Once arrested and had police physically assault, sexual abuse (inappropriate touching, removing my clothing in front of other inmates) and repeatedly threaten to rape me, due to my ambiguous gender presentation. (Kidd & Witten, 2007a, p. 39)

As is often the case among their transwomen peers, many study participants chose not to report these crimes. One respondent simply stated, "It felt pointless. I don't think they could've really done anything except make me feel worse about it" (Kidd & Witten, 2007b).

Rubenstein (2002) also highlights the underreporting of anti-LGBT hate crimes. He points out that, unlike victims of hate crimes based on race or (normative) gender, LGBT victims must essentially "come out" to law enforcement to report the crime. This can be extremely stressful for persons who are already in emotional distress from the aftermath of the crime. Public openness regarding one's transgression of society's gender and sexuality norms can also carry additional risks and increase the likelihood of future hate crime victimization (Kidd & Witten, 2007a), as some "nontraditional" victims receive little public sympathy and may become targets for additional abuse.

As is the case for many of their LGB peers, members of the transgender community often exist in a social environment that carries with it implicit concerns about violence and abuse or the fear thereof. These concerns must be managed on a day-to-day basis. This burden, and other problems that affect physical and mental health, all have an effect on the life course of transgender persons and affect the generative processes of aging. Further, the concerns of transgender persons must, by their nature, influence the lives of others that they touch, as well as others in the community (Witten, 2006b, 2009). Thus, the well-being of gender minority persons, and the protection of their rights, affects the fabric of society, because of the "connectedness of human social networks" (Barabási, 2009) and because good treatment of persons lower in the power hierarchy bodes well for the culture as a whole. (See Cronin & King, 2010, for a discussion of power, inequality, and identification among LGB adults.)

Human social progress, worldwide, is impeded by tolerance of hate crimes and suppression of members of minority groups, including sexual and gender minorities. According to the Human Rights Watch, hate crime victimization not only threatens the safety of transgender people but also detrimentally affects the greater pursuit of civil liberties, public health, and democratic governance, both by gender minority persons and by others in the larger society. In their online information about the Matthew Shepard and James Byrd, Jr. Hate Crimes Prevention Act, the Human Rights Campaign (2010, www.hrc.org) notes that "a hate crime occurs when the perpetrator of the crime intentionally selects the victim because of who the victim is. Hate crimes rend the fabric of our society and fragment communities because they target an entire community or group of people, not just the individual victim."

The legacy of stigmatization, prejudice, and victimization can have a profound negative impact on the well-being of transgender older adults, including physical and mental health, social success, and financial stability. Witten (2011) found much higher rates of financial distress than would be expected in her sample of transgender older adults, including among respondents who identified as white/European American and had had fairly normative work histories. In addition, some elderly transgender people also suffer abuse during later life, and their access to medical and mental health services may be reduced because of their transgender status (Bradley, 1996; Cahill, South, & Spade, 2000; Cook-Daniels, 1995; Cook-Daniels & Munson, 2008; Witten, 2002a, 2003, 2004; Witten & Whittle, 2004) or ability to afford care. Many transgender older adults consider suicide (Witten, 2011) as a result of these factors, particularly if they perceive the future as likely to be even harsher or more problematic than the present.

The health professions, including medicine, nursing, psychology and social work, and the system of health care delivery, are not immune from participating in antitransgender prejudice and mistreatment and sometimes fail to take an active role in ameliorating the many problems faced by transgender older adults. Many transgender-identified individuals have experienced subtle discrimination or more overt abuse by health care professionals. Mistreatment reported by the current cohort of transgender older adults includes traumatic mental health treatment during childhood or adolescence aimed at eliminating the gender variance; traumatic mental health treatment in adulthood, in which the person seeking treatment developed worsened emotional distress because of the beliefs of the therapist about gender identity or roles; denial of needed health care services, including care that was not related to the gender variance, due to anti-transgender (or anti-homosexual) bias; and pediatric surgery with subsequent problematic consequences (in cases with both an intersex [disorder of sexual development, or DSD] physical condition and transgender identification; Greenberg, 1998; Intersex Society of North America, 2007).

Problems with physical and mental health care reflect the larger societal dynamics and prejudices of the era in which they occur. Transgender older adults were children and adolescents during times when it was considered caring and appropriate for parents, therapists, and others to attempt to increase gender conformity and eliminate nonconformity in gender presentation and gendered behavior, largely due to the belief that this would prevent the child from growing up to be homosexual—a dreaded outcome. However, sexuality and gender identity are frequently less malleable than was believed, and people experiencing these interventions often developed increased shame regarding personal difference and guilt over the inability to change. The following are examples from Witten (2008):

> Went to counseling—and was taken out of the home at age 15 to mental hospital—Went back home for 5 months—went back to hospital and then to foster parents.

> They [my therapists] would try to convince me to remain a man (biological sex) as it would be the most healthful and totally discourage any cross dressing.

Cultural and subcultural beliefs and biases also influence the experience of gender minority persons across the life span, with additional health consequences occurring during older adulthood. For example, one FTM TLAR survey respondent stated,

> It is always important to realize that, within the trans-population, different sub-populations will have different health care related problems . . . Add to this the difficulty of FTMs who have taken only hormones but could not afford or do not want surgeries [and therefore are identifiable whenever they seek services]. Billy Tipton [the famous jazz vocalist who transitioned female-to-male without treatment in the 1930s] comes to mind as one who never accessed health care in his lifetime and probably died prematurely because of it.

System-based change during very recent years has improved health and mental health data gathering on behalf of LGBT persons, including transgender older adults, at least to a degree. For example, the Gay and Lesbian Medical Association stated in a 2000 report that the federal government routinely renders the LGBT population "invisible" through lack of data gathering, legal recognition, and other policies. Belongia and Witten (2006) pointed out that practices such as these implicitly sanction anti-LGBT behaviors. However, LGBT health concerns have been included in recent governmental and other policy papers (e.g., *Healthy People 2020*), including some that specifically address the experiences, needs, and resiliency of older adults (Institute of Medicine, 2011; MetLife, 2010). The last decade has shown substantial progress in both health services and health research on behalf of transgender older adults, though much more is needed in order to bring health care options and health outcomes up to standards expected in majority culture.

SOCIAL INFLUENCES ON TRANSGENDER OLDER ADULT WELL-BEING

From a sociological perspective, it is well documented that "health" is positively correlated with position in the societal power hierarchy. For example, Marmot and McDowall's (1986) Whitehall study of more than 10,000 British civil servants over a two-decade period demonstrates an obvious "'gradient' in mortality from top to bottom" of the study hierarchy (Evans, Barer, & Marmor, 1994; Marmot, Kogevinas, & Elson, 1987). Hertzman (2001) further notes that "examples show that major shifts in the health status of whole populations over time do not necessarily depend upon the implementation of public health or medical control measures against specific diseases." They point, instead, to a profound linkage between health and the social environment, including levels and distribution of prosperity in a society. Hence, social environment as mediated by position in the power hierarchy profoundly affects health status. Currently, many, though by no means all, sexuality and gender minority persons are occupying positions low in the social hierarchy or lower than their educational attainments or birth status would predict.

Demographic variables such as socioeconomic status and race also influence the aging experience of transgender persons. A National Gay Task Force–commissioned study (Battle, Cohen, Warren, Ferguson, & Audam, 2002) provides one of the first glimpses into a national, multicity sample of black gay, lesbian, bisexual, and transgender people. This study examines family structure, sexual identity, political behavior, racism and homophobic bias, and policy priorities of more than 2,500 African-American LGBT people that attended Black Gay Pride celebrations in nine cities during the summer of 2000. The effects of racial identification and racism can also be found in the data of the Washington Transgender Needs Assessment Study (Xavier & Simmons, 2000). Results from this survey research document significantly lower levels of educational attainment, gainful employment, and income among minority-identified transgender persons. As is often the case, the effects of multiple minority identifications and poverty are synergistic with regard to increasing risk status and promoting poorer outcomes in older years. Additional research on behalf of specific racial and cultural groups within the larger population of gender minority persons is needed, though some progress has been made during recent years.

Advantages most often enjoyed in majority culture also benefit transgender older adults who share similar histories. Careful study of both the TLARS and the Trans-MetLife Survey data (Witten, 2011) indicate that elders who responded positively about their aging and transition experiences had higher overall incomes, were most often white/European ancestry and MTF, had higher educational attainment, and had come out later in life—and therefore had enjoyed the benefits of being perceived as white men with education for a greater proportion of their lives. Respondents who transitioned later in life would also have had greater opportunity to build up a savings cushion and gain access to retirement benefits, and to finish child rearing, before experiencing the discrimination that often accompanies gender transition or transgender status.

Recent data (Witten, 2011) suggest that transgender older adults share many concerns with their non-transgender peers, including worries about future financial support, later-life care, loss of family and friends, and access to spiritual and religious support. In addition, transgender elders, particularly those who have not enjoyed many advantages earlier in life, often describe a more pervasive and profoundly fearful perspective about the future. Concerns include being mistreated because of anti-transgender bias in the context of incapacity and loss of control, lack of privacy as a transperson, and loss of family and religious support:

> If I am placed in a care facility, being mistreated by staff, including not being humanely cared for as a transsexual female, not being properly prepared for burial as a Jewish female.

> . . . in what ward would they put me, male of female?

> Having genitals that don't fit my external appearance and being abused, mistreated or neglected as a result.

> I am afraid of being separated from my partner and of being forcibly "de-transitioned" if my care providers are transphobic.

> Having care givers shave my face and put me in a dress because I have not had lower surgery.

Some survey respondents (Witten, 2011) were so deeply concerned that they were considering suicide prior to the onset of debility to avoid these outcomes.

Transgender older adults who had not yet completed gender transition some-times also expressed the fear that they would never be able to do so prior to the end of life.

Resilience is also evident in this population. Many respondents reported rely-ing on religious faith or on the wisdom gained during a challenging life to manage these concerns. One transgender elder reported that "belief in Christ Jesus . . . gives me peace and purpose to carry on to the end and faithfully finish the course." Another offered this advice: "Be who you are and enjoy life because its [sic] way too short. I have been every where in the world and American [sic] is a great place. We still have a ways to go when it comes to equal rights . . . I chose to focus on the good and positive of life. I do a lot of outreach, speaking at universi-ties about transgender and crossdressing . . ." Pervasive worry regarding legitimate concerns, and substantial coping abilities, are both apparent in the perspectives of the current cohort of transgender older adults.

Despite the difficult lives of many gender minority persons, health and ser-vice professionals and social scientists must remain cognizant of the spectrum of possible outcomes for this population. Although many transgender persons in the United States are crushed with the burdens of poverty, multiple victimiza-tions, and HIV, gender minority people with higher educational attainment and financial resources frequently age successfully, and many who have not had these advantages also live into the older adult years and often do surprisingly well. In addition, young persons who are currently transitioning gender sometimes re-port much better life experiences than their older peers.

The concerns of transgender persons in midlife and the older adult years are considered next. A recent large study of the concerns of Americans in the midlife years, *Still Out, Still Aging: The MetLife Study of Lesbian, Gay, Bisexual and Transgender Baby Boomers*, found that "LGBT Boomers are much like the rest of the population," in their concerns and challenges (MetLife, 2010, p. 2), but spe-cific differences exist and warrant examination.

MIDLIFE TRANSGENDER CONCERNS

Middle adulthood is a time in which some tasks of adulthood are completed and other new challenges faced. However, individual paths vary greatly and tasks can overlap. For example, many people in their 40s, 50s, and 60s complain that they have become responsible for elderly parents at a time when their adult children are not yet fully emotionally and financially independent. One traditional life cycle task of this period is "launching" adult children and realigning family roles

(Carter & McGoldrick, 1999, p. 287). Tasks of this phase include negotiating new relationships with elderly parents, assisting parents during old age and eventually adjusting to their passing. Middle adults who are in long-term couple relationships and who have children may experience the challenges of returning to the primary social identity of being a couple, rather than parents of young or school-aged children, developing adult relationships with grown children, and accepting new family members through marriage and birth.

Although some authors writing about life cycle events have mentioned gay and lesbian concerns (including Carter & McGoldrick, 1999, pp. 302–303, chap. 20; Smith, Eyler, & Peters-Golden, 1995), most discussions are predicated on the model of the family composed of couples who are heterosexual and non-transgender and their children. (See Hunter, 2005, for an excellent review of LGBT midlife.) Family constructs of transgender middle adults are more diverse, and are often more complex. Children may or may not have relationships with the trans-parent; former spouses may intersect with the new family or not. Many trans-identified middle adults live by themselves, others with a partner of the same sex, different sex, or a partner who is also trans-identified. Family structures evolve over time. Traditional assumptions are often incorrect.

People who publicly transition gender in older adulthood may experience a normative midlife course in many respects. However, most who are out about the transgender identity, or who transition before or during midlife, will experience some significant differences relative to their non-transgender peers. In essence, the transgender community can serve as a countersystem (Lyng, 2001) for examining the underlying definitions of the life cycle roles and concerns presented in discussions of normative aging. The literature in this regard is currently scant. The available evidence indicates that the concerns of gender minority persons in midlife often center on the themes of financial stability, social isolation or connectedness (e.g., to partner and community), personal safety, health and health care, independence, and maintaining an adequate living environment. These concerns are important to the aging majority population as well, though the desire to finish their lives in the habitus that is most true to themselves adds a layer of complexity to midlife for transgender adults. The following discussion of the salient aspects of life experience as a gender minority person in midlife is illustrated with comments from a recent group interview (conducted by TMW) with members of the mid- to late-life transgender-identified community and some of their gay and lesbian peers.

Social Stress and Coping

Transgender persons in midlife sometimes express dissatisfaction with social isolation and sadness, and fear being targeted for criticism and bigotry. For example, one panel respondent (transwoman, age 58) reported intergenerational tension, exemplified by this comment: "The young ones don't want to talk to you. They feel that you are not knowledgeable. You haven't been Queer long enough." Another (51-year-old transwoman) recounted an experience in which a teenager at the local grocery store had called her an "old tranny hag." While some older transpersons report a positive experience in the middle years, including good relationships with youth, recognizing stresses created by current episodes of harassment, combined with lingering negative effects of past discrimination, prejudice, and abuse, is critical to understanding midlife for many transgender persons.

Despite the difficulties, many older sexual and gender minority persons report reasonable life satisfaction and optimism. Older persons employ a variety of coping strategies to manage the challenges of the later years. Social network participation, faith and spirituality (with or without formal religious affiliation; Kidd & Witten, 2007a, 2009), and wisdom gained across the life span can help mitigate problems posed by declining abilities, financial limitations, and loss of regular activity. The emotional effects of earlier mistreatment and current uncertainty can also be reduced with social support. There is currently little formal research regarding specific coping strategies used by transgender middle and older adults.

Gerontological and geriatric research regarding resilience in middle and later life has often centered on peer relationships and peer network support, friendship circles, network structure, and related constructs. Little transgender-specific research has been performed in these areas. While it is clear that the transgender, or gender minority, population is epidemiologically difficult to sample in a meaningful way (either cross-sectionally or longitudinally), it is critical that the social dynamics of the transgender community receive additional research attention. Such information could benefit service professionals who are attempting to strengthen the abilities of older persons who are struggling to cope with the difficulties of life, and techniques derived from this new knowledge might inform the geriatric and gerontological communities as a whole. Until a more robust research base is available, results of small studies, case reports, and clinical experience must inform this discussion. Fortunately, current evidence suggests that central concerns of midlife are similar, regardless of the gender identity or sexual orientation of the individual (MetLife, 2010).

Social Networks and Connectedness

Social support networks contribute greatly to the potential for aging well (Ajrouch, Blandon, & Antonucci, 2005; Lang & Baltes, 1997). Loneliness and loss of members of one's network (partners, friends, pets) can negatively affect self-esteem, positive outlook, sense of well-being, and other important aspects of older adult life (Hawkley & Cacioppo, 2007; Pudrovska, Scheiman, & Carr, 2006; Van Baarsen, 2002; Williams, 2004; Wilson et al., 2007). Regardless of the minority status of the older person, membership in a strong social circle implies less worry about a central concern of midlife and later years: "Who would take care of me if something were to happen?" Participants in the panel interview echoed this need for connectedness, in part as a self-protective strategy. Some also expressed the specific desire for a partner—someone who could advocate effectively for them if they became ill or were hospitalized or incapacitated, and someone who could also share the joys and struggles of daily life. However, for couples that cannot legally marry, fear of destruction of the relationship and joint assets lingers, even if they are fortunate to form a strong relationship in midlife or to be settled in a partnership of long duration. Fear of loss due to lack of rights was frequently mentioned. A middle-aged gay male peer of the transgender panel members emphatically stated, "I have a great fear of being wiped out by biological family [if one partner were to become incapacitated or die], even though my partner and I have sewed everything up with legal documents. They [the biological family] could just back a truck up to the house and empty it. And that scares me to death." Similar sentiments were echoed by the MTF transgender and MTF cross-dressing members of the panel.

Social connectedness (or isolation), both in terms of couple relationships and as a member of a larger community, is crucially important to middle and older adults. Community is a complex interaction of friendship circles, social support networks, and a more generalized "ecological" community. For older adults who are transgender, the lack of social interaction is often one of the greatest sources of difficulty. Most transgender people have a personal story about rejection by a spouse or partner, sibling, parent, or child, usually when they came out or began transition, or they know a peer who has suffered such a loss. For some, entering a family situation as the "new" self can be frightening or problematic. Midlife is often the time of life when the peer group diminishes through death and dislocation, and members of minority groups are often more vulnerable because of smaller community size. This comment by a 48-year-old gay man expresses the angst of many transgender elders: "Loss of friends to death or to moving away from the area is gut-wrenching. It represents a loss of safety and companionship as well as diminishing the chances to find a partner. It is like being in a closet with the walls closing in."

Transgender (and LGB-identified) older adults are developing means of combating loneliness and increasing connectedness. Some join transgender activist groups and find a sense of community there. Support groups are becoming more common but are still relatively rare outside urban areas. Consequently, some transgender adults use internet chat rooms to derive a sense of community, kinship, friendship, and social support. Unfortunately, electronic interactions are usually less satisfying than face-to-face connections, and internet friends are rarely available to provide direct assistance when practical difficulties arise. The Maine Approach of community-based, technology-enhanced elder support (Teel, 2011) offers new means of increasing social and practical resources and may become an effective tool for helping transgender (and other) older adults to remain in their own homes. Pilot projects are in development, including at least one that may be LGBT focused.

Family

Although members of sexual and gender minorities are often stereotyped as promiscuous and lacking family connections or loyalty, this is not reflected in the realities of life in LGBT communities. Transgender adults in midlife have the same family constellations as their majority peers: some are single, some partnered without children, some have grown children, some are raising children currently or caring for elderly parents. Many have a variety of positive and mutually supportive relationships. However, transgender experience is associated with certain family challenges, particularly if transition occurs in midlife, after entering a marriage or partnership in which the transgender was unacknowledged, or perhaps unknown, even to the transgender individual, who had not yet come out to herself or himself.

When persons in middle adulthood transition gender within a long-term couple or married relationship, the partners reconsider the relationship, and in some ways, redefine it. Some people are able to adapt to being perceived as being in a same gender relationship (gay or lesbian) when the couple was previously seen as heterosexual, and others are not. Similarly, some people are uncomfortable with being newly regarded as heterosexual, such as after years in a lesbian community.

Some partners draw this distinction when describing their relationship to others, such as, "I am a lesbian. My partner is FTM." "My husband is becoming a woman, and we are going to stay married." Some may regard the reassessment of the relationship, and how society regards it, as an enriching experience. For example, one heterosexually identified, married young woman became an ardent advocate of same-gender marriage and other LGBT causes when her husband transitioned from male to female. She was incensed by the awareness that she and her husband (now wife) were often the objects of "dirty looks" when they held hands in public, though this had previously brought pleasant smiles from passersby, and considered the difference "ridiculous." Existing, initially heterosexual marriages likely maintain their legal validity when one party transitions gender, though this has not been well tested in the courts. One of Witten's (2011) respondents reported the following:

> My biggest concern is probably that my marriage, which was hetero pre-transition, and is now same-sex (and so recognized in California) will in some way get annulled by legislative or administrative changes. This might have adverse effects on either my or my wife's financial future, or my immigration status, since I am a green-card holding UK citizen living in the US. For example, if I die first, the Federal government may not honour my wife's entitlement to (say) social security benefits which I have earned.

Persons who transitioned gender early in life often do not have children, although some have formed parental relationships with the children of their spouse or partner or entered parenting relationships in other ways. Some people who transitioned in midlife have children from earlier coupled relationships and marriages. When there are children, the construct of the family also must be re-defined (Boenke, 1999), particularly if the children are adolescents or adults. What does it mean for the former "Dad" to now be female, and how does the adult child create an adult relationship with the person who is now "Dad and yet not Dad"? Some transgender adults are pleased to allow their adolescent children to address them by the endearments that they have always used in private, though they may ask them not to do so in public (e.g., "Dad" or "Daddy" in private, "Mom" or "Joan" in public). One 48-year-old transwoman reassured her adolescent daughters that, "I've been your Dad all your lives, and will be til I die."

If divorce ensues, the person who once was Dad and is now female, or the person who once was Mom and is now male, may choose to re-partner with someone of the same or other gender, thereby creating the appearance of a new sexuality in the eyes of the adolescent or adult child. For example, if Dad transitions to female, and forms a relationship with a woman, she will now be regarded by society as a lesbian, although he was previously seen as heterosexual, and the direction of attraction has not changed. Marriage of the adult child will also now involve not only asking parents to accept the new partner but also helping the partner to accept entry into a family with a transgender "parent-in-law." Some transgender adults also partner with another person who is transgender and open about the transition history (e.g., an FTM-FTM couple), which can add another layer of complexity to these discussions.

The launching phase may be disrupted for both the young adult child and the middle adult parent if the child rejects the transitioning parent, thereby cutting each of them off from the mutual support that parents and maturing children can offer one another. However, many adolescents and young adults make it clear that they love the parent, regardless of gender identity or sexual orientation. Problems with acceptance by grandchildren are rare unless their parents disapprove of the grandparent. Young children tend to accept and love their grandparents regardless of "details," such as gender identity, and young children usually do not have many concerns about gender transition, as a child's world is often still heavily influenced by imagination and magical thinking (Ettner, 1999).

Sexuality and Intimacy

Intimacy remains important to personhood across the life course. Intimacy can include physical contact and closeness, such as holding or being held by another person, whether the other person is a romantic partner or a caregiver. It can involve friendship, manifested in person, or via letters, e-mails, phone conversations or media such as Skype (Teel, 2011). Intimacy allows the individual to feel wanted, supported, and cared for.

Sexuality in mid- and later life is often dynamic, evolving, and complex. Older adults are usually stereotyped as lacking in sexual interest, and this is often not the case (Thomsen, 2001). Sexuality and sexual expression among older adults is a relatively new field of study, though some very helpful work has been done. Lindau et al. (2007) provide an excellent discussion of older adult sexuality in the United States; a comprehensive review regarding sexual orientation and aging is found in Fredriksen-Goldsen and Muraco (2010). Few large surveys have included questions regarding transgender or gender-queer sexualities (Sell & Becker, 2001) though interest in this field is growing.

Interpretation of sexuality is usually based on the individual's gendered presentation, from which assumptions are made regarding gender identity, gender role, and sexuality. Ambiguous or inconsistent presentation, such as is the case for a transgender identified middle adult who is in the process of gender transition or who does not have genital surgery, can result in confusion on the part of caregivers, manifested as hostility. One of the most frequently expressed worries in the Trans-MetLife (Witten, 2011) survey was the preservation of privacy, well-being, and patient rights in caregiving environments.

Regardless of the setting, assumptions and inferences are often incorrect or incomplete, as described by another survey respondent (Witten, 2011):

> I was a heterosexual male before my genital surgery and I liked women then. I am a female now (after my surgery) and I still like women. I don't think of myself as a lesbian because nothing changed except my body. However, the world thinks of me as a lesbian. Some of my other MTF trans-friends started off liking women early in their transition and ended up liking men. Still others are with trans-persons. You cannot assume anything when it comes to sexuality in this community.

Some transgender persons find that a bisexual identity best describes their sexuality (Alexander & Yescavage, 2004). Defining oneself as bisexual can render the individual even more societally invisible, as both "transgender" and "bisexual" are terms that are poorly understood and accepted in majority culture. Couples sometimes define their relationship in ways that are inconsistent with their (current) genital status. For example, a transman who has not had genital surgery and a nontrans man may regard themselves as a gay couple and present socially as such—whether they engage in penis-in-vagina intercourse or not. Care must be taken to make sure that inequities based on sexuality "labels" do not impinge on the care of the transgender or queer-identified individual or couple (McNair, 2003; McNair & Hegarty, 2010; Solarz, 1999).

Spirituality and Religion

Gerontology research has demonstrated a strong correlation between faith, spirituality or religiosity and reduced morbidity and enhanced sense of well-being (Hill, Burdette, Angel, & Angel, 2006; Krause & Ellison, 2003; Krause, Ingersoll-Dayton, Ellison, & Wulff, 1999; MacKinlay & McFadden, 2004; Moberg, 2001). Transgender adults in the middle years sometimes experience distress related to religion. During the launching phase, spirituality and religiosity (Jones, 1996) of the midlife parent often increase. Many transgender parents no longer have access to the traditional spiritual dwellings and rituals of earlier times of their lives, as many religions regard nonnormative sexualities and gender identities as not only unacceptable but also sinful. However, LGBT persons of many faiths have formed support organizations without sanctioning from larger religious bodies. For example, although the Vatican still condemns homosexuality, Dignity USA has been providing affiliation and support for gay (subsequently, LGBT) Catholics for decades. Some local congregations accept transgender persons, even if the authority figures of the faith do not. Also, some religious groups, such as the United Church of Christ and the Unitarian Universalist Association of Congregations, are openly welcoming of sexuality and gender minority persons and have made inclusiveness a matter of policy. Many people manage their need for spiritual study or practice individually, without formal religious affiliation. Rationalist and humanist traditions also fill this need for many adults.

Professionals who work with transgender middle and older adults should be aware that many of these individuals transitioned faiths as they transitioned genders. For example, in the TLARS study, over half of respondents had moved from one of the more traditional Western religions to a more personalized spiritual perspective, often considered a fusion of the best principles of the faiths in which the individual believes. As additional faith communities become welcoming of transgender and gender atypical members, this trend may lessen in future cohorts, though reassessment of life's meaning and its reflection in spiritual belief is likely fostered by the profoundly personal journey of gender transition.

Finances

Financial concerns are also important to transgender persons in midlife and are often inseparable from independence, health, and decisions about transition. Most middle-adult transgender persons who have health insurance receive this as a benefit of employment and will lose this coverage if the job is lost, which may occur when the individual begins transition. Many states and jurisdictions still have no antidiscrimination protections for LGBT persons, and employees who begin gender transition can be fired with no other cause. Further, many services related to the physical aspects of transition, particularly surgeries, are not covered by most health plans. Thus, many people who gender transition during midlife use years of savings to cover these expenses. In the words of one 58-year-old transwoman, "I am lucky. I have my healthcare benefits through the VA. It isn't great, but at least I have them . . . [but] I will have to worry about making a decision. Do I save for surgery or for retirement?"

These decisions also affect family members. For example, a married woman in middle adulthood who was fully emotionally supportive of her husband's MTF transition—and had known at the time of the marriage that he was planning to do so—declined to cash in her retirement savings to fund the genital surgery. Although this was a wise decision, his (her) repeated requests created marital strain that would not have arisen if nondiscriminatory, adequate insurance coverage had been available to them. The concerns of spouses, partners, and children of midlife transgender persons (Cook-Daniels, 1995; Witten, 2004) clearly merit additional research and support.

These difficulties are compounded for older persons who are living on fixed incomes or are only able to work part time. Financial duress in midlife also occurs when a chronic illness develops. By age 60, most American adults are taking three to six prescription medications per day for treatment of aging-related conditions, and many take more (Morley, 2002). Most transgender adults also take hormonal medications or medications to suppress hormone production (e.g., antiandrogens). This adds to the total individual financial burden of health maintenance, particularly if insurance does not cover these prescription costs. Nontransgender adults delay obtaining needed medications because of cost (Klein, Turvey, & Wallace, 2004), and it is likely that this occurs even more commonly among their transgender peers.

Health Care

Robust evidence regarding health care for transgender middle and older adults is currently not available for most aspects of physical and mental health. The Institute of Medicine (2011) report, *The Health of Lesbian, Gay, Bisexual, and Transgender People: Building a Foundation for Better Understanding,* includes an agenda for future research. Some recommendations for transgender health care can be extrapolated from the non-transgender population or from the experience of the larger population of LGBT adults. Some of the most important health concerns of transgender persons in middle adulthood—privacy, health maintenance, and HIV, are considered below.

Privacy. Health privacy is a concern of transgender persons across the life span. Questions regarding confidentiality of medical records and pharmacy records remain problematic. In addition, although reconstructive surgical techniques are improving, the surgical history is often evident because of the presence of scars, and many transgender people do not receive genital surgery, either because of personal preference or because of expense. In the words of one 43-year-old trans-man, "Either his chest scars are obvious, or his genitals give him away. Thus, accessing normatively sexed and gendered health care services is nearly impossible . . . There are scads of FTMs who suffer in isolation because they refuse to subject themselves to medical scrutiny, possible mistreatment, and ridicule."

Lack of privacy regarding life history and personal identity becomes more problematic as need for medical services increases, which often occurs in midlife. For example, the colonoscopy at age 50 has become a rite of passage among middle adults with health benefits and carries different implications for those whose genitals "match" their general appearance and those whose genitals do not. MTF cross-dressers and drag queens sometimes attempt to postpone needed medical services until the male body hair can be allowed to grow out to avoid questions regarding personal identity and way of life. One 55-year-old described his life as an MTF cross-dresser as like walking the line between heterosexual and trans-gender, and noted, "As long as I live as a 'het,' I'm okay." However, maintaining that boundary is not always possible when receiving medical or nursing care, and being outed as a cross-dresser can be damaging to the individual and his or her family.

The need for privacy affects all those with nonnormative bodies that they cannot hide and all gender minority persons regardless of whether surgery has been performed. All panel discussants placed a high priority on the ability to maintain secrecy in order to receive appropriate health care, and to maintain employment and, hence, financial stability. These concerns were echoed in the TLARS and Tran-MetLife surveys. The lack of protection from discrimination, particularly in employment, in most jurisdictions, makes these concerns particularly acute.

Health maintenance. Recommended health services for persons in midlife are similar, in most respects, regardless of the gender identity of the individual, with some significant differences. A thorough discussion of this subject is beyond the scope of this book. A number of useful reviews and clinical recommendations for transgender adult health care have been produced in recent years, including the Center of Excellence for Transgender Health (2011); Dahl, Feldman, Goldberg, and Jaberi (2006); Eyler (2007); Eyler and Feldman (2008); Feldman (2007, 2008); Feldman and Goldberg (2006); Feldman and Safer (2009); Gorton, Buth, and Spade (2005); Hembree et al. (2009); Witten and Eyler (2007); WPATH (2011).

Unfortunately, although evidence from large sample studies (e.g., Asscheman, 2011) is increasing, most study populations do not include large numbers of older adults, particularly those who have used hormonal medications for long periods of time. The clinical evidence is therefore not robust for many aspects of transgender health care, and recommendations will likely be revised as additional data become available. Health care professionals are therefore advised to follow the clinical recommendations that are applicable for all adults in midlife and older adulthood, and to incorporate additional evidence-based recommendations that are transgender specific as these are developed or refined.

Health screening and counseling services that should be offered to all adults, aged 25–64 years include the following (adapted from the U.S. Preventive Services Task Force, www.arhg.gov and www.uspreventiveservicestaskforce.org, which provides recommendations on a variety of health maintenance and preventive health care topics):

- Assessment of height, weight, blood pressure, serum lipids (cholesterol)
- Screening for sexually transmissible and bloodborne infections
- Colon cancer screening, particularly by age 50
- Assessment of smoking and assistance with quitting
- Evaluation of physical activity and recommendations regarding safe increase
- Dietary assessment and advice (calcium sources, vegetables, limiting fats and sweets)
- Injury prevention (seat belts, smoke and carbon monoxide alarms, firearm storage)
- Prevention of sexually transmissible infections, including HIV, and unwanted pregnancy
- Dental evaluation
- Assessment for depression and other mental health concerns
- Assessment of problem drinking and drug use
- Recommendation or low-dose aspirin for preventing cardiac disease if indicated; other cardiac evaluation as needed

In addition, other health assessments should be considered for persons who have taken transgender hormonal supplementation or had surgical procedures. The following are offered as suggestions based on current information, with the caution that all clinical care should be individualized and that transgender health maintenance is an evolving field within which there are differences of opinion. Transgender middle adults should work closely with a physician, a physician assistant, or a nurse practitioner who can access updated information from the medical literature as this field continues to advance.

- Breast cancer screening may benefit both transwomen (MTF) and transmen (FTM) who have not had chest surgery. Transmen who have not had chest surgery should follow the guidelines for non-trans women, including for mammography. Indications for screening mammography for transwomen are less clearly defined, though it should be considered over age 50, particularly if other risks are present, such as use of estrogen and progestin for more than 5 years, overweight, or family history of breast cancer. Some transwomen prefer to have mammographic screening even without these risks, using the same guidelines as non-trans women.
- Cytologic (Pap) cancer screening should be considered for transwomen who have had vaginoplasty and who have a history of human papillomavirus infection, or if the glans penis was used in the vaginoplasty. Transmen who have not had the cervix removed should have Pap testing according to recommendations for non-trans-women.
- FTM persons who have used testosterone and who have not had removal of the ovaries should be evaluated for symptoms and signs of polycystic ovaries; hysterectomy and oophorectomy (removal of the ovaries) should be considered, particularly after age 40, or if tolerating gynecological exams is psychologically difficult and fertility is not desired.
- Prostate cancer can occur in MTF transwomen, even after gender confirmation surgery, because the prostate is not removed. However, PSA testing is not reliable if estrogen is being used. Digital rectal examinations can be performed. Transwomen should discuss prostate cancer with their physicians, nurse practitioners and physician assistants, as recommendations for early detection may continue to evolve.
- Osteoporosis screening may be particularly important for both transwomen and transmen who have had their testes or ovaries removed, especially if not taking estrogen or testosterone consistently, older than age 60, or both. Some sources recommend baseline bone mineral density testing, or earlier testing if other risk factors are present.
- Persons who take testosterone should have the hemoglobin level assessed to evaluate for developing polycythemia (elevated hemoglobin or thickening of the blood) especially early in treatment.

- *It is particularly important that anyone who is taking hormonal medications not smoke or use other tobacco products.* Smoking while taking estrogen increases the risk of developing thrombotic disease (blood clots and emboli); smoking with androgen use increases the risk of polycythemia and stroke among persons taking testosterone, particularly among older adults (Wald et al., 2006). Professionals in medicine, nursing, and the mental health fields can assist the transgender adults in their practices by asking about tobacco use and assisting in smoking cessation.

The use of supplemental estrogens or androgens in midlife and later years is based on several principles (adapted from the above sources):

- The use of estrogen or testosterone conveys certain health benefits and is associated with significant medical risks. These should be discussed in detail with patients who wish to use these medications, particularly at the start of treatment (see WPATH, 2011, pp. 97–104).
- A thorough medical evaluation should be undertaken before beginning hormone supplementation, with particular attention to conditions that may be influenced by hormone use.
- For estrogen use, transdermal estradiol patches, at the lowest effective dose, are probably safer for older persons than many other estrogen preparations.
- Testosterone should also be used at the lowest effective dose during midlife and older age, and preferably administered by topical gel or patch.
- Appropriate laboratory monitoring should be performed.
- *Some of the risks of concurrent smoking and hormone use rise with age.*

Although research regarding specific health effects of hormonal preparations among middle-adult and older persons, particularly long-term use, is strongly needed, many transgender people take estrogens or androgens in the fifth decade and beyond, often for decades. This should be done with medical assistance and monitoring to enhance health status and reduce complications. Persons taking "natural hormones," such as those obtained over the internet, should also be reminded that any preparation that produces masculinization or feminization of the body can potentially produce undesirable effects and health risks and should be used with medical consultation, if at all possible. (A discussion of hormonal use without medical or nursing assistance, as is often done due to economic constraints or other difficulties, is beyond the scope of this chapter. The "informed consent model" [see WPATH, 2011, p. 35, for a description] is used in some public health settings to make medical and nursing care more accessible to homeless or low-income transpersons who take hormonal preparations.)

HIV and AIDS. HIV is a particular concern in the health care of persons in middle and older adulthood, as persons older than age 50 years (Emlet, 2004; Lee, 2006; Sanchez Rodriguez & Rodriguez Alvarez, 2003; Whipple & Scoura, 1989) represent the fastest growing segment of the American population with respect to new cases of HIV and AIDS (through the numeric majority of new cases occurs among young adults). HIV among older adults has been referred to as a "double jeopardy" stigmatizing situation (Emlet, 2006) due to speculation regarding how older persons would acquire HIV infection, when persons in middle and older adulthood are stereotyped as sexless. For individuals who are transgender or gender-queer identified, the double jeopardy can become "triple jeopardy" because of the stigma associated with their gender identity or transgender status.

Cultural, racial, and ethnic factors must also be taken into account when interacting with persons who are transgender and HIV positive (Muñoz-Laboy & Dodge, 2007). HIV is a particular burden for low-income transgender individuals, especially those involved, or previously involved, in sex work (Bockting & Kirk, 2002; Bockting, Rosser, & Coleman, 1999). Finding supportive environments for HIV positive transgender adults can be difficult, and the dual stigma keeps many from seeking appropriate care (Melendez et al., 2006; Schwarz & Scheer, 2004).

More people living with HIV or AIDS are living longer, more active lives. This improvement in quality and quantity of life has brought with it the higher risk of exhausting financial resources and of impoverishment in the older adult years. The combination of the physiologic changes of aging, the chronic illnesses that occur in later life, and the biological burden of HIV infection can make care of HIV more complicated in middle and older adulthood (Manfredi, 2002; Marzolini et al., 2011).

Many people living with HIV in middle and older adulthood age successfully (Kahana & Kahana, 2001) despite these challenges, and spirituality (Vance et al., 2011) can be a vital resource. Anecdotal evidence suggests that transgender adults with HIV often also do well, though additional research is needed.

LATER-LIFE TRANSGENDER EXPERIENCES AND CONCERNS

The mature years are a time of continued growth and development. They are not only "quantitatively an important part of the lifespan, they are and have always been an essential and meaningful part. It is not necessary for everyone to reach this stage of life, but it has probably been important for the stability and vitality of human culture that a significant minority of society do so in every period of history" (Coleman & O'Hanlon, 2004).

The later stages of life are often characterized by *generativity* (Erikson, Erikson, & Kivnick, 1986) and a desire to contribute to the well-being of future generations, as well as to the principles and causes one holds dear. Individuals at this stage of life are often contributing members of society; in contemporary times, many are still gainfully employed or significantly involved in the lives of children or grandchildren. This is often a time of life characterized by reflecting on life experience, which can generate fresh understandings. Some older adults report that they have become more fully integrated, more true to themselves. Older survey respondents (Witten, 2011) reflected these experiences in their comments:

> I have come to admit that I am transgender & am not concerned really with who knows . . . I can deal with God as I know I have tried to help everyone in my life . . . GOD BLESS.

> I consider whatever the going semantical definition of what I am (TS/TG/CD, GQ, etc.) I consider it a gift. One that I am glad I found. I would have loved to have determined it at an earlier age, but I will take what I have . . . I can only hope that anyone else who discovers that they have this "gift." That they can accept it for the beauty that it can provide during this "trip around the sun."

The final stage of life, which Erikson characterized as the conflict between *integrity and despair,* is in some ways a natural outgrowth of the previous life stages, including the generative years. The personal lessons and insights gained during midlife and later years can serve to ease the fear of death, as life is reconsidered at the time when it must soon be given up.

Counterbalancing the positive aspects of this time of life is the diminishment in physical and mental abilities, and the development or acceleration of chronic illnesses, including those that will eventually result in death. Physical changes range from relatively insignificant (presbyopia) to those requiring significant lifestyle changes (diabetes) to permanent loss of abilities (consequences of stroke) (Beers, Jones, Berkwitz, Kaplan, & Porter, 2004). Some changes interfere with the ability of the older person to maintain independent living in the community, resulting in the need for assistance, including temporary or permanent services funded through insurance or public means. For older persons who are transgender or members of other gender minorities, this stage is characterized by normative changes of aging and the effects and social consequences of the gendered identity (Gooren, Giltay, & Bunck, 2008). In the words of one older transman (Witten, 2011): "[I am afraid of] Being trapped in a nursing home and forced to live on an institutional schedule with bigoted attendants who try to treat me like a woman or harass me about my gender, out me to the other residents . . ."

Quality of life for older adults often centers on social integration achieved earlier in life and carried forward, and on personal flexibility and resilience that can foster the development of new relationships during the later years. Community resources can also be crucial, although some are more welcoming of members of sexual and gender minorities than others. Stallings, Dunham, Gatz, Baker, and Bengtson (1997) address these concerns with regard to the normative elderly (see also Magai & McFadden, 1996; Thompson, 1996; Turner, 1996). The experience of transgender older adults requires additional research attention, though some recent work (MetLife, 2010) represents a good beginning.

Significant life transitions of the elder years are similar for all older adults. Personal control is eroded by loss of the strength, mobility, and organizational skills needed to maintain a private residence and to operate a motor vehicle. In-home assistance and support services, such as Meals on Wheels, can help to keep older persons in their own homes for a time, though needs often eventually become more fundamental, necessitating transitioning to assisted living and, eventually, dependent nursing care. Sadly, elder care organizations in many areas are unaware that they have transgender clients in their service areas (Belongia & Witten, 2006), suggesting that they are not equipped to provide appropriate care for this population. One of the greatest challenges of the current era is enabling older adults to remain at home throughout their lives; some recent technological developments are making this a more feasible possibility. The community-based Maine Approach (Teel, 2011) has potential for application in the LGBT communities, particularly in areas with higher numbers of out LGBT older adults.

The concerns and challenges of older adulthood are similar in many respects to those of middle adulthood, though often amplified by diminishment in resources and acuity of need. Some differences also reflect generational, cohort effects.

Social Support and Connection

Loss of social support through loss of the spouse or partner, and diminishment of the friendship circle through death and dementia, further erode the ability of older persons to manage their lives and cope emotionally. For members of gender minorities, this can be more problematic than for the normative population. Transgender older adults have, on average, fewer friends whose gender identity is similar to their own than their majority culture peers and may be deeply affected by the loss of the empathic connection and understanding that these relationships provide.

Some transgender elders have also been estranged from siblings or children because of the coming-out process and gender transition, although others have continued these mutually supportive relationships. This is significant, as grown children are still one of the principal sources of emotional, material, and practical support for older adults. Grandchildren often provide emotional warmth, acceptance, and connectedness to the future during the elder years. Elders who no longer have contact with friends from early in life miss the benefit these relationships provide when they reflect on their life history. Siblings, particularly sisters, are often helpful in this regard. The personal "summing up" that is often a feature of older adulthood (Erikson et al., 1986; Viederman, 2003) can be difficult when the "fault line" between the pre- and posttransition lives has no bridging relationships.

Most transgender elders have transitioned gender during the early adult years or middle adulthood and are no longer struggling with the immediate implications of coming out during the later years. However, some who did not have the opportunity to transition earlier in life do so during their 60s, 70s, or later. This affects relationships with siblings, children, grandchildren, and other members of the extended family. Although "blood is thicker than water" and most families will eventually accept the gender transition, some will not, thereby depriving the older person of necessary emotional connections later in life. Rejecting relatives usually offer religious or moralistic reasons for their decision, although some eventually overcome or modify these beliefs to allow for reconciliation with the transgender family member. When this does not occur, some transgender older adults find that the strengths that they have developed during the difficulties they have already faced are sustaining, such as the (Witten, 2011) survey respondent who reported no significant concerns about aging, stating, "I came into this world alone, had to deal with my issues alone . . . and I plan to go out alone." However, such stoicism and resolve may erode late in life, and LGBT-identified or -allied volunteers may provide some measure of needed support.

Some older transgender persons find companionship in LGBT organizations, though, as has been discussed elsewhere in this volume, most organizations maintain a youth-oriented focus. Social and support organizations for male-to-female transgender and cross-dressing adults often have more older adult and elderly members, including some who have transitioned gender, or who have come out as cross-dressers, later in life. Membership in gender minority, or LGBT, organizations can also provide an opportunity for generative activities, giving time and resources to benefit the next generation:

> Ronnie is a 65-year-old retired businessman who became aware of the impor-
> tance of her female self seven years ago, after decades of cross-dressing on an
> intermittent basis. "He" sought psychotherapy when the awareness of the
> transgender identity could no longer be denied. She now takes estrogen ther-
> apy and lives true to her female self much of the time, but has decided not to
> publicly transition gender, due to the complications that would arise, particu-
> larly in her rural community. She and her wife frequently travel to a larger city to
> attend social events for MTF transgender and cross-dressing persons and their
> partners, which they both enjoy. Ronnie has recently assumed a leadership role
> in this organization, as a way of giving back to the community, and helping oth-
> ers who are beginning their journey of gender self-discovery. (Eyler, 2011)

Identifiable (out) FTM older adults have thus far been less numerous or less visible in many areas, but this is changing, as the next generation matures. The stigma that accompanies minority gender identification has also reduced some-what over time. It is to be hoped that the next generation of transgender elders will experience a higher level of peer support, as a greater number of older adults feel secure enough to be open about their life histories, gender transition, and true gender identity, and the larger culture becomes more accepting of gender-variant persons.

Spirituality

Spirituality often provides insight and strength for older persons, regardless of gender identity. Many elders report an increased sense of spirituality, whether they participate in organized religion or not (T. M. Witten, personal communi-cations, 1997, 2004). Rationalist, nontheistic traditions also fill this need for many elderly persons who are in the process of evaluating life's experiences and mean-ings. Most transgender elders are associated with a traditional religion or identify themselves as being highly spiritual (Witten, 2004). In addition to providing an opportunity for community, religious bodies sometimes sponsor other services that can be useful to older persons, though specific attention to the needs of sexual and gender minority persons is uncommon. Still, feeling welcome and supported can make it easier for older persons to access other services that they need. Many transgender older adults find alternative means of expressing their faith and receiving religious support, if their traditional religious body is unwelcoming (Kidd & Witten, 2007a, 2007b; Witten, 2004).

Privacy

As transgender elders develop a greater need for supportive services, the process of obtaining these services is complicated by the decision of whether to come out to the professionals involved at each new step in this process. In some cases, this is unavoidable. For example, when composing a will or durable power of attorney, the nature of the relationship between the parties must be shared with the attorney. If the gender transition occurred in the context of a legal marriage, and the spouses decided to remain married, the elderly couple would be in the unusual position of enjoying a legal same-gender marriage, which confers certain legal protections—and the need to be out about the gender transition to claim these protections. If the couple has a two-gender, heterosexual marriage, but entered into this relationship after the gender transition, it may still be subject to legal challenge, as in a well-known case in Texas (*Littleton v. Prange*, 2000). Legal services will likely be needed to ensure that the rights of the transgender elder and his or her spouse or partner are protected, and this will involve coming out about the transition, even if the older adult has been living "stealth" with regard to the natal sex and assigned gender for decades. This is an evolving field of case law, and transgender older adults are not yet in a position to count on accessing any civil rights that have not been explicitly established.

Situations requiring medical or nursing care or physical assistance can be significantly more complicated because of the loss of bodily privacy. Although this is a concern for transgender persons at every age, concerns intensify as the need for help increases and becomes less discretionary. Older adults who cross-dress (MTF) must decide how to balance the need for care with the discomfort of letting the male body hair grow out, or be open about cross-dressing (Witten, Eyler, & Weigel, 2000). If services are provided in the home, the recipient must consider whether to hide female garments and cosmetics. The position of older transmasculine adults (transgender, gender nonconforming, or cross-dressing) who are still presenting socially as women is analogous. Persons who have transitioned gender may face a different level of disclosure and explanation. Most elderly persons who are transsexual or transgender use hormone supplementation, sometimes at doses that would be unusual for an older person who is not transgender, and this is usually discussed early in any clinical relationship. If genital surgery has not been performed, the (often vulnerable) elderly person will have no option but to disclose the transgender identity early in any clinical or physically assistive relationship.

Health

Health care needs of older adults are similar to the needs of middle adults, discussed earlier in this chapter. In addition, services that should be considered for persons older than age 65, regardless of gender identity or hormonal status, include the following (adapted from the *Guide to Clinical Preventive Services*, report of the U.S. Preventive Services Task Force, www.ahrg.gov or USPreventiveServicesTaskForce.org):

- Elder safety, including fall prevention and reduction in the hot water heater temperature
- CPR training for household members, if not already done
- Immunizations for tetanus-diphtheria, influenza, pneumococcal pneumonia, and others as per local guidelines
- Reassessment of living will and durable power of attorney documentation

Health care professionals should also remain aware of the potential for substance abuse later in life (Wu & Blazer, 2011) and its associated medical complications. Use of substances, especially alcohol, is prevalent among older adults, and there is no evidence to suggest that transgender elders experience fewer problems in this regard than their non-transgender peers.

Transgender elders who take estrogens or androgens must share this information with their health professionals, as many risks associated with hormone use increase with age. Clinical care should be individualized and will likely follow general guidelines regarding physical examination and laboratory monitoring. (For additional details regarding use of hormonal medication, see Center of Excellence for Transgender Health, 2011; Dahl et al., 2006; Eyler, 2007; Eyler & Feldman, 2008; Feldman, 2007, 2008; Feldman & Goldberg, 2006; Feldman & Safer, 2009; Gorton et al., 2005; Hembree et al., 2009; Witten & Eyler, 2007; WPATH, 2011.) Evidence for specific guidance regarding hormone dosage in late life is currently lacking, but consideration should be given to using the lowest possible effective dose, as both androgen and estrogen levels decline with age in non-transgender women and men (Darby & Anawalt, 2005; Snyder, 2004), and it seems unlikely that transgender older adults require the same levels of hormonal support as their young adult peers. However, osteoporosis risk rises with age for both women and men, so hormonal support sufficient to prevent this complication should be continued unless contraindicated.

The elder years are a time of further adjustment to declining physical and mental abilities, changing family relationships, and diminishing peer group and social circle. Family and social support and assistive services can play crucial roles in assisting transgender elders in maintaining quality of life. Spirituality, introspection, and reminiscence are also critically important as life is reevaluated in the final years. In the words of one older adult survey respondent (Witten, 2011):

> Aging and end of life issues are extremely important for people. Many draw final emotional and spiritual conclusions about our lives from how we experience those final days. For all of us who have outlived our partners and friends we need others in the LGBTIQ community who accept us to be the family we have outlived and creating alternative formal relationships to supplant the ones society denies us is all important. Old age is a time of extreme vulnerability to the same degree that infancy is, but the elderly lives are devalued in comparison. We need to change this, along with far more cultural competency demands and trainings for health care and mental health providers for the services we cannot provide in the LGBTIQ community.

Professionals who work with gender-variant patients and clients can improve services available to them, and the manner in which they are delivered, by sharing their knowledge through presentations at local and regional professional societies, including medical and nursing grand rounds; advising service organizations, and, most important, by remaining involved in the lives of their clients and patients as they require additional assistance during later years.

GRACEFUL EXITS

More than 2.4 million people die each year in the United States. About half of deaths of Americans aged 65 or older occur in hospitals, approximately one-fourth take place in nursing homes, and approximately one-fourth happen at home. Dignity, comfort, and respect are central aspects of quality of life, as life draws to an end (Hermann & Looney, 2011). Elder survey respondents in Witten (2011) echoed those hopes for their own deaths.

End-of-life experiences are multifaceted. Complex interactions ensue, involving the individual at the end of life, family, friends and significant others, health care professionals, and legal representatives. Other cultural entities and organizations become involved, such as the armed forces, if the deceased is in active duty or is a veteran. If the individual is transgender, these dynamic interactions can become even more complex at a time when this is neither necessary nor desirable. Persons who transitioned gender decades ago are now elderly, and many have died, making clear the importance of end-of-life care for the transgender community (Witten, 2003).

End-of-life stages can be roughly categorized as follows: (1) predeath, (2) imminent death, (3) death, and (4) postdeath (Witten, 2009). The beginning of the predeath phase is often difficult to characterize, particularly when death is expected but not predictable, such as in cases of chronic illnesses (e.g., many cancers and AIDS) or in a hospice environment.

Predeath and Imminent Death

Reminiscing, finding life closure, and preparing to face death are important during predeath. Spiritual, interpersonal, legal, and financial concerns must be faced, unless they are deliberately avoided. Reminiscing can create emotional stress and grief for transgender persons who are facing death because of both the normative concerns common to this stage of life and the reasons specific to gender minority persons. These can center on conflicts created by the reminiscence process (i.e., between life experiences in the natal sex and its assigned gender and those later in life, after the transition process). Many people who have transitioned gender wish to forget, or at least suppress, details of life before they lived in their chosen (true) gender, but the process of reminiscence—a summing up of what life has been and has meant—will bring focus back to early memories, as well as more recent events.

For everyone at this stage of life, the principal questions are likely to be, "Who have I been in this life, and what has it meant to me?" (as described in Viederman, 2003). Gender minority persons may have unresolved concerns in this regard, but have often already faced these questions more thoroughly than have their nontransgender peers. Many also have more experience with medical treatments and have had more opportunity to work out family conflicts during coming out and the gender transition process—though many have "unfinished business" with family and friends from earlier in life.

Significant aspects of these stages include both internal processes and practical concerns. Legal documents must be completed. This is of paramount importance. The medical durable power of attorney and living will provide guidance about medical care and decision making in case of incapacity; guardian of person documentation provides for survivor rights to the body after death, so that funerary preferences can be carried out. General power of attorney, will or living trust, guardian over assets, and definition of beneficiaries protect assets and define last wishes. Documentation such as a personal property list, special requests list, and record of burial arrangements and desires, will help the surviving significant others, family, and friends to manage the time immediately following death. Some people also create family love letters and ethical wills. These are not legal documents but are intended for the benefit of loved ones, providing information about personal values, hopes, most important lessons learned in life, and advice for the future. Ethical wills can amplify the spirit of the living will, addressing questions about care in case of coma, brain death, and other possible scenarios in more detail.

Wills, durable powers of attorney, and advance directives are important for all older adults but are crucial if the dying person is transgender, especially as some states do not recognize marriages that take place following gender change, and the federal government has historically not allowed changes in formal documents (such as passports) unless surgery has been performed—though this is being challenged. Therefore, documentation procedures can be complex, but surviving spouses and partners may have no legal standing unless wills and related documents have been completed. They may lose even jointly acquired property if the transgender person dies intestate, and may not be able to carry out the wishes of the deceased with regard to burial and memorial practices. This is particularly burdensome for low-income gender minority persons, who may already be spending their limited funds on medical treatments and family necessities.

As death becomes not only realistic but also inevitable, the dying person will need to face his or her fears about dying, define and honor spiritual beliefs about life and death, accept that the hospital or care facility may be the final home, use remaining time wisely, learn to remain in the moment and create positive times, maintain hope, preserve dignity, and live fully until the last moments of life— with varying levels of engagement and success. These emotional tasks are addressed during a time when many practical and immediate considerations consume personal energy. These include preserving autonomy and a sense of personal control as decisions are made about pursuing or discontinuing medical treatments, managing pain and other symptoms, putting legal affairs in order, resolving differences with family and friends, making amends to the extent that this will ever be done, minimizing stress for loved ones, ensuring family support, and maintaining working relationships with the health care team and practical assistants (Witten, 2008).

Nonnormative gender identification influences and modifies these events and tasks. Isolation from peers is a burden too often borne by transgender elders, and is a great fear for many, as this minority community social system is further decimated by aging and death of its members. Other common concerns include disclosure, privacy, and potentially difficult interactions with care providers (Witten, 2008, 2011). Problems can occur when health care professionals and caregivers do not understand the effect of the transgender identity on the predeath experience. Clinical situations arise that violate the dignity of the transgender person, often because of ignorance rather than willful intent. For example, one nursing home facility director referred to transgender as "a homosexual thing" (Belongia & Witten, 2006), and a 22-year-old student nurse stated, "I would not be willing to treat a transsexual client. It's a sin!" (Witten, 2009). A number of survey respondents (Witten, 2011) specifically reported fears of being mistreated in faith-based care settings because of religiously based negative perceptions of their gender identity. The following cases illustrate the concerns of transgender older adults in care settings.

Jane is an 87-year-old male-to-female transsexual woman who transitioned gender more than 15 years ago and is now in hospice care for a malignancy that has entered the terminal stage. She was rejected by her family when she came out about her transgender identity and is dependent on the hospice staff for care and support. Recently, problems with incontinence have become difficult to manage, and the nurses have decided that a Foley (indwelling) catheter would be the best solution. Jane has been resistant to this and to accepting any help in changing her underpants. Though she has not admitted this, she is ashamed of the fact that, despite her feminine persona, her genitalia are male in appearance. She is also worried about the potential responses of some members of the staff to her body. (Witten & Whittle, 2004)

James, a 71-year-old transman who transitioned gender 30 years ago, with chest surgery but not genital reconstruction, was experiencing Alzheimer dementia. He was placed in a local authority care home [a nursing home in the United Kingdom] where every other client was female. He had no family and no visitors. The staff at the care home complained about his removal of his incontinence pads. They had also been withholding his mail, which included a support group magazine, deciding that he was not able to read and understand it. A local volunteer visitor contacted a transgender support group after discovering James very distressed. On further discussion, he revealed that he regarded the incontinence aids as "sanitary towels" such as women would use to manage menstruation, not something that he, as a man, would be comfortable using. (Witten & Whittle, 2004)

Honoring the identity of the transgender elder during the last stage of life can present practical challenges and the need for health care and social service providers to learn about the realities of life as a gender minority person, which many caring people are willing to do. But until education and clinical competence in this regard become more widespread, transgender older adults will remain fearful: "Will I be treated with dignity? Will I be respected? Will I be in a defenseless situation at the mercy of those that do not understand me being trans, or are unwilling to try?" (Witten, 2011).

Further complications can arise if the transgender patient or client becomes cognitively impaired. Persons who have delirium or dementia often speak of events from earlier in life as though they are current and may believe that they are back in those situations. It is not unusual for women who changed their names at the time of marriage to refer to themselves by their birth name and for persons who are multilingual to revert to their "mother tongue" even if others do not understand this. Sometimes elders who have transitioned gender will mix in recalled material from time lived in the other gender or use a birth name. This can be confusing to new or part-time members of the care staff but can be managed with education about delirium and dementia and their effects. Cognitive impairment also interferes with the ability of the transgender elder to articulate effectively personal needs and preferences with regard to privacy, toileting, and hygiene.

The predeath stage can be particularly harsh in environments not organized to respect individual identity, self-perception, autonomy, and dignity. The federal correctional system and state penal systems provide care to inmates who have become terminally ill while serving a sentence; however, transgender inmates often have not been able to obtain basic transgender health services, including hormone supplementation, though this deprivation is not consistent with current practice (Brown, 2009; WPATH, 2011, pp. 67–68). It is doubtful that end-of-life care in these environments is consistently affirming of the transgender identity. The armed services provide medical services to men and women in active service and to veterans. Policies concerning transgender are currently repressive and unhelpful to enlisted personnel (Witten, 2007b) but, as noted previously, in 2011 were greatly improved with regard to care of veterans—a very positive development for older adults with histories of military service.

Family dynamics develop over many years and often manifest in uncomfortable ways during family crises (Haley et al., 2002), such as the impending death of a member of the family. When the dying person is transgender, another level of complexity can be introduced. If the gender minority person has been estranged from children or grandchildren, the predeath period provides a last chance for rapprochement. In some cases, the imminence of death will prompt reunions with estranged family, which can be helpful, stressful, or both. Some adult children have unresolved feelings of loss, grief, and betrayal at the loss of the "original" parent through gender transition. When confronted with the impending loss of the transgender parent to death, they may behave in unsupportive ways; others will "rise to the occasion" and behave graciously. These situations should be managed in the same way as other "deathbed conflicts" by medical, nursing, and mental health professionals.

Regardless of whether the family is empathic and helpful, many transgender older adults are possessed of significant resilience, having learned to manage the storms of life during years or decades of living without many of the privileges and supports of majority society. In addition, some receive emotional support and companionship in the last stages of life through LGBT organizations, as was the case for James, described earlier. Some gender minority persons also find that the spiritual wisdom they have acquired during years of questioning and introspection serves them well, regardless of whether they have been accepted, or rejected, by the religion of their childhood.

The possibility of dying alone is a serious worry for many people, regardless of gender identity. If family members are not supportive and no friends are available, volunteers—often LGBT-identified or allies—can provide support in life's final moments. No one should be forced to die alone.

DEATH AND ITS AFTERMATH

Transgender elders who make their wishes clear regarding funeral and burial rites may have their choices thwarted by family members who are ambivalent or hostile regarding gender transition, unless these are legally documented and a sympathetic friend or relative has the legal authority to enforce them. Even such simple matters as the name to be inscribed on the grave marker can be contested. As is the case for persons who are members of other sexual and gender minorities, many transgender individuals have led, in a sense, two lives. (See Isherwood, 1996, pp. 199–203, for a striking example of this phenomenon in the death of a young, gay man.) Relatives who were estranged by the gender transition, or who simply did not remain in touch, may be confronted with the realities of the loved one's life in the true psychological gender during the mourning process. An open casket funeral will leave little doubt regarding the gender identity of the deceased and may be shocking to anyone who did not participate in the life of the individual during, or after, the transition process. Important persons in the posttransition life may also not be accepted by the family of origin, resulting in friction with the partner and posttransition family. The importance of legal preparation for end-of-life and postmortem concerns, for persons who transition gender and their spouses and partners, cannot be overemphasized.

The transgender identity and gender-transitioned life of the deceased also often affect spouses and significant others during the period following death, which is when they are also least likely to be prepared to manage these difficulties and insults. For example, transgender persons can be "outed" during the mortuary process, when incongruities of public presentation and genital anatomy are observed by the mortician. The case of Billy Tipton, whose FTM status was sensationally revealed by a family member after death, is well known among gender minority persons. Public response can have serious ramifications for the lives of the bereaved partner and family. The coroner's office may also record the deceased's natal sex on the death record, resulting in additional family embarrassment and practical difficulties due to the mismatch between the death certificate and other important documents (Witten, 2009).

Insurance payments, Social Security claims, military death benefits, and other economic matters of import to the spouse, partner, or family may be delayed because of lack of documentation establishing the identity continuity of the deceased (i.e., that the person who purchased the policy is, in fact, the deceased, despite the change of name and sex). In states and countries that grant no recognition to same-sex relationships, regardless of import or duration, lack of legal preparation can cause serious problems for the surviving family, who may not be able to prove that the joint property is theirs, and who are at risk from claims by biological kin of the deceased. The burden of this cultural system falls disproportionately on lower-income transgender elders and their families, who may not have been able to afford attorney's fees, though families with more resources, but inadequate documentation, may also suffer these losses. Inheritance laws vary by state and country and are often problematic for gender minority persons, their partners, and their families.

The life course of the transgender-identified person is a complex tapestry of interacting normative and nonnormative processes. Gerotranscendence (Tornstam, 2005) and dying well, for gender minority persons, are profoundly tied to the integration of the gendered self, in the context of the normative aging processes. Cultural factors also may promote acceptance of gender minority persons or may enforce marginalization and maltreatment. However, many older transgender persons have acquired personal resilience, wisdom, and spirituality during their life journey, with the challenges and accomplishments that it has offered in the struggle to live true to the truest self.

The transgender identity can often add social and practical complexities to the end-of-life processes, for both the transgender person and for her or his spouse, partner, and other family members. Professionals who work with people at the end of life are advised to remain mindful of the concerns commonly experienced by gender minority persons and their loved ones.

Death awaits each of us. May we all come to a place of peace with the lives we have lived and paths we have chosen, and may our departures from life be filled with dignity and grace.

CONCLUSION

Gender minority persons make up a growing but largely still epidemiologically invisible minority group within the worldwide elderly population (Witten, 2003, 2007a). Persons who transition gender, who do not self-identify as a member of either normative gender, who identify strongly with the gender not usually associated with their natal sex, or who cross-dress or transgress gender norms in other significant ways, are referred to as transgender, though many other terms are used as well. Some transgender elders transitioned gender in young or middle adulthood, some within recent years. Information about the lives of these older adults is just beginning to enter the scientific literature, although many professionals have clinical experience with older transgender persons. Gender identities other than woman or man are traditional within many indigenous cultures, although at present little information is available regarding the status of elders of these populations.

Quality of life is an important aspect of scholarship on behalf of older persons, and as yet there has been little research attention paid to this aspect of aging among transgender adults (Docter, 1985; Whittle, 2007; Witten, 2010, p. 154; Witten & Eyler, 2007). There is now a strong need for obtaining rigorous data on behalf of transgender and gender-variant older adults as they age. Elder health surveillance methods must be put in place for these populations in much the same way as for other populations (Maylahn, Alongi, Alongi, Moore, & Anderson, 2005), including for subgroups within the transgender communities. Research is also needed with regard to aspects of successful aging, such as creativity, generativity, resilience, self-efficacy, usefulness, forgiveness and optimism, and other facets of personal resilience, among transgender older adults.

There is also a strong need for health and social policy development on behalf of transgender elderly persons, including with respect to privacy, confidentiality, and protection from discrimination in health care, palliative care and end-of-life services, as well as availability of appropriate supportive elder care services when these are needed (Belongia & Witten, 2007; Witten & Whittle, 2004). Transgender older adults also have the same needs as their younger peers for personal safety and nondiscrimination in the legal arena. It is also to be hoped that education of professionals in physical and mental health care, social services, and law enforcement will promote tolerance of gender minority identification and behavior and reduce stigma and potential abuse.

Cohort and intergenerational effects are also important, as each group of older adults has perceptions and needs unique to their life course trajectories, as influenced by time-bound cultural experience. Older adults are often called on to serve as a source of wisdom (Holkup, Salois, Tripp-Reimer, & Weinert, 2007) and experience for younger members of the community, thereby increasing the social capital (Hunter, Neiger, & West, 2011; Viswanath, Steele, & Finnegan, 2006) of the group as a whole, and the self-identity of both older and younger members. This also promotes positive aging experience and the sense of self-worth, usefulness, and satisfaction (Ardelt, 1997). These processes are likely also occurring in the transgender community, though they remain to be effectively studied, along with concepts such as transgender gerotranscendence (Wadensten & Carlsson, 2003) and the meaning of elder wisdom in this population.

Members of sexual and gender minority groups stigmatized in majority culture have often survived many challenging experiences before entering the elder years. In the normative elderly population, older adults strive to survive and find quality of life under less than ideal conditions, while facing the stigma and discrimination that often accompanies aging in contemporary society. Transgender older adults have usually had similar experiences, as well as enduring discrimination and sometimes abuse that is frequently coupled to perceptions about their bodies, gender expression, and sexuality. Further study of the resilience of transgender older adults would have potential benefit for the non-transgender population as well.

The experiences of individuals who transition gender during the elder years demonstrate that they can maintain personal dignity, autonomy, and positive social connections while seeking integration of the physical and psychological elements of the authentic self. Persons who transition during youth or middle adulthood and subsequently reach the elder years in the chosen gender face similar challenges in some ways, such as maintaining privacy in care settings, and different challenges in others ways, because of the emotional effect of having come out or transitioned in different eras. Our research and professional experience suggest that members of the health care and helping professions can assist in this actualizing process and in helping older gender minority persons live more comfortably and age more successfully.

It is hoped that, joint efforts between transgender persons and organizations, and members of the health care, social services, and caring professions, will assist in improving the lives of older gender minority persons as they move through midlife, the elder years, and the final stages of life.

It is also hoped that international organizations such as the World Health Organization will recognize the health needs of gender minority persons as deserving of study and practical assistance, and that human rights organizations will regard the gender-variant population as an often suppressed or violated global minority in need of protection and support (Kidd & Witten, 2007b). The June 2011 United Nations resolution is a hopeful sign in that regard. They will also have an important role to play in countries in which customs and myths regarding gender variance continue to excuse the persecution of gender minority persons. Moreover, global aging organizations, such as the Gerontological Society of America, the International Gerontological Association, and the American Gerontological Society, are encouraged to work with WHO and other organizations to develop policies to address the needs of elders of this global community.

Gender identity is a fundamental aspect of the human psyche, and persons of any gender group—women, men, persons with other gender identifications or who transition gender—should have the same rights to personal safety, dignity and opportunity throughout life, and peaceful existence in later years.

> You matter because you are you. You matter to the last
> moment of your life and we will do all we can not only
> to help you die peacefully but to live until you die.
>> —*Dame Cicely Saunders,*
>> *a founder of modern palliative care*

> They are not dead who live in the hearts they leave
> behind . . .
>> *Tuscarora saying.*

ACKNOWLEDGMENTS

Tarynn M. Witten

I would like to thank the numerous respondents to the past and ongoing TLARS and Trans-MetLife surveys. Their participation has greatly enhanced the understanding of this topic. Most of the quotations in this chapter are drawn from the more than 1,800 global respondents to the Trans-MetLife survey, and I would like to express my profound respect for all of the respondents who took the time and effort to provide the information I needed to concretize the concepts this portion of the chapter. Without your energy, I would not have been able to speak as accurately as I have. It is your words that give power to what I have to say.

A. Evan Eyler

Many thanks to my students, colleagues, patients, family, and friends, whose insights, questions, reflection, and revelations have so often made transgender clinical and academic work so interesting and worthwhile. Thank you for sharing your journeys with me.

We would also like to thank our colleagues and friends, transgender, "cisgender," and "none of the above," for their feedback on our work, and for the many useful discussions on this and related topics.

All research related to this chapter was performed under human subjects protection and institutional review board approval from the University of Michigan, Ann Arbor, the University of Texas Health Science Center at San Antonio, and Virginia Commonwealth University.

Identifying information and personal details of included life stories have been changed to honor privacy concerns.

CONTACTING THE PROJECT

All of the authors' published joint research papers, reviews, and citations, as well as Dr. Witten's work in this area, are available by request directly from Tarynn M. Witten at tmwitten@vcu.edu. Dr. Witten is actively seeking participants, on an ongoing basis, for her research survey projects about aging in the transgender and intersex/DSD communities. If you are interested in contacting Dr. Witten, please send an e-mail to either tmwitten@vcu.edu or tarynngeek@gmail.edu.

REFERENCES

Adler, L. (Ed.). (1993). *International handbook of gender roles*. Westport, CT: Greenwood Press.

Agrawal, A. (1997). Gendered bodies: The case of the "third gender" in India. *Contributions to Indian Sociology, 31*(2), 273–297.

AIDS Alert. (2004). The aging AIDS epidemic. More normal lifespans present next hurdle: Experts discuss longevity with HIV infection [Special report]. *AIDS Alert,* 19(9), 101–102.

Ajrouch, K. J., Blandon, A. Y., & Antonucci, T. C. (2005). Social networks among men and women: The effects of age and socioeconomic status. *Journal of Gerontology, Series B, Psychological Sciences and Social Sciences,* 60B(6), S311–S317.

Alexander, J., & Yescavage, K. (Eds.). (2004). *Bisexuality and transgenderism: Inter-SEXions of the others.* Binghamton, NY: Haworth Press.

Alexander, R., & Meshelemia, J. C. A. (2010). Gender identity disorders in prisons: What are the legal implications for prison mental health professionals and administrators. *Prison Journal,* 90, 269–287.

Almack, K., Seymour, J., & Bellamy, G. (2010). Exploring the impact of sexual orientation on experiences and concerns about end of life care and on bereavement for lesbian, gay and bisexual older people. *Sociology,* 44, 908–924.

American Psychiatric Association. (2000). *Diagnostic and statistical manual of mental disorders* (4th ed., text rev., DSM IV-TR). Washington, DC: Author.

Anderson, B. (1996). "Bullshit!" S/He said: The happy, modern, sexy, Indonesian married woman as transsexual. In L. Sears (Ed.), *Fantasizing the feminine in Indonesia.* Durham, NC: Duke University Press.

Anderson, N. B., Bulatao, R. A., & Cohen, B. (2004). *Critical perspectives on racial and ethnic differences in health in late life.* Washington, DC: National Academy Press.

Ardelt, M. (1997). Wisdom and life satisfaction in old age. *Journal of Gerontology, Series B, Psychological Sciences and Social Sciences,* 52B, P15–P27.

Ardelt, M. (2000). Antecedents and effects of wisdom in old age: A longitudinal perspective on aging well. *Research on Aging,* 22, 360–394.

Assscheman, H., Giltay, E. J., Megens, J. A., de Ronde, W. P., van Trotsenburg, M. A., & Gooren, L. J. (2011). A long-term follow-up study of mortality in transsexuals receiving treatment with cross-sex hormones. *European Journal of Endocrinology,* 164(4), 635–642.

Associated Press State and Local Wire. (2006, August 19). San Diego man sentenced to 206 years in sex assaults.

Atamer, Y. (2005). The legal status of transsexuals in Turkey. *International Journal of Transgenderism,* 8(1), 65–71.

Bakshi, S. (2004). A comparative analysis of hijras and drag queens: The subversive possibilities and limits of parading effeminacy and negotiating masculinity. *Journal of Homosexuality,* 46(3/4), 211–213.

Balzer, M. (1996). Sacred genders in Siberia: Bear festivals and androgyny. In S. Ramet (Ed.), *Gender reversals and gender cultures.* London: Routledge.

Baqi, S., Shah, S. A., Baig, M. A., Mujeeb, S. A., & Memon, A. (1999). Seroprevalence of HIV, HBV, and syphilis and associated risk behaviours in male transvestites (Hijras) in Karachi, Pakistan. *International Journal of STD and AIDS,* 10(5), 300–304.

Barabási, A.-L. (2009). *Linked: How everything is connected to everything else and what it means for business, science and everyday life.* New York: Plume.

Baskaran, S. (2004). *Made in India: Decolonisations, queer asexualities, trans/national projects.* New York: Palgrave Macmillan.

Basu, A. M. (2000). Gender in population research: Confusing implications for health policy. *Population Studies, 54,* 19–38.

Basu, J. (2001). Some social and legal difficulties of treatment of transsexuals in India. *Social Science International, 17*(1), 74–81.

Battle, J., Cohen, C. J., Warren, D., Fergerson, G., & Audam, S. (2002). *Say it loud: I'm black and I'm proud.* New York: National Gay and Lesbian Task Force Press. Retrieved from www.ngltf.org

Belongia, L., & Witten, T. M. (2006, Fall). We don't have that kind of client here: Institutionalized bias against and resistance to transgender and intersex aging research and training in elder care facilities. *American Public Health Association Gerontological Health Section Newsletter.* Retrieved from www.transcience.org

Bengtsson, T., & Lindstrom, M. (2000). Childhood misery and disease in later life: The effects on mortality in old age of hazards experienced in early life, southern Sweden, 1760–1894. *Population Studies, 54,* 263–277.

Beyrer, C. (1998). Other genders: Kathoeys, waria, hijras, toms and dees. In *War in the blood: Sex, politics and AIDS in Southeast Asia.* Bangkok: White Lotus.

Blackwood, E. (1984). Sexuality and gender in certain Native American tribes: The case of cross-gender females. *Signs, 10*(1), 27–42.

Blackwood, E., & Wieringa, S. (Eds.). (1999). *Female desires: Same-sex relations and transgender practices across cultures.* New York: Columbia University Press.

Bockting, W., Robinson, B., Benner, A., & Scheltema, K. (2004). Patient satisfaction with transgender health services. *Journal of Sex and Marital Therapy, 30*(4), 277–294.

Bockting, W. O. (1999). From construction to context: Gender through the eyes of the transgendered. *Siecus Report, 28*(1), 3–7.

Bockting, W. O., & Coleman, E. (2007). Developmental stages of the transgender coming out process: Toward an integrated identity. In R. Ettner, S. Monstrey, & A. E. Eyler (Eds.), *Principles of transgender medicine and surgery* (pp. 185–208). New York: Haworth Press.

Bockting, W. O., & Kirk, S. (2000). *Transgender and HIV.* Binghamton, NY: Haworth Press.

Bockting, W. O., Rosser, S., & Coleman, E. (1999). Transgender HIV prevention: Community involvement and empowerment. *International Journal of Transgenderism, 3*(1/2). Retrieved from http://symposion.com/ijt/hiv_risk/bockting.htm

Boellstorff, T. (2001). Playing back the nation: Waria, Indonesian transvestites. *Cultural Anthropology, 19*(2), 159–195.

Boenke, M. (Ed.). (1999). *Trans forming families: Real stories about transgendered loved ones.* Imperial Beach, CA: Walter Trook.

Bowles, S. (1995, December 10). A death robbed of dignity mobilizes a community. *Washington Post,* p. B01.

Bradley, M. (1996). Caring for older people: Elder abuse. *BMJ, 313,* 548–550.

Broom, A. W., Bramson, I., van Tiberg, T. G., van der Ploeg, H. M., & Deeg, D. J. H. (2006). Cosmic transcendence and framework of meaning in life: Patterns among older adults in The Netherlands. *Journal of Gerontology, Series B, Psychological Sciences and Social Sciences*, 61B(3), S121–S128.

Brown, G., Wise, T. N., Costa, P. T., Herbst, J. H., Fagan, P. J., & Schmidt, C. W. (1996). Personality characteristics and sexual functioning of 188 cross-dressing men. *Journal of Nervous and Mental Disorders*, 184(5), 265–273.

Brown, G. R., & McDuffie, E. (2009). Health care policies addressing transgender inmates in prison systems in the United States. *Journal of Correctional Health Care*, 15, 280–291.

Brown, N. (2007). Stories from outside the frame: Intimate partner abuse in sexual-minority women's relationships with transsexual men. *Feminism and Psychology*, 13(3), 373–393.

Browning, F. (1993). *The culture of desire: Paradox and perversity in gay lives today*. New York: Crown Publishing.

Bullough, V., & Bullough, B. (1993). *Cross dressing, sex, and gender*. Philadelphia: University of Pennsylvania Press.

Cahill, S., South, K., & Spade, J. (2000). *Outing aging: Report of the NGLTF Task Force on Aging*. Washington, DC: National Gay and Lesbian Task Force. Retrieved from www.ngltf.org

Carter, B., & McGoldrick, M. (Eds.). (1999). *The expanded family life cycle: Individual, family and social perspectives*. Needham Heights, MA: Allyn & Bacon.

Center of Excellence for Transgender Health, University of California, San Francisco. (2011). *Primary care protocol for transgender health care*. Retrieved from http://transhealth.ucsf.edu/ and http://transhealth.ucsf.edu/trans?page=protocol -agingtrans?page=protocol-oo-oo

Chong, J. (1990). Social assessment of transsexuals who apply for sex reassignment therapy. *Social Work in Health Care*, 14(3), 87–105.

Chong, J. (1991). Transsexualism: A challenge to social work practice. *Hong Kong Journal of Social Work*, 23, 2–9.

Chrissy Lee Polis, victim in Maryland McDonald's attack, alleges hate crime. (2011, April 24). *Huffington Post*. Retrieved from www.huffingtonpost.com/2011/04/24 /chrissy-lee-polis-victim-mcdonalds-beating_n_852962.html

Clements-Nolle, K., Marx, R., Guzman, R., & Katz, M. (2001). HIV prevalence, risk behaviors, health care use, and mental health status of transgender persons: Implications for public health intervention. *American Journal of Public Health*, 91, 915–921.

Cole, S. S., Dallas, D., Eyler, A. E., & Samons, S. (2000). Issues of transgender. In L. T. Szuchman & F. Muscarella (Eds.), *Psychological perspectives on human sexuality* (pp. 149–197). New York: John Wiley & Sons.

Coleman, E., Cogan, P., & Gooren, L. (1992). Male cross-gender behavior in Myanmar (Burma): A description of the Acault. *Archives for Sexual Behavior*, 21(3), 313–332.

Coleman, P. G., & O'Hanlon, A. (2004). *Ageing and development*. New York: Oxford University Press.

Cook-Daniels, L. (1995). *Lesbian, gay male, and transgender elder abuse*. Retrieved from www.amboyz.org/articles/elderabuse.html

Cook-Daniels, L. (2006). Trans aging. In D. Kimmel, T. Rose, & S. David (Eds.), *Lesbian, gay, bisexual and transgender aging: Research and clinical perspectives* (pp. 21–35). New York: Columbia University Press.

Cook-Daniels, L., & Munson, M. (2008). *Sexual violence, elder abuse, and sexuality of transgender adults age 50+: Results of three surveys*. Retrieved from www.forge -forward.org/docs/APA2008_trans_elders_3surveys.pdf

Coppin, A. K., Ferrucci, L., Lauretani, F., Phillips, C., Chang, M., Bandinelli, S., & Guralnik, J. M. (2006). Low socioeconomic status and disability in old age: Evidence from the InChianti Study for the mediating role of physiological impairments. *Journal of Gerontology, Series A, Biological Sciences and Medical Sciences*, 61A(1), 86–91.

Costa, L., & Matzner, A. (2006). *Male bodies, women's souls: Personal narratives of Thailand's transgendered youth*. Binghamton, NY: Haworth Press.

Cronin, A., & King, A. (2010). Power, inequality and identification: Exploring diversity and intersectionality amongst older LGB adults. *Sociology*, *44*, 876–892.

Cui, Y. H., Ren, G. Y., Fang, M. Z., & Xia Y. (1998). The MMPI results in 54 transsexuals. *Chinese Mental Health Journal*, 12(3), 138–139, 144. (In Chinese.)

Currah, P., & Minter, S. (2000). *Transgender equality*. New York: National Gay and Lesbian Task Force Policy Institute.

Dahl, M., Feldman, J. L., Goldberg, J. M., & Jaberi, A. (2006). Physical aspects of transgender endocrine therapy. *International Journal of Transgenderism*, 9(3), 111–134. doi:10.1300/J485v09n03_06.

Darby, E., & Anawalt, B. D. (2005). Male hypogonadism: An update on diagnosis and treatment. *Treatments in Endocrinology*, 4(5) 293–309.

D'Augelli, A. R., & Grossman, A. H. (2001). Disclosure of sexual orientation, victimization, and mental health among lesbian, gay, and bisexual older adults. *Journal of Interpersonal Violence*, 16(10), 1008–1102.

Davis, D. L., & Whitten, R. G. (1987). The cross-cultural study of human sexuality. *Annual Review of Anthropology*, 16, 69–98.

Department of Veterans Affairs, Veterans Health Administration. (2011). *Providing health care for transgender and intersex veterans*. VHA Directive 2011-024. Retrieved from http://www.va.gov/vhapublications/ViewPublication.asp?pub_ID=2416

Depp, C. A., & Jeste, D. V. (2006). Definitions and predictors of successful aging: A comprehensive review of large quantitative studies. *American Journal of Geriatric Psychiatry*, *14*, 6–120.

Devor, H. (1989). *Gender blending: Confronting the limits of duality*. Bloomington: University of Indiana Press.

Dittman, R. J. (2003). Policing hate crime. From victim to challenger: A transgendered perspective. *Probation Journal*, 50, 282–288.

Docter, R. F. (1985). Transsexual surgery at 74: A case report. *Archives of Sexual Behavior*, 14(3), 271–277.

Dunbar, E. (2006). Race, gender, and sexual orientation in hate crime victimization: Identity politics or identity risk? *Violence and Victims*, 23(3), 323–337.

Earth, B. (2006). Diversifying gender: Male to female transgender identities and HIV/AIDS programming in Phnom Penh, Cambodia. *Gender and Development*, 14(2), 259–271.

Eddie Izzard: The tough transvestite who can take care of himself. (2004, May 23). *The Independent*. Retrieved November 22, 2008, from www.independent.co.uk /news/people/profiles/eddie-izzard-the-tough-transvestite-who-can-take-care-of -himself-564108.html

Elkins, R., & King, D. (Eds.). (1996). *Blending genders: Social aspects of cross-dressing and sex-changing*. New York: Routledge.

Ellison, J. (2008, February 19). Free to be female. *Newsweek*. Retrieved from www .newsweek.com/id/109565

Ellison-Loschmann, L., & Pearce, N. (2006). Improving access to health care among New Zealand's Maori population. *American Journal of Public Health*, 96(4), 612–617.

Emerton, R. (2004a). Neither here nor there· The current status of transsexual and other transgender persons under Hong Kong law. *Hong Kong Law Journal*, 34(2), 245–277.

Emerton, R. (2004b). Time for change: A call for the legal recognition of transsexual and other transgender persons in Hong Kong. *Hong Kong Law Journal*, 34(3), 515–555.

Emerton, R. (2006). Finding a voice, fighting for rights: The emergence of the transgender movement in Hong Kong. *Inter-Asia Cultural Studies*, 7(2), 243–269.

Emlet, C. A. (2004). HIV/AIDS and aging: A diverse population of vulnerable older adults. *Journal of Human Behavior in a Social Environment*, 9(4), 45–63.

Emlet, C. A. (2006). "You're awfully old to have this disease": Experiences of stigma and ageism in adults 50 years and older living with HIV/AIDS. *Gerontologist*, 46, 781–790.

Epple, C. (1998). Coming to terms with Najajo nádleehí: A critique of berdache, "gay," "alternate gender," and "two spirit." *American Ethologist*, 25(2), 267–290.

Erikson, E. H., & Erikson, J. M. (1997). *The life cycle completed*. New York: W. W. Norton Press.

Erikson, E. H., Erikson, J. M., & Kivnick, H. Q. (1986). *Vital involvement in old age: The experience of old age in our time*. New York: W. W. Norton.

Ettner, R. (1999, August 20). XVI International Meeting, Harry Benjamin International Gender Dysphoria Association, London.

Ettner, R., Mostrey, S., & Eyler, A. E. (Eds.). (2007). *Principles of transgender medicine and surgery*. New York: Haworth Press.

Evans, R. G., Barer, M. L., & Marmor, T. R. (Eds.). (1994). *Why are some people healthy and others not? The determinants of health of populations*. Hawthorne, NY: Aldine de Gruyter.

Everard, K. M., Lach, H. W., Fisher, E. B., & Baum, M. C. (2000). Relationship of activity and social support to the functional health of older adults. *Journal of Gerontology, Series B, Psychological Sciences and Social Sciences,* 55B(4), S208–S12.

Eyler, A. E. (2007). Primary medical care of the gender-variant patient. In R. Ettner, S. Monstrey, & A. E. Eyler (Eds.), *Principles of transgender medicine and surgery* (pp. 15–32). Binghamton, NY: Haworth Press.

Eyler, A. E. (2011). *Transgender aging: Clinical concerns* [Invited plenary session]. The 28th Annual Women in Medicine Conference, Stoweflake Mountain Resort, July 26, 2011, Stowe VT.

Eyler, A. E., & Feldman, J. (2008). The transsexual male. In J. J. Heidelbaugh (Ed.), *Clinical men's health: Evidence in practice* (pp. 561–584). Philadelphia: Saunders/ Elsevier.

Eyler, A. E., & Wright, K. (1997, July–September). Gender identification and sexual orientation among genetic females with gender-blended self-perception in childhood and adolescence. *International Journal of Transgenderism,* 1(1). Retrieved from www.symposion.com/ijtc0101.htm

Fahrenthold, D. A. (2002, August 13). Transgender teens killed on D.C. street. *Washington Post,* p. B01.

Feldman, J. (2007). Preventive care of the transgendered patient: An evidence-based approach. In R. Ettner, S. Monstrey, & A. E. Eyler (Eds.), *Principles of transgender medicine and surgery* (pp. 33–72). Binghamton, NY: Haworth Press.

Feldman, J. (2008). Medical and surgical management of the transgender patient: What the primary care clinician needs to know. In H. J. Makadon, K. H. Mayer, J. Potter, & H. Goldhammer (Eds.), *Fenway guide to lesbian, gay, bisexual, and transgender health* (pp. 365–392). Philadelphia: American College of Physicians.

Feldman, J., & Bockting, W. (2003, July). Transgender health. *Minnesota Medicine,* 86(7), 25–32. Retrieved from www.mmaonline.net/publications/MNMed2003 /July/Feldman.html

Feldman, J., & Goldberg, J. (2006). Transgender primary medical care. *International Journal of Transgenderism,* 9(3), 3–34. doi:10.1300/J485v09n03_02.

Feldman, J., & Safer, J. (2009). Hormone therapy in adults: Suggested revisions to the sixth version of the standards of care. *International Journal of Transgenderism,* 11(3), 146–182. doi:10.1080/15532730903383757.

Ferron, P., Young, S., Boulanger, C., Rodriguez, A., & Moreno, J. (2010). Integrated care of an aging HIV-infected male-to-female transgender patient. *Journal of the Association of Nurses in AIDS Care,* 21(3), 278–282.

Finlon, C. (2002). Substance abuse in lesbian, gay, bisexual and transgender communities. *Journal Gay and Lesbian Social Services,* 14(4), 109–116.

Finnegan, D. G., & McNally, E. B. (2002). *Counseling lesbian, gay, bisexual, and transgender substance abusers: Dual identities.* Binghamton, NY: Haworth Press.

Ford, N., & Kittisuksathit, S. (1994). Destinations unknown: The gender construction and changing nature of the sexual expressions of Thai youth. *AIDS Care,* 6(5), 517–530.

Franks, J. (2004). Sunset Pink Villa: A home for gay and lesbian elders. *Gerontologist*, *44*, 856–857.

Fredriksen-Goldsen, K. I., & Muraco, A. (2010). Aging and sexual orientation: A 25-year review of the literature. *Research on Aging, 32*, 372–413.

Fruhoff, G. A., & Mahoney, D. (Eds.). (2010). Older GLBT family and community life. New York: Routledge.

Fulton, R., & Anderson, S. W. (1992). The Amerindian "man-woman": Gender, liminality, and cultural continuity. *Current Anthropology, 33*(5), 603–610.

Furth, C. (1993). Androgynous males and deficient females: Biology and gender boundaries in sixteenth- and seventeenth-century China. In H. Abelove, M. Barale, & D. Halperin (Eds.), *The lesbian and gay studies reader*. New York: Routledge Press.

Garner, B. A. (1999). *Black's law dictionary* (2nd ed.). St. Paul, MN: Thomson West.

Gay and Lesbian Medical Association. (2000). *Healthy People 2010: Companion document for lesbian, gay, bisexual, and transgender (LGBT) health*. San Francisco: Gay and Lesbian Medical Association. Retrieved from www.glma.org

Gender Education and Advocacy. (2005). Transgender Day of Remembrance: About DOR. Retrieved from www.gender.org/remember/day/what.html

George, L. K. (2005). Socioeconomic status and health across the life course: Progress and prospects [Special issue 2]. *Journal of Gerontology, Series B, Psychological Sciences and Social Sciences, 60B*, 135–139.

Gfroerer, J., Penne, M., Pemberton, M., & Folsom, R. (2003). Substance abuse treatment need among older adults in 2020: The impact of the aging baby-boom cohort. *Drug and Alcohol Dependence, 69*(2), 127–135.

Ghilarducci, T. (2007). Pressures on retirement income security. *Public Policy and Aging Report, 17*(2), 8–12.

Godlewski, J. (1988). Transsexualism and anatomic sex ratio reversal in Poland. *Archives of Sexual Behavior, 17*(6), 547–548.

Goldman, D. P., Joyce, G. F., & Zheng, Y. (2007). Prescription drug cost sharing: Associations with medication and medical utilization and spending and health. *JAMA, 298*(1), 61–69.

Gooren, L. J., Giltay, E. J., & Bunck, M. C. (2008). Long-term treatment of transsexuals with cross-sex hormones: Extensive personal experience. *Journal of Clinical Endocrinology and Metabolism, 93*, 19–25. doi:10.1210/jc.2007-1809.

Gorton, R. N., Buth, J., & Spade, D. (2005). *Medical therapy and health maintenance for transgender men: A guide for health care providers*. San Francisco: Lyon-Martin Women's Health Services.

Green, A. F., Rebok, G., & Lyketsos, C. G. (2008). Influence of social network characteristics on cognition and functional status with aging. *International Journal of Geriatric Psychiatry, 23*(9), 972–978.

Green, L., & Grant, V. (2008). "Gagged grief and beleaguered bereavements?" An analysis of multidisciplinary theory and research related to same sex partnership bereavement. *Sexualities, 11*, 275–300.

Greenberg, J. A. (1998). Defining male and female: Intersexuality and the collision between law and biology. *Arizona Law Review*, 41(2), 265–328.

Gruenewald, T. L., Karlamangla, A. S., Greendale, G., Singer, B. H., & Seeman, T. E. (2007). Feelings of usefulness to others, disability and mortality in older adults: The MacArthur Study of Successful Aging. *Journal of Gerontology, Series B, Psychological Sciences and Social Sciences*, 62B(1), P28–P37.

Gupta, S. C., Singh, H., & Rastogi, S. N. (1998). Gender identity disorder: A case report with twelve years follow-up. *Indian Journal of Clinical Psychology*, 15(1), 50–55.

Guralnick, J. M., Butterworth, S., Wadsworth, E. J., & Kuh, D. (2006). Childhood socioeconomic status predicts physical functioning a half century later. *Journal of Gerontology, Series A, Biological Sciences and Medical Sciences*, 61A(7), 694–701.

Haley, W. E., Allen, R. S., Reynolds, S., Chen, H., Burton, A., & Gallagher-Thompson, D. (2002). Family issues in end-of-life decision making and end-of-life care. *American Behavioral Sciences*, 46(2), 284–298.

Harcourt, J. (2006). *Current issues in GLBT health*. Binghamton, NY: Haworth Press.

Hawkins, B. A. (2005). Aging well: Toward a way of life for all people, preventing chronic disease-public health research. *Practice and Policy*, 2(3), 1–3. Retrieved from www.cdc.gov/issues/2005/jul/05_0018.htm

Hawkley, L. C., & Cacioppo, J. T. (2007). Aging and loneliness: Downhill quickly? *Current Directions in Psychological Science*, 16, 187–191.

Hembree, W. C., Cohen-Kettenis, P., Delemarre-van de Waal, H. A., Gooren, L. J., Meyer, W. J., III, Spack, N. P., . . . Montori, V. M. (2009). Endocrine treatment of transsexual persons: An Endocrine Society clinical practice guideline. *Journal of Clinical Endocrinology & Metabolism*, 94(9), 3132–3154. doi:10.1210/jc.2009-0345.

Herek, G. (1989). Hate crimes against lesbians and gay men. *American Psychologist*, 44(6), 948–955.

Herek, G., Cogan, J. C., & Gillis, J. R. (2002). Victims' experiences in hate crimes based on sexual orientation. *Journal of Social Issues*, 58(2), 319–339.

Herek, G. M. (2009). Hate crimes and stigma-related experiences among sexual minority adults in the United States: Prevalence estimates from a national probability sample. *Journal of Interpersonal Violence*, 24, 54–74.

Herek, G. M., Gillis, J. R., Cogan, J. C., & Glunt, E. K. (1997). Hate crime victimization among lesbian, gay, and bisexual adults: Prevalence, psychological correlates, and methodological issues. *Journal of Interpersonal Violence*, 12, 195–215.

Hermann, C. P., & Looney, S. W. (2011). Determinants of quality of life in patients near the end of life. *Oncological Nursing Forum*, 38(1), 23–31.

Hertzman, C. (2001). Health and human society. *Scientific American*, 89(6). Retrieved from www.americanscientist.org/articles/01articles/Hertzman.html

Higashi, Y., Nomiya, A., & Morino, H. (2000). Transgenderism in Japan: Past, present and future. In M. L. Ng, M. Perez-Conchillo, & E. Coleman (Eds.), *Sexuality in the new millennium: Proceedings of the 14th World Congress on Sexology*. August 1999, Hong Kong SAR, China.

Hill, T. D., Burdette, A. M., Angel, J. L., & Angel, R. J. (2006). Religious attendance and cognitive functioning among older Americans. *Journal of Gerontology, Series B, Psychological Sciences and Social Sciences*, 61B(1), P3–P9.

Hines, S. (2006). Intimate transitions: Transgender practices of partnering and parenting. *Sociology*, 40(2), 353–371.

Hines, S. (2007). Transgendering care: Practices of care within transgender communities. *Critical Social Policy*, 27, 462–486.

Hoenig, J., & Kenna, C. (1974). The prevalence of transsexualism in England and Wales. *British Journal of Psychiatry*, 124, 181–190.

Holkup, P. A., Salois, E. M., Tripp-Reimer, T., & Weinert, C. (2007). Drawing on wisdom from the past: An elder abuse intervention with tribal communities. *Gerontologist*, 47(2), 248–254.

Human Rights Campaign. (2010). Matthew Shepard and James Byrd, Jr. Hate Crimes Prevention Act. Public Law No. 111-84. Retrieved from www.hrc.org/laws_and_elections/5660.htm

Human Rights Watch. (2006, May 18). *Nepal. "Sexual cleansing" drive continues: New arrests of transgender people/HIV workers*. Retrieved from http://hrw.org/english/docs/2006/03/17/nepal13020.htm

Humes, C. (1996). Becoming male: Salvation through gender modification in Hinduism and Buddhism. In S. Ramet (Ed.), *Gender reversals and gender cultures*. London: Routledge.

Hunter, B. D., Neiger, B., & West, J. (2011). The importance of addressing social determinants of health at the local level: The case for social capital. *Health Social Care Community*, 19(5), 522–530.

Hunter, S. (2005). *Midlife and older LGBT adults*. Binghamton, NY: Haworth Press.

Institute of Medicine. (2011). *The health of lesbian, gay, bisexual, and transgender people: Building a foundation for better understanding* [Prepublication e-copy, uncorrected proofs]. Washington, DC: National Academies Press. Retrieved from www.nap.edu/catalog/13128.html

Intersex Society of North America. (2006). Retrieved from www.isna.org

Iran executes two gay teens in public hanging. (2005, July 21). *UK Gay News*. Retrieved from www.ukgaynews.org.uk/Archive/2005july/2101.htm

Isherwood, C. (1996). *Diaries: Vol. 1. 1939–1960*. London: Meuthen London.

Jackson, N. C., Johnson, M. J., & Roberts, R. (2008). The potential impact of discrimination fears of older gays, lesbians, bisexuals, and transgender individuals living in small- to moderate-sized cities on long-term health care. *Journal of Homosexuality*, 54(3), 325–339.

Jackson, P. (1995a). Kathoey: The third sex. In P. Jackson (Ed.), *Dear Uncle Go: Male homosexuality in Thailand*. Bangkok, Thailand: Bua Luang Books.

Jackson, P. (1995b). Thai Buddhist accounts of male homosexuality and AIDS in the 1980s. *Australian Journal of Anthropology*, 6(3), 140–153.

Jackson, P. (1997). Kathoey-gay-man: The historical emergence of gay male identity in Thailand. In L. Manderson & M. Jolly (Eds.), *Sites of desire, economies of pleasure: Sexualities in Asia and the Pacific*. Chicago: University of Chicago Press.

Jackson, P. (1998). Male homosexuality and transgenderism in the Thai Buddhist transition. In W. Leyland (Ed.), *Queer Dharma: Voices of gay Buddhists*. San Francisco: Gay Sunshine Press.

Jackson, P. (1999). Tolerant but unaccepting: The myth of a Thai "gay" paradise. In P. Jackson & N. Cook (Eds.), *Gender and sexualities in modern Thailand*. Chiangmai: Silkworm Books.

Jacobs, S. E., & Cromwell, J. (1992). Visions and revisions of reality: Reflections on sex, sexuality, gender, and gender variance. *Journal of Homosexuality, 23*(4), 43–69.

Jacobs, S. E., Thomas, W., & Lang, S. (Eds.). (1997). *Two-Spirit people: Native American gender identity, sexuality, and spirituality*. Urbana: University of Illinois Press.

Jaffrey, Z. (1997). *The invisibles: A tale of the eunuchs of India*. London: Weidenfeld and Nicolson.

Jenness, V. (2003). Engendering hate crime policy: Gender, the "dilemma of difference," and the creation of legal subjects. *Journal of Hate Studies, 2*, 73–97.

Jenness, V. (2010). From policy to prisoners to people: A "soft mixed methods" approach to studying transgender prisoners. *Journal of Contemporary Ethnography, 39*, 517–553.

Johnson, M. (1997). *Beauty and power: Transgendering and cultural transformation in the southern Philippines*. Oxford: Berg.

Johnson, M. (1998). Global desirings and translocal loves: Transgendering and same sex sexualities in the southern Philippines. *American Ethnologist, 25*(4), 695–711.

Johnson, M., Jackson, P., & Herdt, G. (2000). Critical regionalities and the study of gender and sexual diversity in South East and East Asia. *Culture, Health and Sexuality, 2*(4), 361–375.

Kahana, E., & Kahana, B. (2001). Successful aging among people with HIV/AIDS. *Journal of Clinical Epidemiology, 54*(Suppl. 1), S53–S56.

Kameya, Y., & Norita, V. (2000). Clinical and psychosociological case study on gender identity disorder in Japan. In M. L. Ng, M. Perez-Conchillo, & E. Coleman, & E. (Eds.), *Sexuality in the new millennium: Proceedings of the 14th World Congress on Sexology*. August 1999, Hong Kong SAR, China.

Kaufman, R. (2008). Introduction to transgender identity and health. In H. J. Makadon, K. H. Mayer, J. Potter, & H. Goldhamer (Eds.), *Fenway guide to lesbian, gay, bisexual, and transgender health* (pp. 331–364). Philadelphia: American College of Physicians.

Kidd, J. D., & Witten, T. M. (2007a). Assessing spirituality, religiosity, and faith in the transgender community: A case study in violence and abuse—implications for the aging transgender community and for gerontological research. *Journal of Religious Gerontology, 20*(1/2), 29–62.

Kidd, J. D., & Witten, T. M. (2007b). Transgender and transsexual identities: The next strange fruit—hate crimes, violence and genocide against the trans-communities. *Journal of Hate Studies*, 6(1), 31–63.

Kidd, J. D., & Witten, T. M. (2009). Methods for understanding spirituality and religiosity in the transgender community. In J. W. Ellor (Ed.), *Methods in religion, spirituality and aging*. London: Routledge.

Kimmel, D., Rose, T., & David, D. (2006). *Lesbian, gay, bisexual, and transgender aging: Research and clinical perspectives*. New York: Columbia University Press.

Klein, D., Turvey, C., & Wallace, R. (2004). Elders who delay medication because of cost: Health insurance, demographic health, and financial correlates. *Journal of Gerontology, Series B, Psychological Sciences and Social Sciences*, 44B(6), 779–787.

Knodel, J., Watkins, S., & VanLandingham, M. (2002). *AIDS and older persons: An international perspective* (PSC Research Report No. 02-495). Retrieved from Population Studies Center at the Institute for Social Research, University of Michigan www.psc.isr.umich.edu/pubs/

Kockett, G., & Fahrner, E.-M. (1988). Male-to-female and female-to-male transsexuals: A comparison. *Archives of Sexual Behavior*, 17(6), 539–546.

Kok, L. P. (1993). Management of sexual disorders. *Singapore Medical Journal*, 34(6), 553–556.

Kraaij, V., Arensman, E., & Spinhoven, P. (2002). Negative life events and depression in elderly persons: A meta-analysis. *Journal of Gerontology, Series B, Psychological Sciences and Social Sciences*, 57B(1), P87–P94.

Krause, N. (2002). Church-based social support and health in old age: Exploring variations by race. *Journal of Gerontology, Series B, Psychological Sciences and Social Sciences*, 57B, S263–S274.

Krause, N. (2003). Religious meaning and subjective well-being in late life. *Journal of Gerontology, Series B, Psychological Sciences and Social Sciences*, 58B, S160–S170.

Krause, N. (2006a). Church-based social support and mortality. *Journal of Gerontology, Series B, Psychological Sciences and Social Sciences*, 61B(3), S1140–S1146.

Krause, N. (2006b). Exploring the stress-buffering effects of church-based and secular social support on self-rated health in late life. *Journal of Gerontology, Series B, Psychological Sciences and Social Sciences*, 61B(1), S35–S43.

Krause, N., & Ellison, C. G. (2003). Forgiveness by God, forgiveness of others, and psychological well-being in late life. *Journal of the Scientific Study of Religion*, 42, 77–93.

Krause, N., Ingersoll-Dayton, B., Ellison, C. G., & Wulff, K. M. (1999). Aging, religious doubt, and psychological well-being. *Gerontologist*, 39, 525–533.

Krause, N., & Shaw, B. A. (2000). Role-specific feelings of control and mortality. *Psychology and Aging*, 15(4), 617–626.

Kröhn, K., Bertermann, H., Wand, H., & Wille, R. (1981). Nachtuntersuchung bei operierten Transexuellen. *Nervenarz*, 52, 26–31.

Kubzansky, L. D., Berkman, L. F., & Seeman, T. E. (2000). Social conditions and distress in elderly persons: Findings from the MacArthur Studies of Successful

Aging. *Journal of Gerontology, Series B, Psychological Sciences and Social Sciences,* 55B(4), P238–P246.

Kulick, D. (1998a). Fe/male trouble: The unsettling place of lesbians in the self-images of Brazilian travesti prostitutes. *Sexualities,* 1, 299–312.

Kulick, D. (1998b). Transgender in Latin America: Persons, practices and meanings. *Sexualities,* 1, 259–260.

Kurtz, M. (2000, September 7). Lesbian wedding allowed in Texas by gender loophole. *Seattle Post-Intelligencer.*

Kuyper, L., & Vanwesenbeeck, I. (2011). Examining sexual health differences between lesbian, gay, bisexual and heterosexual adults; the role of sociodemographics, sexual behavior characteristics and minority health. *Journal of Sexuality Research,* 48(2/3), 263–274.

Lal, V. (1999, Winter). Not this, not that: The Hijras of India and the cultural politics of sexuality. *Social Text,* no. 61, 119–140.

Lancaster, R. N. (1998). Transgenderism in Latin America: Some critical introductory remarks on identities and practices. *Sexualities,* 1, 261–274.

Lang, F. R., & Baltes, M. M. (1997). Being with people and being alone in late life: Costs and benefits for every day functioning. *International Journal of Behavioral Development,* 21, 729–746.

Lang, S. (1990). Traveling women: Conducting a fieldwork project on gender variance and homosexuality among North American Indians. In E. Lewin & W. L. Leap (Eds.), *Out in the field: Reflections of lesbian and gay anthropologists.* Urbana: University of Illinois Press.

Langevin, R. (1983). *Sexual strands: Understanding and treating sexual anomalies in men.* Hillsdale, NJ: Lawrence Erlbaum.

Lee, S. (2006). Women and HIV: Aging with HIV. *Beta,* 18(2), 33–35.

Leupp, G. (1995). *Male colors: The construction of homosexuality in Tokugawa Japan.* Berkeley: University of California Press.

Lev, A. (2004). *Transgender emergence.* Binghamton, NY: Haworth Press.

Levin, J. S. (Ed.). (2001). *Religion in aging and health.* Thousand Oaks, CA: Sage.

Li, F., Fisher, K. J., Bauman, A., Ory, M. G., Chodzkp-Zajko, W., Harmer, P., . . . Cleveland, M. (2005). Neighborhood influences on physical activity in middle-aged and older adults: A multilevel perspective. *Journal of Aging and Physical Activity,* 13, 87–114.

Li, S. L. (2003). *Cross-dressing in Chinese opera.* Hong Kong: Hong Kong University Press.

Lindau, S. T., Schumm, L. P., Laumann, E. O., Levinson, W., O'Muircheartaigh, C. A., & Waite, L. J. (2007). A study of sexuality and health among older adults in the United States. *New England Journal of Medicine,* 356(8), 22–34.

Linder, J. F., Enders, S. R., Craig, E., Richardson, J., & Meyers, F. J. (2002). Hospice care for the incarcerated in the United States: An introduction. *Journal of Palliative Medicine,* 5, 4549–4552.

Littleton v. Prange. (2000). Court of Appeals of Texas, San Antonio, TX. No. 04-99-00010-CV. October 27, 1999.

Locke, M. (2006, January 28). Three sentenced in transgender killing in U.S. Associated Press Worldstream.

Lombardi, E. L., Wilchins, R. A., Priestling, D., & Malouf, D. (2001). Gender violence: Transgender experiences with violence and discrimination. *Journal of Homosexuality*, 42(1), 89–101.

Los Angeles County Commission on Human Relations. (2006). *2005 hate crime report*. Los Angeles: Author.

Lunsing, W. (2003). What masculinity? Transgender practices among Japanese "men." In J. Roberson & N. Suzuki (Eds.), *Men and masculinities in contemporary Japan: Dislocating the salaryman Doxa*. London: Routledge Curzon.

Luo, Y., & Waite, L. J. (2005). The impact of childhood and adult SES on physical, mental, and cognitive well-being in later life. *Journal of Gerontology, Series B, Psychological Sciences and Social Sciences*, 60B, S93–S101.

Lyng, S. (2000). *Class lecture notes in medical sociology*. Virginia Commonwealth University, Richmond.

Lyyra, T.-M., & Heikkinen, R.-L. (2006). Perceived social support and mortality in older people. *Journal of Gerontology, Series B, Psychological Sciences and Social Sciences*, 61B(3), S147–S152.

Ma, J. L. C. (1997). A systems approach to the social difficulties of transsexuals in Hong Kong. *Journal of Family Therapy*, 19(1), 71–88.

Ma, J. L. C. (1999). Social work practice with transsexuals in Hong Kong who apply for sex reassignment surgery. *Social Work in Health Care*, 29(2), 85–103.

Mackie, V. (2002). Citizenship, embodiment, and social policy in contemporary Japan. In R. Goodman (Ed.), *Family and social policy in Japan: Anthropological approaches*. Cambridge: Cambridge University Press.

MacKinlay, E., & McFadden, S. H. (2004). Ways of studying religion, spirituality, and aging: The social scientific approach. *Journal of Religious Gerontology*, 16(3/4), 75–90.

Magai, C., & McFadden, S. H. (1996). *Handbook of emotion, adult development, and aging*. San Diego, CA: Academic Press.

Mahalingam, R. (2003). Essentialism, culture, and beliefs about gender among the Aruvanis of Tamil Nadu, India. *Sex Roles*, 49(9/10), 489–496.

Manfredi, R. (2002). HIV disease and advanced age: An increasing therapeutic challenge. *Drugs and Aging*, 19(9), 647–669.

Mansey, K. (2006, November 9). Sex-change woman to advise on hate crime. *Dairy Post (Liverpool)*.

Manton, K. G., Singer, B. H., & Suzman, R. M. (1993). *Forecasting the health of elderly populations*. New York: Springer.

Marmot, M., Wilkinson, R., & Wilkinson, R. G. (2006). *The social determinants of health*. Oxford: Oxford University Press.

Marmot, M. G., Kogevinas, M., & Elston, M. A. (1987). Social/economic status and disease. *Annual Review of Public Health*, 8, 111–135.

Marmot, M. G., & McDowall, M. E. (1986). Mortality decline and widening social inequalities. *Lancet*, 2(8501), 274–276.

Marzolini, C., Back, D., Weber, R., Furrer, H., Cavassini, M., Calmy, A., . . . Elzi, L.; on behalf of the Swiss HIV Cohort Study. (2011). Aging with HIV: Medication use and risk for potential drug-drug interactions. *Journal of Antimicrobial Chemotherapy*. doi:10.1093/jac/dkr248.

Mason, G. (2005). Being hated: Stranger or familiar? *Social and Legal Studies*, 14(4), 585–605.

Matzner, A. (2001a). The complexities of acceptance: Thai students attitudes towards kathoey. *Crossroads: An Interdisciplinary Journal of South East Asian Studies*, 15(2), 71–93.

Matzner, A. (2001b). *O Au No Keia: Voices from Hawai'i's Mahu and transgender communities*. Xlibris.

Maylahn, C., Alongi, S., Alongi, J., Moore, M. J., & Anderson, L. A. (2005). Data needs and uses for older adult health surveillance: Perspectives from state agencies. *Preventing Chronic Disease—Public Health Research, Practice, and Policy*, 2(3), 1–5. Retrieved from www.cdc.gov/pcd/issues/2005/jul/05_0020.htm

McGhee, D. (2003). Joined-up government, "community safety" and lesbian, gay, bisexual and transgender "active citizens." *Critical Social Policy*, 23, 245–274.

McLelland, M. J. (2004). From the stage to the clinic: Changing transgender identities in post-war Japan. *Japan Forum*, 16(1), 1–20.

McNair, R. P. (2003). Lesbian health inequalities: A cultural minority issue for health professionals. *Medical Journal of Australia*, 178(12), 643–645.

McNair, R. P., & Hegarty, K. (2010). Guidelines for the primary care of lesbian, gay and bisexual people: A systematic review. *Annals of Family Medicine*, 8, 533–541.

McPhail, B. A. (2002). Gender-bias hate crimes: A review. *Trauma Violence Abuse*, 3, 125–143.

McPhail, B. A., & DiNitto, D. M. (2005). Prosecutorial perspectives on gender-bias hate crimes. *Violence against Women*, 11(9), 1162–1185.

Meadow, T. (2010). "A rose is a rose": On producing legal gender classifications. *Gender & Society*, 24(6), 814–837.

Meezan, W., & Martin, J. I. (2003). *Research methods with GLBT populations*. Binghamton, NY: Haworth Press.

Melendez, R. M., Exner, T. A., Erhart, A. A., Dodge, B., Remien, R. H., Rotheram-Borus, M. J., . . . Hong, D. (2006). Health and healthcare among male-to-female transgender persons who are HIV positive. *American Journal of Public Health*, 96(6), 1034–1037.

MetLife. (2010). *Still out, still aging: The MetLife Study of Lesbian, Gay, Bisexual, and Transgender Baby Boomers*. Westport, CT: MetLife Mature Market Institute.

Meyer, W., Bockting, W. O., Cohen-Kettenis, P., Coleman, E., DiCeglie, D., Devore, H., . . . Wheeler, C. C. (2001). *The standards of care for gender identity disorders*. 6th Version. Harry Benjamin International Gender Dysphoria Association (later the World Professional Association for Transgender Health). Retrieved from the World Professional Association for Transgender Health www.wpath.org/documents2/socv6.pdf

Moberg, D. O. (Ed.). (2001). *Aging and spirituality*. Binghamton, NY: Haworth Pastoral Press.

Monro, S. (2003). Transgender politics in the UK. *Critical Social Policy, 23*, 433–452.

Moran, L. J., & Sharpe, A. N. (2004). Violence, identity and policing: The case of violence against transgender people. *Criminal Justice, 4*, 395–417.

Moreno-John, G., Gachie, A., Fleming, C. M., Napoles-Springer, A., Mutran, E., Manson, S. M., & Perez-Stable, E. J. (2004). Ethnic minority older adults participating in clinical research: Developing trust. *Journal of Aging and Health, 16*(5), 93S–123S.

Morgan, J. J., Mancl, D. B., Kaffar, B. J., & Ferreira, D. (2011). Creating safe environments for students who identify as lesbian, gay, bisexual or transgender. *Intervention in School and Clinic, 47*, 3–13.

Morley, J. E. (2002). Drugs, aging, and the future. *Journal of Gerontology, Series A, Biological Sciences and Medical Sciences, 57A*(1), M2–M6.

Morris, R. C. (1997). Educating desire: Thailand, transnationalism and transgression. *Social Text, 52/53*, 53–79.

Mukasa, J. V. (2006). *On transgender human rights issues in Africa*. Retrieved from www.pambazuka.org/en/category/comment/38727

Muñoz-Laboy, M., & Dodge, B. (2007). Bisexual Latino men and HIV and sexually transmitted infections risk: An exploratory analysis. *American Journal of Public Health, 97*(6), 1102–1106.

Murray, S., & Roscoe, W. (Eds.). (1998). *Boy-wives and female husbands: Studies in African homosexualities*. New York: Palgrave.

Murray, S. O. (1994). On subordinating Native American cosmologies to the empire of gender. *Current Anthropology, 35*(1), 59–61.

Nakamura, K., & Matsuo, H. (2003). Female masculinity and fantasy spaces: Transcending genders in the Takarazuka theatre and Japanese popular culture. In J. Roberson & N. Suzuki (Eds.), *Men and masculinities in contemporary Japan: Dislocating the salaryman doxa*. London: Routledge Curzon.

Nanda, S. (1990). *Neither man nor woman: The Hijras of India*. Belmont, CA: Wadsworth Press.

Nanda, S. (1997). The Hijras of India. In M. Duberman (Ed.), *A queer world: The Center for Lesbian and Gay Studies reader*. New York: New York University Press.

Nanda, S. (2000). *Gender diversity: Cross-cultural variations*. Prospect Heights, IL: Waveland Press.

National Coalition of Anti-Violence Programs. (2009). *Hate violence against lesbian, gay, bisexual and transgender people in the United States, 2008*. Retrieved from http://ncavp.org/common/document_files/Reports/2008%20HV%20Report%20/maller%20file.pdf

National Coalition of Anti-Violence Programs. (2011). *Hate violence against lesbian, gay, bisexual, transgender, queer and HIV-affected communities: A report from the National Coalition of Anti-Violence Programs*. Retrieved from http://www.avp.org/documents/NCAVPHateViolenceReport2011Finaledjlfinaledits.pdf

National Gay and Lesbian Task Force. (2005). *Make room for all: Diversity, cultural competency and discrimination in an aging America*. Retrieved from www.thetask force.org/reslibrary/list.cfm?pubTypeID=2#pub304

Nemoto, T., Operario, D., Keatley, J., Han, L., & Soma, T. (2004a). HIV risk behaviors among male-to-female transgender persons of color in San Francisco. *American Journal of Public Health, 94*, 1193–1199.

Nemoto, T., Operario, D., Keatley, J., Nguyen, H., & Sugano, E. (2005). Promoting health for transgender women: Transgender resources and neighborhood space (TRANS) program in San Francisco. *American Journal of Public Health, 95*, 382–384.

Nemoto, T., Operario, D., Keatley, J., & Villegas, D. (2004b). Social context of HIV risk behaviours among male-to-female transgenders of colour. *AIDS Care, 16*(6), 724–735.

Ng, M. L., Wong, K. K., Chow, S. K., Tang, S. K., Leung, A., & Chan, M. M. (1989). Transsexualism: Service and problems in Hong Kong. *Hong Kong Practitioner, 11*(12), 591–602.

Nichols, A. (2010). Dance ponnaya, dance! Police abuses against transgender sex workers in Sri Lanka. *Feminist Criminology, 5*, 195–222.

Nolan, J. J., Akiyama, Y., & Berhanu, S. (2002). The hate crime statistics act of 1990: Developing a method for measuring the occurrence of hate violence. *American Behavioral Scientist, 46*(1), 136–153.

Nummela, O., Seppanen, M., & Uutela, A. (2011). The effect of loneliness and change in loneliness on self-rated health (SRH): A longitudinal study among aging people. *Archives of Gerontology and Geriatrics, 53*(2), 163–167.

O'Connell, H., Chin, A.-V., Cunningham, C., & Lawlor, B. C. N. (2003). Alcohol use disorders in elderly people: Redefining an age-old problem in old age. *BMJ, 327*(7416), 664–667.

Olson, J., Forbes, C., & Belzer, M. (2011). Management of the transgender adolescent. *Archives of Pediatric Adolescent Medicine, 165*, 171–176.

Oslin, D. W. (2005). Treatment of late-life depression complicated by alcohol dependence. *American Journal of Geriatric Psychiatry, 13*(6), 491–500.

Otis, M. D. (2007). Perceptions of victimization risk and fear of crime among lesbians and gay men. *Journal of Interpersonal Violence, 22*, 198–217.

Patton, C. (2006). *Anti-lesbian, gay, bisexual and transgender violence in 2005: A report of the National Coalition of Anti-Violence Programs*. Retrieved from www .ncavp.org

Perrin, E. C. (2002). *Sexual orientation in child and adolescent health care*. New York: Kluwer Academic / Plenum.

Perry, B. (2005–2006). A crime by any other name: The semantics of "hate." *Journal of Hate Studies, 4*(1), 120–137.

Pinquart, M., & Sorenson, S. (2000). Influences of socio-economic status, social network, and competence on subjective well-being in later life: A meta-analysis, *Psychology and Aging, 14*(2), 187–224.

Poasa, K. H., & Blanchard, R. (2004). Birth order in transgendered males from Polynesia: A quantitative study of Samoan Fa'afāfine. *Journal of Sex and Marital Therapy, 30,* 13–23.

Preves, S. E. (2000). Negotiating the constraints of gender binarism: Intersexuals' challenge to gender categorization. *Current Sociology, 48,* 27–50.

Prince-Hughes, T. (1999). A curious double insight: The well of loneliness and Native American alternative gender traditions. *Rocky Mountain Review, 53*(2), 31–43.

Pryzgoda, J., & Chrisler, J. C. (2000). Definitions of gender and sex: The subtleties of meaning. *Sex Roles, 43*(7/8), 553–569.

Puar, J. L. (2001). Global circuits: Transnational sexualities and Trinidad. *Signs, 26*(4), 1039–1065.

Pudrovska, T., Schieman, S., & Carr, D. (2006). Strains of singlehood in later life: Do race and gender matter? *Journal of Gerontology, Series B, Psychological Sciences and Social Sciences, 61B*(6), S315–S322.

Rautio, N., Heikkinen, E., & Heikkinen, R.-L. (2001). The association of socioeconomic factors with physical and mental capacity in elderly men and women. *Archives of Gerontology and Geriatrics, 33,* 163–178.

Redman, D. (2011). Fear, discrimination and abuse: Transgender elders and the perils of long-term care. *Aging Today, 32*(2), 1–2.

Reitzes, D. C., & Mutran, E. J. (2006). Self and health: Factors that encourage self-esteem and functional health. *Journal of Gerontology, Series B, Psychological Sciences and Social Sciences, 61B*(1), S44–S51.

Remembering Our Dead. (2007). Retrieved from www.rememberingourdead.org

Rikard, R. V., & Rosenberg, E. (2007). Aging inmates: A convergence of trends in the American criminal justice system. *Journal of Correctional Health Care, 13,* 150–162.

Robert, S. A., Cherepanov, D., Palta, M., Dunham, N. C., Feeny D., & Fryback, D. G. (2009). Socioeconomic status and age variations in health-related quality of life: Results from the National Health Measurement Study. *Journal of Gerontology B Psychological Science and Social Science, 64B,* 378–389.

Rodgers, R. G., Hummer, P. A., & Nam, C. B. (2000). *Living and dying in the USA: Behavioral, health and social differentials of adult mortality.* San Diego, CA: Academic Press.

Rosebury, B. (2003). On punishing emotions. *Ratio Juris, 16*(1), 37–55.

Rosnick, C. B., Small, B. J., McEvoy, C. L., Borenstein, A. R., & Mortimer, J. A. (2007). Negative life events and cognitive performance in a population of older adults. *Journal of Aging & Health, 19,* 612–629.

Ross, N. A., Garner, R., Bernier, J., Feeny, D. H., Kaplan, M. S., McFarland, B., . . . Oderkir, J. (2011). Trajectories of health-related quality of life by socio-economic status in a nationally representative Canadian cohort. *Journal of Epidemiology Community Health.* doi:10.1136/jech.2011.115378.

Roughgarden, J. (2005). *Evolution's rainbow: Diversity, gender and sexuality in nature and people.* Berkeley: University of California Press.

Ruan F. F. (1991). Transvestism and transsexualism. *In Sex in China: Studies in sexology in Chinese culture* (pp. 145–158). New York: Plenum Press.

Ruan, F. F., Bullough, V., & Tsai, Y. M. (1989). Male transsexualism in mainland China. *Archives of Sexual Behavior*, 18(6), 517–522.

Rubenstein, W. B. (2002). Do gay rights laws matter? An empirical assessment. *Southern California Law Review*, 75(65), 65–120.

Rubenstein, W. B. (2004). The real story of U.S. hate crimes statistics: An empirical analysis. *Tulane Law Review*, 78, 1213–1246.

Sambamoorthi, U., Shea, D., & Crystal, S. (2003). Total and out-of-pocket expenditure for prescription drugs among older persons. *Gerontologist*, 43, 345–359

Sanchez Rodriguez, J. L., & Rodriguez Alvarez, M. (2003). Normal aging and AIDS. *Archives of Gerontology and Geriatrics*, 36(1), 57–65.

Satterfeld, S. B. (1988). Transsexualism. The sexually unusual: Guide to understanding and help [Special issue]. *Journal of Social Work and Human Sexuality*, 7(1), 77–87.

Schmidt, J. (2003). Paradise lost? Social change and the Fa'afafine in Samoa. *Current Sociology*, 51, 417–432.

Schrank, D. (2007, September 25). Police investigate as a hate crime attack on man leaving nightclub. *Washington Post*, p. B04.

Schwarz, S., & Scheer, S. (2004). HIV testing behaviors and knowledge of HIV reporting regulations among male-to-female transgenders. *Journal of Acquired Immune Deficiency Syndromes*, 37(2), 1326–1327.

Seelau, S. M., & Seelau, E. P. (2005). Gender-role stereotypes and perceptions of heterosexual, gay, and lesbian domestic violence. *Journal of Family Violence*, 20(6), 363–371.

Sell, R. L., & Becker, J. B. (2001). Sexual orientation data collection and progress toward *Healthy People 2010. American Journal of Public Health*, 91, 876–882.

Servicemembers Legal Defense Network. (2011). About "Don't Ask, Don't Tell." Retrieved from www.sldn.org/pages/about-dadt

Shankle, M. D. (Ed.). (2006). *The handbook of lesbian, gay, bisexual, and transgender public health: A practitioner's guide to service.* New York: Harrington Park Press.

Shankle, M. D., Maxwell, C. A., Katzman, E. S., & Landers, S. (2003). An invisible population: Older lesbian, gay, bisexual, and transgender individuals. *Clinical and Regulatory Affairs*, 20(2), 159–182.

Sigusch, V. (1991). Die Transsexuellen und unser nosomorpher Blick. *Zeitschrift für Sexualforschung*, 4, 225–256.

Sims, A. M. (2007). *Gender non-conformists: Male and female reconsidered.* Retrieved from www.gpac.org/press/asap_2007.01.24.html

Sinnott, M. (2000). The semiotics of transgendered sexual identity in the Thai print media: Imagery and discourse of the sexual other. *Culture Health and Sexuality*, 2(4), 425–440.

Sinnott, M. (2004). *Toms and dees: Transgender identity and female same-sex relationships in Thailand.* Honolulu: University of Hawai'i Press.

Sisk, J. (2006a, May/June). Fear and loathing: Hate crimes against LGBT individuals. *Social Work Today*, pp. 22–26.

Sisk, J. (2006b, May/June). Sexuality in nursing homes: Preserving rights, protecting well-being. *Social Work Today*, pp. 14–20.

Smith, M., Eyler, A. E., & Peters-Golden, H. (1995). The family life cycle: Practical applications for the primary care physician. In J. Nobel (Ed.), *Textbook of primary care medicine* [CD-ROM version]. St. Louis: Mosby-Year Book.

Snyder, P. J. (2004). Hypogonadism in elderly men—what to do until the evidence comes. *New England Journal of Medicine, 350*(5), 440–442.

Solarz, A. L. (Ed.). (1999). *Lesbian health: Current assessment and directions for the future*. Washington, DC: National Academy Press.

Staley, M., Hussey, W., Roe, K., Harcourt, J., & Roe, K. (2001). In the shadow of the rainbow: Identifying and addressing health disparities in the lesbian, gay, bisexual and transgender population—a research and practice challenge. *Health Promotion Practice, 2*, 207–211.

Stallings, M. C., Dunham, C. C., Gatz, M., Baker, L. A., & Bengtson, V. L. (1997). Relationships among life events and psychological well-being: More evidence for a two-factor theory of well-being. *Journal of Applied Gerontology, 16*(1), 104–119.

Steckley, R. G. (2009). Gay, lesbian, bisexual and transgender people: An introductory discussion of terminology and demographics. *Communication Disorders and Sciences in Culturally and Linguistically Diverse Populations, 16*, 4–10.

Stevenson, J. S. (2005). Alcohol use, misuse, abuse, and dependence in later adulthood. *Annual Reviews of Nursing Research, 23*, 245–280.

Stringer, J. (2000). Two Japanese variants of the absolute transvestite film. *Journal of Homosexuality, 39*(3/4), 111–126.

Sugihara, Y., & Katsurada, E. (1999). Masculinity and femininity in Japanese culture: A pilot study. *Sex Roles, 40*(7/8), 635–646.

Summerhawk, B., McMahill, C., & McDonald, D. (1998). Who's a lesbian? The story of a male-to-female transsexual lesbian: An interview with Mako. In B. Summerhawk, C. McMahill, & D. McDonald (Eds.), *Queer Japan: Personal stories of Japanese lesbians, gays, bisexuals and transsexuals*. Norwich, Canada: New Victoria.

Tait, R. (2009, September 11). Iran set to allow first transsexual marriage. *The Guardian*. Retrieved from www.guardian.co.uk/world/2009/sep/11/iran-transexual-marriage

Tate, R. B., Lah, L., & Cuddy, T. E. (2003). Definition of successful aging in elderly Canadian males: The Manitoba follow-up study. *Gerontologist, 43*, 735–744.

Taylor, M. G., & Lynch, S. M. (2004). Trajectories of impairment, social support, and depressive symptoms in later life. *Journal of Gerontology, Series B, Psychological Sciences and Social Sciences, 59B*, 238–246.

Teel, A. S. (2011). *Alone and invisible no more: How grassroots community action and 21st-century technologies can empower elders to stay in their homes and lead healthier, happier lives*. White River Junction, VT: Chelsea Green.

Teh, Y. K. (1998). Understanding the problems of mak nyahs (male transsexuals) in Malaysia. *South East Asia Research, 6*(2), 165–180.

Teh, Y. K. (2001). Mak myahs (male transsexuals) in Malaysia: The influence of culture and religion on their identity. *International Journal of Transgenderism*, 5(3). Retrieved from www.symposion.com/ijt/ijtvoo5noo3_04.htm

Teh, Y. K. (2002). *The mak nyahs: Malaysian male to female transsexuals*. Singapore: Eastern Universities Press.

ten Brummelhuis, H. (1999). Transformations of transgender: The case of the Thai kathoey. In P. Jackson & G. Sullivan (Eds.), *Lady boys, tom boys, rent boys: Male and female homosexualities in contemporary Thailand*. Binghamton, NY: Haworth Press.

Tengan, T. (2002). (En)gendering colonialism: Masculinities in Hawai'i and Aotearoa. *Cultural Values*, 6(3), 239–256.

Thompson, E. H. (1996). *Men and aging: A selected, annotated bibliography*. Westport, CT: Greenwood Press.

Thomsen, S. (2001, June 30). Sex and the seniors: Frisky and risky. *Plain Dealer*, p. E1:9.

Tolentino, R. B. (2000). Transvestites and transgressions: Panggagaya in Philippine gay cinema. *Journal of Homosexuality*, 39(3/4), 325–337.

Tomsen, S., & Mason, G. (2001). Engendering homophobia: Violence, sexuality, and gender conformity. *Journal of Sociology*, 37(3), 257–273.

Tornstam, L. (2005). *Gerotranscendence: A developmental theory of positive aging*. New York: Springer.

Totman, R. (2003). *The third sex: Kathoey—Thailand's ladyboys*. London: Souvenir Press.

Transgender Asia. (2006). Retrieved from http://web.hku.hk/~sjwinter/Transgender ASIA/index.htm

Transgender Law and Policy Institute. (2006, October 22). *Hate crimes laws*. Retrieved from www.transgenderlaw.org/hatecrimeslaws/index.htm

TranScience Longitudinal Aging Research Study. (1999). Retrieved from www .transcience.org

Tsoi, W. F. (1980). Female transsexualism in Singapore a report on 20 cases. *Australian and New Zealand Journal of Psychiatry*, 14(2), 141–143.

Tsoi, W. F. (1988). The prevalence of transsexualism in Singapore. *Acta Psychiatrica Scandinavia*, 78(4), 501–504.

Tsoi, W. F. (1993). Follow-up study of transsexuals after sex-assignment surgery. *Singapore Medical Journal*, 34(6), 515–517.

Tsoi, W. F., Kok, L. P., & Long, F. Y. (1977). Male transsexualism in Singapore: A description of 56 cases. *British Journal of Psychiatry*, 131, 405–409.

Tsoi, W. F., Kok, L. P., Yeo, K. L., & Ratnam, S. S. (1995). Follow-up study of female transsexuals. *Annals of the Academy of Medicine, Singapore*, 24(5), 664–667.

Turner, J. S. (1996). *Encyclopedia of relationships across the lifespan*. Westport, CT: Greenwood Press.

Turrell, G., Lynch, J. W., Kaplan, G. A., Everson, S. A., Helkala, E. L., Kauhanen, J., & Salonen, J. T. (2002). Socioeconomic position across the lifecourse and cognitive function in late middle age. *Journal of Gerontology, Series B, Psychological Sciences and Social Sciences,* 57B(1), S43–S51.

Ulrich, L. (2011). *Bisexual invisibility: Impacts and recommendations.* www.sf-hrc.org /Modules/ShowDocument.aspx?documentid=989

United States Army Standards of Fitness. (2002). Retrieved from www.apd.army.mil /pdffiles/r40_501.pdf

United States Government Printing Office. (2009). Public Law No. 111-84, October 28, 2009. Retrieved from http://frwebgate.access.gpo.gov/cgi-bin/getdoc.cgi?db name=111_cong_public_laws&docid=f:publ084.111.pdf

UN rights body hits out against violence based on sexual orientation. (2011, June 17). *UN News Centre.* Retrieved from http://www.un.org/apps/news/story.asp?NewsID= 38762&Cr=prejudice&Cr1

U.S. Department of Health and Human Services, Office of Disease Prevention and Health Promotion. (2010, November). *Healthy People 2020.* ODPHP Publication B0132. Retrieved from http://www.healthypeople.gov/2020/about/default.aspx

U.S. v. Guerrero, 33 M.J. 295, 297–298 (C.M.A. 1991).

U.S. v. Modesto, 39 M.J. 1055 (A.C.M.R. 1994).

Valentine, D. (2000). *"I know what I am": The category "transgender" in the construction of contemporary United States American conceptions of gender and sexuality* (unpublished doctoral dissertation), New York University.

Valliant, G. E. (2002). *Aging well: Surprising guideposts to a happier life from the landmark Harvard Study of Adult Development.* Boston: Little, Brown.

Van Baarsen, B. (2002). Theories of coping with loss: The impact of social support and self-esteem on adjustment to emotional and social loneliness following a partner's death in later life. *Journal of Gerontology, Series B, Psychological Sciences and Social Sciences,* 57B(1), S33–S42.

Vance, D. E., Brennan, M., Enah, C., Smith, G. L., & Kaur, J. (2011). Religion, spirituality, and older adults with HIV: Critical personal and social resources for an aging epidemic. *Clinical Interventions in Aging,* 6, 101–109.

Van Kesteren, P. J., Gooren, L. J., & Megens, J. A. (1996). An epidemiological and demographic study of transsexuals in the Netherlands. *Archives of Sexual Behavior,* 25(6), 589–600.

Vasey, P. L., & Bartlett, N. H. (2007). What can the Samoan "Fa'afafine" teach us about the Western concept of gender identity disorder in childhood? *Perspectives in Biology and Medicine,* 50(4), 481–490.

Viederman, M. (2003). *Life passages in the face of death. Psychological engagement of the physically ill patient: Pt. 2* [Videotape]. Washington, DC: American Psychiatric Publishing.

Virginia Transgender Health Initiative Study. (2007). Retrieved from www.vdh.virginia .gov/epidemiology/DiseasePrevention/documents/pdf/THISFINALREPORTVol1 .pdf

Viswanath, K., Steele, W. R., & Finnegan, J. R. (2006). Social capital and health: Civic engagement, community size, and recall of health messages. *American Journal of Public Health,* 96(8), 1456–1461.

Wadensten, B., & Carlsson, M. (2003). Theory-driven guidelines for practical care of older people based on the theory of gerotranscendence. *Journal of Advanced Nursing, 41*(5), 462–470.

Walinder, J. (1971). Incidence and sex ratio of transsexualism in Sweden. *British Journal of Psychiatry, 118*, 195–196.

Walinder, J. (1972). Transsexualism: Definition, prevalence, and sex distribution. *Acta Psychiatrica Scandinavica, 44*(Suppl.), 255–257.

Wallace, S. P., Cochran, S. D., Durazo, E. M., & Ford, C. L. (2011). *The health of aging lesbian, gay and bisexual adults in California*. Policy Brief CLA Center for Health Policy Research (PB2011-2), pp. 1–8.

Weitze, C., & Osburg, S. (1996). Transsexualism in Germany: Empirical data on epidemiology and application of the German transsexual's act during the first ten years. *Archives of Sexual Behavior, 25*(4), 409–425.

Welle, D. L., Fuller, S. S., Mauk, D., & Clatts, M. C. (2006). The invisible body of queer youth: Identity and health in the margins of lesbian and trans communities. *Journal of Lesbian Studies, 10*(1/2), 43–71.

Whipple, B., & Scoura, W. K. (1989). HIV and the older adult. *Journal of Gerontological Nursing, 15*, 15–18.

Whittle, S. (1996). Gender fucking or fucking gender? Current cultural contributions to theories of gender blending. In R. Ekins & D. King (Eds.), *Blending genders: Social aspects of cross-dressing and sex-changing*. New York: Routledge.

Whittle, S. (2007). *The aging trans-person*. Presented as a talk at the World Professional Association for Transgender Health, Chicago.

Wikan, U. (1977). Man becomes woman: Transsexualism in Oman as a key to gender roles. *Man, 12*(2), 304–319.

Wikan, U. (1991). The xanith: A third gender role? In U. Wikan (Ed.), *Behind the veil in Arabia: Women in Oman*. Chicago: University of Chicago Press.

Wilhelm, A. D. (2004). Tritiya-Prakriti: People of the third sex. Understanding homosexuality, transgender identity and intersex conditions. In *Through Hinduism*. Philadelphia: Xlibris Corporation.

Williams, K. (2004). The transition to widowhood and the social regulation of health: Consequences for health and health risk behavior. *Journal of Gerontology, Series B, Psychological Sciences and Social Sciences, 54B*(6), S343–S49.

Williams, L., Labonte, R., & O'Brien, M. (2003). Empowering social action through narratives of identity and culture. *Health Promotion International, 18*(1), 33–40.

Wilson, R. S., Krueger, K. R., Arnold, S. E., Schneider, J. A., Kelly, J. F., Barnes, L. L., . . . Bennett, D. A. (2007). Loneliness and risk of Alzheimer disease. *Archives of General Psychiatry, 64*, 234–240.

Winter, S. (2005). Heterogeneity in transgender: A cluster analysis of a Thai sample. *International Journal of Transgenderism, 8*(1), 31–42.

Winter, S. (2006a). Language and identity in transgender: Gender wars and the Thai kathoey. In A. Lin (Ed.), *Everyday struggles in language, culture, and education: Problematizing identity*. Mahwah, NJ: Lawrence Erlbaum.

Winter, S. (2006b). Thai transgenders in focus: Demographics, transitions, and identities. *International Journal of Transgenderism*, 9(1), 15–27.

Witten, T. M. (2001). *The transgender/intersex experience: Living in the quantum shadow.* Presentation at the International Lesbian and Gay Conference, Oakland, CA.

Witten, T. M. (2002a). Midlife issues of aging in the LGBT community: A roundtable discussion. *Outword*, pp. 98–97.

Witten, T. M. (2002b). *On the epidemiology and demography of transgender and intersex: A white paper.* TranScience Research Institute Preprint Series, 2. WP-2002-01. Retrieved from www.transcience.org

Witten, T. M. (2002c). Geriatric care and management issues for the transgender and intersex populations. *Geriatric Care and Management Journal*, 12(3), 20–24.

Witten, T. M. (2003). Transgender aging: An emerging population and an emerging need. *Review Sexologies*, 12(4), 15–20.

Witten, T. M. (2004). Issues of transgender and intersex middle adulthood life course analysis. The courage to search for something more: Middle adulthood issues in the transgender and intersex community. *Journal of Human Behavior in the Social Environment*, 8(3–4), 189–224.

Witten, T. M. (2005). Birth sex is not gender: Comments on "Efforts to address gender inequalities must begin at home." *Lancet*, 366(9496), 1505. Retrieved from www.thelancet.com/journals/lancet/article/PIIS0140673605676052/comments?action=view&totalComments=1

Witten, T. M. (2006a). *Gender identity and the military. Transgender, transsexual, and intersex-identified individuals in the armed forces: Pt. 1.* Center for the Study of Sexual Minorities in the Military, University of California, Santa Barbara. Retrieved from www.gaymilitary.ucsb.edu/

Witten, T. M. (2006b, Winter). Transgender aging: The graying of transgender. American Public Health Association. *Gerontological Health Section Newsletter.* Retrieved from www.apha.org/newsletter/index.cfm?fuseaction=newsletter&secid=7#Transgender%20Aging

Witten, T. M. (2007a). End-of-life concerns for transgender elders and their caregivers: Graceful exits. American Society on Aging, *Outward.* Retrieved from www.transcience.org

Witten, T. M. (2007b). *Gender identity and the military: Transgender, transsexual, and intersex-identified individuals in the U.S. Armed Forces.* Retrieved from www.palmcenter.org/press/dadt/releases/palm_center_releases_study_on_gender_identity_in_u_s_military

Witten, T. M. (2008). Transgender bodies, identities, and healthcare: Effects of perceived and actual violence and abuse. In J. J. Kronenfeld (Ed.), *Research in the sociology of healthcare: Inequalities and disparities in health care and health: Vol. 25. Concerns of patients* (pp. 225–249). Oxford: Elsevier JAI.

Witten, T. M. (2009). Graceful exits: III. Intersections of aging, transgender identities, and the family/community. *Journal of LGBT Family Studies*, 5, 36–63. doi:10.1080/15504280802595378.

Witten, T. M. (2010). Graceful exits: III. Intersections of aging, transgender identities, and the family/community. In C. A. Fruhauf & D. Mahoney (Eds.), *Older GLBT family and community life*. London: Routledge.

Witten, T. M. (2011). *Results from the Trans-MetLife online survey of aging*. Manuscript in preparation.

Witten, T. M., Ekins, R. J. M., Ettner, R., Harima, K., King, D., Landén, M., . . . Sharpe, A. N. (2003). Transgender and transsexuality. In C. R. Ember & M. Ember (Eds.), *The encyclopedia of sex and gender: Men and women in the world's cultures* (pp. 216–229). New York: Kluwer/Plenum.

Witten, T. M., & Eyler, A. E. (1999). Hate crimes against the transgendered: An invisible problem. *Peace Review, 11*(3), 461–468.

Witten, T. M., & Eyler, A. E. (2007). Transgender aging and care of the elderly transgendered patient. In R. Ettner, S. Monstrey, & A. E. Eyler (Eds.), *Principles of transgender medicine and surgery* (pp. 285–310). Binghamton, NY: Haworth Press.

Witten, T. M., Eyler, A. E., & Weigel, C. (2000, Winter). Transsexuals, transgenders, cross-dressers: Issues for professionals in aging. *OutWord*. Retrieved from www.asaging.org/LGAIN/outword-063.htm

Witten, T. M., & Whittle, S. P. (2004). TransPanthers: The graying of transgender and the law. *Deakin Law Review, 9*(2), 503–522. Retrieved from www.deakinlawreview.org/currentIssue.php

World Health Organization. (2007). Gender-based violence. Retrieved from www.who.int/gender/violence/en

World Professional Association for Transgender Health (WPATH). (2011). *Standards of care for the health of transsexual, transgender, and gender nonconforming people*. 7th Version. Retrieved from www.wpath.org

Wu, L.-T., & Blazer, D. G. (2011). Illicit and nonmedical drug use among older adults: A review. *Journal of Aging and Health, 23*, 481–504.

Xavier, J. M., & Simmons, R. (2000). *The Washington Transgender Needs Assessment Survey* [Personal communication].

Xu, K. T. (2003). Financial disparities in prescription drug use between elderly and nonelderly Americans. *Health Affairs, 22*, 210–221.

Yueksel, S., Kulaksizouglu, I., Tuerksoy, N., & Sahin, D. (2000). Group psychotherapy with female to male transsexuals in Turkey. *Archives of Sexual Behavior, 29*(3), 279–290.

Yueksel, S., Yuecel, B., Tuekel, R., & Motavalli, N. (1992). Assessment of 21 transsexual cases in group psychotherapy admitted to hospital. *Nordisk Sexologi, 10*(4), 227–235.

Zhang, Z., & Hayward, M. D. (2001). Childlessness and the psychological well-being of older-persons. *Journal of Gerontology, Series B, Psychological Sciences and Social Sciences, 56B*(5), S311–S320.

Zucker, K. J. (2004). Gender identity development and issues. *Child and Adolescent Psychiatric Clinics of North America, 13*, 551–568.

Zucker, K. J. (2005). Gender identity disorder in children and adolescents. *Annual Review of Clinical Psychology, 1*, 467–492.

Zucker, K. J. (2007). Gender identity disorder in children, adolescents and adults. In G. O. Gabbard (Ed.), *Gabbard's treatments of psychiatric disorders* (4th ed., pp. 2069–96). Washington, DC: American Psychiatric Press.

Zucker, K. J., & Blanchard, R. (2003). Birth order in the Fakafefine. *Journal of Sex and Marital Therapy, 29*(4), 251–253.

CHAPTER SEVEN

Intersex and Aging

A (Cautionary) Research Agenda

HEATHER LAINE TALLEY, PH.D.,
AND MONICA J. CASPER, PH.D.

When we were first asked to write a chapter about intersex* and aging, we thought, "How hard can it be?" Surely, with all the social, political, psychological, and biomedical focus on intersex issues in recent decades, including national attention sparked by publication of Jeffrey Eugenides' novel *Middlesex* (2002) and John Colapinto's nonfiction *As Nature Made Him*, it would be relatively easy to pull together everything known about intersex and aging. We planned to conduct a literature review; interview activists, clinicians, and scientists; and analyze relevant policy documents. But we quickly discovered, to paraphrase Gertrude Stein, that *there is no there there*. That is, very little published material exists on intersex and aging. Intersex activism focused on the *beginnings* of life has largely ignored aging, while researchers and policy makers in the field of aging and life course studies have generally excluded intersex as a category. The topic appears to be on nobody's scholarly radar, with the exception of a very few recent articles (e.g., Gedro, 2009; Witten, 2007).

---

* See appendix, page 285, for discussion about terminology of *intersex*.

Further, much to our chagrin, our efforts to research this topic were met with skepticism, silence, and even hostility, especially from self-identified intersex respondents. They are, quite predictably, fed up with being "subjects" of scholarly investigation, poked and prodded biologically and theoretically to serve varied agendas. While our political sentiments and prior affiliations with the intersex patient rights movement have sensitized us to these silences,* ethnographic myopia occasionally prompted unwelcome resentment and hubris. One of us would ask, "Don't they know we're trying to be helpful?" The other would reply, "Don't they know we're not like those other researchers, unsympathetic to the needs of people with intersex conditions?" Thereby we illustrated exactly what is wrong with much of the research on people with intersex conditions, namely, that research questions are typically not generated from within affected communities but rather are pursued by scholars with multiple commitments and affiliations who may or may not be *centrally* committed to the topic (or people) in question. Rather than emphasizing our good intentions—which are true, but it seems trite to say so—we peremptorily ask forgiveness for any intellectual and political trespasses herein and invite critical commentary of our work.

It is particularly important to signal our cautionary approach here; in the process of crafting this research agenda, new language has emerged. Specifically, the very category we were charged with interrogating has been radically critiqued. In 2006, a Consensus Statement on Management of Intersex Disorders was published in the journal *Pediatrics*. Notably, the statement called for a dramatic rethinking of terminology stating:

> Terms such as "intersex," "pseudohermaphroditism," "hermaphroditism," "sex reversal," and gender-based diagnostic labels are particularly controversial. These terms are perceived as potentially pejorative by patients and can be confusing to practitioners and parents alike. We propose the term "disorders of sex development" (DSD), as defined by congenital conditions in which development of chromosomal, gonadal, or anatomic sex is atypical. (Lee et al., 2006, p. e488)

The statement recommends the deferral of routine methods of childhood intervention until later in life when patients can be actively engaged in the decision-making process. To be sure, these developments remain in the most embryonic stages. The term *intersex* remains widely used for reasons we discuss later, and the treatment suggestions outlined in the statement are not yet widely implemented.

---

* Casper was executive director of ISNA in 2003.

Ultimately, the issues explored here are unfolding within a changing social and medical context. So if there is no *there* there, and if it is not at all clear that we (the authors, by virtue of our non-intersex status) are well suited to go there anyway, where do we go from here? In lieu of presenting an overview of the (non-existent) literature or a finely grained ethnographic analysis, we opted instead to discuss the reasons why we, as a society, know very little about DSDs/intersex and aging and to offer a research agenda for the twenty-first century. We describe our agenda here as *cautionary* because we are acutely aware that we do not speak for any or all people affected by disorders of sex development, nor do we expect everyone interested in intersex concerns to share our views. Our agenda, such as it is, is meant to serve as a first step in what we hope will be an ongoing conversation among patients, intersex activists, clinicians, scientists, and policy makers about intersex and aging. This conversation is well worth having. Although not much is known about the broad topic of DSDs and aging, two things *are* certain: DSDs are common, affecting approximately 1 in 1,500–2,000 births in the United States (see Blackless et al., 2000; Sax, 2002), and, like all human beings, people who experience DSDs or identify as intersex are aging.

WHO PUT THE "I" IN THE LGBTQ SOUP?

It may seem strange to include DSDs/intersex in this book alongside lesbian, gay, bisexual, transgender, and queer (LGBTQ) identities and concerns. After all, intersex is not a sexual orientation or practice, nor is it a political identity for all but a handful of people. Statistically, based on the limited evidence available, the percentage of intersex people who are gay, lesbian, or bisexual seems to mirror that of the general population, though this varies by diagnosis, as does the rate of gender transition. For some DSDs, such as certain kinds of congenital adrenal hyperplasia (CAH) and partial androgen insensitivity syndrome (PAIS), transition rates are much higher than among the general public (Cohen-Kettenis, 2005; Dessens, Froujke, & Slijper, 2005; Dreger, 2003; Mazur, 2005; Meyer-Bahlburg, 2005; Schober, 1999; Zucker, 2005). There is no unassailable reason why this book, or any LGBTQ reference, should include intersex. Moreover, there is concern among some advocates that folding the "I" into LGBTQ assumes similar needs among all groups and that this may make invisible the needs of intersex people or privilege the political aims of "gay pride" at the expense of the very real psychosocial and clinical needs of people with DSDs.

Yet there are important reasons to talk about DSDs/intersex in relation to LGBTQ priorities and concerns. First, just as sexuality is profoundly shaped in our culture such that LGBTQ concerns are stigmatized, so too is intersex. Homophobia underlies some of the surgical treatments for intersex; what genitals look like matters tremendously in a culture rigidly organized around heterosexuality. Second, the bodies of people with intersex conditions have been pathologized and conceptualized as deviant, as are the bodies of gay, lesbian, and transgendered people (Terry, 1999). Nonconforming bodies can be read as abnormal, as threats to the social order. People with atypical bodies and sexualities must be "fixed," according to this social logic. Therefore, because intersex is related to both genital anatomy and sexual activities (i.e., what one can presumably do with these anatomies), the lives and experiences of people with DSDs, regardless of their sexuality, cannot help but be affected by social hierarchies of sexuality and power in which "LGBTQ" and its fictive kin are marginalized and stigmatized.

WHAT IS INTERSEX? WHAT ARE DSDS?

The term *disorders of sex development* refers to conditions in which an individual's genital or reproductive anatomy, or chromosomal constellation, are defined as "ambiguous," or atypical, or in which there is a specific type of reproductive endocrinological deficiency or imbalance. Alternately, the term *intersex* describes a group of people who identify as intersex because the experience of being born with, and treated for, a DSD has influenced personal experiences and self-perceptions. Of course, the underlying assumption of the DSD aspect of this definition is that chromosomes, genitalia, and reproductive anatomy are always consistent and unambiguous and that "discordance" must mean that a problem *requires* treatment. Ambiguity may appear at birth (and may even be diagnosed before birth) but also can sometimes appear later in the life cycle, particularly at puberty.

Definitions of DSDs/intersex vary considerably among health care professionals, scientists, and laypersons. The intersex patient rights movement (Chase, 1998; Preves, 2003) and some feminist scholars (Fausto-Sterling, 2000; Kessler, 1998) have advanced the idea that intersex, like other concepts related to sex and gender, is constructed and contested. That is, while DSDs may be based in "nature" through the actions of genes and hormones, our understanding of these conditions' significance is social, cultural, and political.

For many decades, the prevailing meaning of intersex has been corporeal deviation. Historically, however, *hermaphrodites*, as intersexed individuals were once called, were viewed alongside other nonnormative humans as "fantastic monsters" (Thomson, 1996), and their bodies were perceived as "signs of wonder and spiritual curiosity" (Daston & Park, 2001). With the development of sophisticated surgical capabilities, people with visible DSDs began to be conceptualized as medical oddities to correct (Dreger, 1998). Beginning in the early twentieth century, atypical genitalia and other physical characteristics were considered not only different but also *abnormal*, a departure from the way human beings were supposed to look and function. While these views have been somewhat tempered, the modern belief that DSDs are pathologic and need repair endures, and intersex has at times been a focus of questionable surgical and psychological normalization for half a century (Dreger, 2004). However, DSDs/intersex is a rubric for many different conditions, each with its own etiology, diagnosis, treatment, degree of impairment (if any), and social meaning.

Professional treatment for DSDs was pioneered in the 1930s by Hugh Hampton Young and Lawson Wilkins in the Pediatric Endocrine Unit at the Johns Hopkins Hospital. Building on this work, psychologist John Money, also at Johns Hopkins, advanced a research and treatment program focused on sex and gender assignment (Bullough, 2003; Colapinto, 2001). The basic premise behind these treatments was that any child could be raised in either gender, provided that the gender assignment was reinforced by appropriate social cues such as dress, toys, and behavior (Money, 1968; Money & Ehrhardt, 1972). At the time, this quite progressive theory was interpreted to mean that regardless of a child's "true" sex, which sometimes could not be determined in a binary conceptual framework, the child could—and indeed should—be raised as *either* a boy *or* a girl *and* that sex could and should be surgically (re)constructed.

The influence of the Johns Hopkins approach, especially Money's articulation of it, was profound. The standard of care for DSDs was, until very recently, widespread cosmetic surgery on infants and children with atypical genitalia to ensure an "appropriate" sex and gender classification. The problem is not that sex and gender are assigned at birth but, rather, that potentially damaging and irreversible surgery is used to buttress the assignment, which may or may not fit the individual in adulthood.

Why do such categories matter? In Western culture, especially in conservative political climates, considerable stigma is attached to bodies and practices that challenge existing heterosexist order. Putatively offensive bodies not only are subject to normalizing and disciplining by social institutions but also are included in a range of queer practices and sexualities. Inhabiting an anatomically correct body with corresponding "legitimate" gender and sexual behavior matters tremendously in a culture organized around inflexible binary categories of sex, gender, and coupling. Like "deviant" sexualities (Terry, 1999), atypical anatomies are conceptualized as capable of harming the social body. Indeed, the American Academy of Pediatrics (AAP) has previously referred to the birth of a child with an intersex condition that causes atypical genitalia as a "social emergency" and recommended urgent treatment on that basis (AAP Committee on Genetics, 2000). More recent statements have been worded more moderately but still communicate a sense of emergency based at least in part on the appearance of the genital anatomy (e.g., Hughes, 2007).

INTERSEX, PATIENT RIGHTS, AND DEMOGRAPHIC MYOPIA

In the 1990s, an alternative meaning of intersex emerged to challenge notions of pathology. Cheryl Chase, founder and first executive director of the Intersex Society of North America (ISNA), drew on her own traumatic experiences to launch a social movement against involuntary "normalizing" treatment and for greater acceptance and understanding.* She had been born with a DSD condition and treated surgically in infancy. As an adult, when Chase learned the truth by recovering her own medical records, she experienced a severe emotional crisis. Over the course of a decade, as she considered her medical history and realized that such damaging treatments persisted, she decided to improve the lives of people with DSDs, first by naming a previously hidden problem cloaked in shame and secrecy, and then by changing treatment practices surrounding variations in sex development.

The resulting patient rights movement has both challenged and transformed the standard of care for children born with DSDs/intersex conditions (Preves, 2003), highlighting problems such as deception, insufficient consent, and negative outcomes of surgery with respect to sexual and urinary function. It also exposed a disparity in treatment: more often than not, children with atypical genitalia have been "turned into" girls rather than boys, in part because the surgery (i.e., removing rather than adding organs) was often technically simpler. However, this perspective is based on the problematic assumptions that it is more important for genitalia to be cosmetically correct than sexually functional, and that sexual (especially orgasmic) ability is not important for girls and women.

In recent years, many physicians and psychologists have recommended genital cosmetic surgery (Baskin, 2004; Baskin et al., 1999), and others have opposed

---

* The history of the intersex patient rights movement, including Chase's decisive role and ISNA's ongoing influence, can be found in Dreger (1999), Preves (2003), and Bloom (2003).

it (Frader et al., 2004; Lee & Gruppuso, 1999). The intersex patient rights perspective, first articulated in the 1990s and now shared by many bioethicists, and medical and mental health professionals (Creighton & Minto, 2001; Navarro, 2004), advocates the following principles:

- Parental and social distress stemming from atypical genitalia should not be treated by surgery on the affected child.
- Parental and family mental health counseling should be provided during the newborn period and longitudinally.
- Variations in sex development should be managed in an atmosphere of appropriate medical disclosure rather than in secrecy and in shame.
- Gender assignment should often proceed without surgical enforcement.
- Persons born with variations in sex development may, or may not, ultimately choose cosmetic genital surgery.
- Surgeries that are not required to correct a functional defect (such as impairment in urinary function) should be deferred until the individual is old enough to understand the nature of the operation and actively choose to have it performed.
- Fully informed consent should be secured before any surgical procedure.

The Consensus Statement (2006) stopped short of full endorsement of these principles, but included some of them at least in part, such as narrowing the indications for early surgery, and recommendations for "open communication with patients and families . . . shared decision-making . . . patient and family concerns should be respected and addressed in strict confidence" (p. e490). However, medical, psychological, sociological, and anthropological literatures on intersex focus primarily on medical and social responses to infants and children with variations in sex development (see Karzakis, 2008). Historically, too, the intersex patient rights movement has articulated a political agenda that questions the effectiveness and ethics of these interventions in early life.

One problem common to the historical clinical approaches to variations in sex development and the intersex patient rights movement is a notable demographic myopia. Attention is focused on the beginning of the life cycle without much attention paid to the difficulties of aging and the later stages of life. In short, sex development is conceptualized as a challenge to be addressed in infancy and early childhood, while questions about intersex conditions *over the life course* remain largely unasked, though there has been some recent progress in this regard. Aging researchers are gradually responding to gaps in our collective knowledge by identifying the significance of understanding LGBTQ and intersex lives in crafting responsive aging policies (Harrison, 2005). Yet as gerontology explores LGBTQ aging, scholars have noted that discussion of DSDs/intersex remains still relatively neglected (Aragon & Gangamma, 2008). At the same time, clinical implications of demographic myopia are increasingly being addressed. For example, the October 2006 Disorders of Sex Development (DSD) Symposium, jointly sponsored by ISNA and the Gay and Lesbian Medical Association, featured presentations on a variety of topics, many of which concerned later-life stages.

In addition, feedback from adults who are dissatisfied with psychosexual quality of life following infant genital surgery underlies some of the current changes in early life treatment (Barthold, 2011) and concerns with long-term support are beginning to enter into the conversation (Brain et al., 2010). In particular, subsequent reviews have placed additional emphasis on long-term outcomes, such as the preservation of orgasmic capacity (Barthold, 2011; Nabhan & Lee, 2007).

So, too, has advocacy evolved. The 2008 formation of Accord Alliance (www .accordalliance.org) focused on "improved quality of life through a patient-centered model of care with an emphasis on an interdisciplinary team approach to health care delivery," signifying an approach that expands on ISNA's original focus on early childhood (www.accordalliance.org/about-accord-alliance.html). Importantly, ISNA's recent closure may well illustrate a growing consensus that advocacy must also address long-term issues.

Indeed, we suggest that the ways in which variations in sex development are managed at the beginning of life have lasting implications for the late-life experience of persons who are born with them. Yet discussion about what it means to be an adult born with a DSD/intersex condition, and the concerns that may emerge during aging, have been limited. References to adults with DSD/intersex conditions are usually made with respect to prior childhood treatments. The following examples from academic, clinical, and political spheres illustrate how sex development has been approached almost exclusively as a beginning-of-life concern, even though questions about later life seem intimately connected to these discussions.

In a *Pediatrics* article titled "Intersex Issues: A Series of Continuing Conundrums," Blizzard (2002) reviews research concerning long-term outcomes of adults with intersex conditions and concludes that medicine can no longer take a "paternalistic" approach to treating variations in sex development. Although his concern with regard to the adult individuals' current satisfaction with *previous* childhood treatments contributes to the evolution of medical practice, he does not inquire about the possible medical concerns of persons born intersexed as they age.

In *Lessons from the Intersexed*, Suzanne Kessler (1998) critiques the medical construction of sex through genital surgery as a "solution" to children with atypical genitals. Kessler concludes that current treatment protocols are unethical because genital surgery is medically unnecessary and is conducted without the consent of the patient. As treatment is overwhelmingly centered on early intervention, Kessler rightly focuses her lens on sex assignment in the neonatal period. However, absent from her multifaceted documentation is clinicians' neglect of issues that emerge throughout the life course. What lessons might adults with intersex conditions have to share?

Similarly, ISNA's agenda was focused on improving the care of intersexed infants, by instituting a patient-centered model (in contrast to what they identified as the concealment-centered model). As described on ISNA's website (www.isna .org), the patient-centered model seems clinically inclusive. It is based on the idea that "children with intersex, parents of those children, and adults with intersex should be treated in an open, shame-free, supportive, and honest way." Yet ISNA's work, valuable as it has been, focused on encouraging preliminary gender assignment at birth while eschewing childhood genital surgery. While ISNA recognized that childhood treatment is connected to adult health and advanced the understanding that intersex is a lifelong issue and that adults, too, have medical needs, the organization did not provide specific guidance about treatments that may be suggested or desired later in life. We were strong supporters of ISNA's mission as it pertains to early life interventions, yet were concerned about the lack of attention to issues concerning "adults with intersex," given the organization's stated goals. It is to be hoped that Accord Alliance, which is in some respects ISNA's successor, will be able to achieve a broader life cycle focus.

In sum, there is currently a serious lack of clinical and scholarly attention paid to the concerns of people with DSDs/intersex conditions over the life course. How do we make sense of this demographic myopia? Why the exclusive focus on infants and children in medical, academic, and political discourse, even though intersex conditions have significant implications for adults across the life course? Academics, clinicians, and activists certainly acknowledge a link between early interventions and adult quality of life (e.g., some forms of early surgery negatively influence adult psychosexual satisfaction), but there are few analyses or agendas grounded in the specificity of young adulthood, middle adulthood, and old age. Infants in particular and children in general have been primary subjects in medical and academic analyses and in political activities. To understand why infancy is so conspicuous and aging so invisible in academic literature and intersex activism, we turn to what babies might mean for health care professionals, for parents, and for society.

With the majority of births occurring in hospitals in the United States, spaces obviously dedicated to by medical knowledge and technology, intervention is likely when an infant is born with atypical genitalia. Treatment has historically assumed that ambiguity with regard to sex or gender necessarily leads to a life of suffering and alienation (Karkazis, 2008; Preves, 2003). But as the intersex patient rights movement pointed out, the infant patient is unable to consent to surgical treatment, and parents who consent on behalf of the child are often unfamiliar with DSDs/intersex conditions. Both infants and parents are thus vulnerable populations (Preves, 2002). Comparatively, physicians, nurses, psychologists, and social workers possess radically disproportionate power relative to the infant patient and knowledge relative to the infant's parents. When surgery is recommended, the infant patient is compliant, and parents are often invested in the procedures for psychosocial reasons of their own (Karkazis & Rossi, 2010). Given that consent for treatment is given by parents rather than by patients, some intersex activism approaches parental consent as intrinsically problematic. If parents' motivations are not congruent with children's needs, the relationship between caregiver and child is tenuous, if not antagonistic.

For families of infants diagnosed with intersex conditions, sex and gender normality are highly desired. In the popular imagination, gender is understood to descend from sex, and gender is a primary way we make sense of who people are and what they should be doing. We understand ourselves, and one another, through gendered identities and representations (Lorber, 1993). At birth, gender is inferred from an infant's phenotypic (genital) sex; thus, unusual sex development may be experienced as a crisis of personhood (and of parenthood) for a child's family. Thus, families who consent to treatment can serve as a method for negotiating stigma. Not surprisingly, intersex advocates highlight how parent-child relationships can be adversarial.

Making an infant's body culturally intelligible is often seen as a prerequisite for a family to make sense of who their baby is and who they are in relation to their baby. Parenting is strongly predicated on a child's gender event—there are "right" ways to raise a girl and "right" ways to raise a boy—although these specifics vary between cultures. "Sexual dimorphism for culture's smooth operation" predominates in Western culture, such that ambiguous sex is not an option and early interventions have been seen as "essential" (Hausman, 2000, p. 1471). However, because health care professionals may convey a sense of emergency, and may conflate medical and psychosocial issues, parents may not understand that procedures to modify atypical genitals may be largely peripheral to immediate medical issues associated with a DSD/intersex condition, such as ensuring adequate urinary functioning.

In the omnipresent focus on the beginnings of life, questions about intersex and aging are often overlooked. We do not mean to imply that questions about the beginnings of life are unimportant, nor are we suggesting that focusing on the beginning of life should be replaced by attention to the life course. Rather, we argue that medical, psychological, sexual, and political issues emerge as people with intersex conditions age that are currently either gravely understudied or remain to be elucidated.

In light of the paucity of literature on DSDs over the life course and with the understanding that most people with intersex conditions are not sick or unwell in the classic sense of the term, we offer the following research agenda. Our hope is that clinicians, academicians, policy makers, and advocates might begin to expand inquiry beyond the beginnings of life and to more fully address sex development from a life cycle perspective.

WHAT DO WE NEED TO KNOW?

As a strategy for thinking beyond the beginning of life, we use a life course framework. The life course comprises many developmental events, including but not limited to birth and death. A life course perspective resists the tendency to divide life into two distinct periods—young and old—preferring to conceptualize the life course as a series of age-related processes that unfold over historical times and places (Elder et al., 2003). In essence, a life course perspective situates aging in sociohistorical contexts. This approach emphasizes that "time operates at both a socio-historical and personal level" (Elder et al., 2003, p. 8). Life course theory emphasizes the importance of the *cohort effect*. Cohorts are defined by birth year so that age *and* history are integrated into life experience and perspectives.

A life course approach is especially crucial for work regarding intersex for two reasons. First, we lack knowledge about sex development across every life stage other than the neonatal period, and second, we need to situate the treatment of DSDs in specific historical contexts. A life course perspective forces us to consider individuals' varying and shifting relationships with biomedical technologies and psychological theories. Treatment approaches to intersex conditions change over time as medical protocols and psychological theories are reevaluated and new techniques are innovated (Karkazis, Tamar-Mattis, & Kon, 2010). As a result, patients with similar variations in sex development may have experienced different treatments depending on when and where they were born and the social (and geographic) contexts in which they were treated.

Finally, the aging process is a significant aspect of any investigation of human life experience. Dramatic demographic shifts in recent decades, including increased longevity and decreased fertility, mean that the populations of the United States and the world are aging. In this context, the concerns of middle adulthood and the older years are receiving greater academic consideration. We hope that the evolving life course research perspective will include the range of questions that remain about sex development and intersex life experience.

SOCIAL

- How do people with intersex conditions experience isolation, stigma, unwanted attention, and objectification? What are the effects of these experiences across the life course?
- What lifelong social support mechanisms exist for people with intersex conditions? What services are required in young adulthood, middle adulthood, and old age?
- How frequently are children and adults with intersex conditions affected by violence and abuse? Is this vulnerability magnified in old age?
- How does the experience of intersex affect interpersonal relationships across the life course?
- How do familial discord and estrangement impact the health and well-being of people with intersex conditions across the life course? How frequently does this occur?
- How are family dynamics affected by the treatment choices of adults with intersex conditions and vice versa?
- What resources are necessary to ensure health and well-being across the life course for people with intersex conditions?

- What limitations do people with intersex conditions encounter in pursuing diagnosis, treatment, care, and social support?
- Does any aspect of any intersex/DSD condition impact a person's ability to maintain continuous, gainful employment, and if so, how does this affect long-term financial security?
- What obstacles do adults with intersex conditions encounter when attempting to establish or change gender identity?
- What obstacles, if any, do adults with intersex conditions encounter when attempting to marry or to adopt children?
- Given the complex role parents of children of children with DSDs play in treatment seeking and consent, how do intersex adults navigate the role of parent?
- What effects do sensationalized images of intersex in popular culture have on adults with intersex conditions?

SEXUAL

- How is sexuality, from childhood through adulthood and into old age, affected by the variations of sex development?
- How do intersex conditions affect sexual identity formation or reassessment processes for intersex persons, and possibly their partners?
- What treatment resources might be useful for people with intersex conditions and their sexual partners?
- How do people with intersex conditions articulate their conditions to potential intimate partners?
- In what ways may intersex conditions or treatment affect a person's ability to find intimate partners?
- How do intersex conditions affect sexual practices?
- How do traumatic treatment experiences affect the desire of people with intersex conditions to engage in sexual and intimate relationships?
- How might clinical treatment in adulthood be developed such that sexual needs and desires are taken into account?
- How might intersex activists best articulate a patient-centered treatment model that identifies positive sexuality in adulthood and old age as an important outcome?
- What kinds of body image concerns do people with intersex conditions experience, and how do these influence sexuality and sexual practices?
- Do current treatments sufficiently take sexuality and sexual functioning into account as an important outcome? If so, how? If not, why not?

- What kind of information regarding contraception, sexually transmitted infection, and other sexual health issues is needed by adults with various intersex conditions?
- What is the incidence of sexual violence experienced by intersexed adults? How often is this violence perpetrated by partners, family members, or strangers?
- What kind of information do adults with intersex conditions receive from their health professionals about reproductive options?
- How will new reproductive technologies affect the definitions and experiences of fertility for people with intersex conditions?

MENTAL HEALTH

- How do traumatic treatment experiences affect intersexed adults' well-being?
- How does shame or secrecy about an intersex condition affect an adult's self-esteem?
- How do people with intersex conditions feel about what happened to their bodies in the process(es) of treatment?
- In what ways is the ability of adults to make choices about future treatment for intersex conditions affected by access to information or the lack of it?
- How do intersexed adults feel about their parents' decisions regarding childhood treatment? If so, how does this affect feelings about one's family of origin?
- What is the incidence of depression, anxiety, and other symptoms among the adult and elderly intersex population? What factors influence adult mental health concerns?
- What kinds of mental health services would assist adults with intersex conditions?
- What kinds of educational resources could be developed for training mental health professionals to assist the intersex population?
- How do feelings about past treatment of intersex conditions affect adults' willingness to seek further mental and physical health services?
- How do intersex conditions affect personal identity over the life course?

BIOLOGICAL/CLINICAL

- What is the effect of hormone use across the life course?
- How should intersex individuals who take hormones manage their treatment as they age? Should they simulate menopause or the age-related decline in androgen production?

- What is the long-term effect of genital surgery on sexual, urinary, and other functioning? How do these effects change over the life course?
- Are people with intersex conditions more susceptible to certain illnesses? If so, how might these be prevented or mitigated?
- How does intersex affect a person's ability or decision to become a parent? What services are available to help people make these decisions?
- What is the short- and long-term effect of infertility in women and men with intersex conditions? What services might be helpful in achieving fertility or managing infertility?
- How are prosthetic body alterations (e.g., breast implants, prosthetic testes) cared for across the life course?
- Are the medical and psychosocial problems commonly experienced by older adults likely to affect people with intersex conditions in different ways? If so, how?
- What assumptions about elderly intersexed persons do clinical and scientific researchers make? If they are not accurate, how might these assumptions be challenged in practice?

ADVOCACY

- How can a patient-centered treatment model that takes life course experiences into account best be defined and put into practice?
- How might activist organizations' agendas be expanded to include more life course concerns?
- What new political goals will emerge as activists broaden their focus to intersex conditions over the life course?
- How might activists communicate their concerns about intersex conditions over the life course to clinicians and to researchers, and vice versa?
- What political liaisons might be productive for intersex activism directed beyond early life treatments?

POLITICAL/LEGAL

- What kinds of legislation would help ensure ethical medical, psychological, and custodial treatment of intersex adults?
- What kinds of legal protections—if any—are needed to combat employment and residential discrimination of people who are intersex identified?
- How might advocacy and information groups for people with intersex conditions and their families be encouraged to expand their agendas to include life course and aging issues?

- How does the "same-sex marriage debate," and its political ramifications, resonate with or affect people who are intersex identified?

POSTSCRIPT

We conclude our agenda with a few practical observations. As with all research regarding sex and sexuality, a research agenda on intersex and aging exists in a political climate. To be carried out, policy makers must support scientists in a variety of disciplines who need both the intellectual freedom and the practical resources to do this work. In addition, the shared experience of aging is both fascinating and unglamorous and often receives less-than-adequate emphasis from scientists, policy makers, advocates, and the general public. And finally, research findings about health and illness across the life course can influence the health of individuals and populations only if the services needed to implement them are available and affordable to those who need them.

APPENDIX

Editor's Afterthoughts on the Politics of "Intersex"

A. Evan Eyler, M.D., M.P.H.

Social science and societal dialogue regarding personal identity and self-perception, including gender and sexuality, continue to evolve. During the last half-century, members of historically disadvantaged, or persecuted, sexual and gender minorities have entered the political arena to claim the benefits available to individuals and couples in majority society.

The relationship between sexual and gender minority persons and the health and social science professions has often been complex, uncomfortable, or problematic. Lesbian, gay, bisexual, and transgender people have invested substantial effort and endured personal risks that accompany loss of invisibility to obtain appropriate health and social services and to stop being the recipients of hazardous ones. For example, treatments designed to "cure" homosexuality or bisexuality, and the research that supports them, are now regarded as ineffective and unethical; mental health care for sexual orientation–questioning youth focuses instead on self-acceptance and healthy social and sexual expression. Similarly, transgender health care is now centered on achieving psychological wholeness and comfort, often through medical treatments that modify the body to promote congruence with internal self-perception, rather than on counseling aimed at eliminating the transgender feelings.

During the 1990s, persons who had been born with variations in sex development often manifested by genital anatomy that was different than the usual female or male, entered the public and political dialogue as visible protagonists, rather than as faceless recipients of medical and psychological intervention and curiosity. The Intersex Society of North America was founded in 1993 with the goals of ending infant surgeries aimed at achieving genital conformity, or cosmesis, and the secrecy and shame that too often accompanied them. For some persons who gravitated to ISNA and other intersex organizations, activism to improve the health care of infants born with atypical genital or reproductive anatomy was the principal focus; for others, the opportunity to be open about their profound personal experiences of difference—to claim an intersex identity—was tremendously important. (The statements of Mani Bruce Mitchell, in the ISNA film *Hermaphrodites Speak!* [Chase, 1997] and Tiger Howard Devore in the Discovery Channel documentary *Is It a Boy or a Girl?* [Ward et al., 2000] provide moving examples in that regard. Both are still active intersex advocates; see www.tigerhowarddevorephd.com; www.ianz.org.nz.)

During the several years that this book has been in preparation, terminology regarding intersex/DSD/variation in sex development has continued to evolve and diversify and has been contested by groups with different constituencies, philosophies, and conclusions regarding this aspect of human experience and its significance at this historical time (Davidson, 2009). It is with some trepidation that we have chosen to include a chapter on intersex and aging, in view of this ongoing process and the weighty implications of these developments. Nonetheless, many adults who were born with a DSD condition or who identify as intersex persons are now entering middle or older adulthood, and the concerns of these individuals, their partners, and their families have not been well addressed. We offer this chapter in the hope of stimulating further dialogue on this important aspect of sexual and gender minority aging.

We have chosen to alternate the use of use "intersex" and "DSD" because many adults, for whom this is a significant aspect of personal identity, continue to use the term *intersex*. DSD has been used occasionally to refer specifically to the associated medical conditions. For those who prefer some other terminology or perspective, we respect diversity in identity and experience, and we mean no harm. We look forward to reading additional scholarship and lived experience in the years ahead.

REFERENCES

American Academy of Pediatrics (AAP) Committee on Genetics. (2000). Evaluation of the newborn with developmental anomalies of the external genitalia. *Pediatrics, 106*(Pt. 1), 138–142.

Aragon, A., & Gangamma, R. (2008). *Intersexuality*. In S. Loue & M. Sajatovic (Eds.), *Encyclopedia of aging and public health* (pp. 475–476). New York: Springer.

Barthold, J. (2011). Disorders of sex differentiation: A pediatric urologist's perspective of new terminology and recommendations. *Journal of Urology, 185*, 383–400.

Baskin, L. S. (2004). Anatomical studies of the female genitalia: Surgical reconstructive implications. *Journal of Pediatric Endocrinology and Metabolism, 17*, 581–557.

Baskin, L. S., Erol, A., Li, Y. W., Liu, W. H., Kurzrock, E., & Cunha, G. R. (1999). Anatomical studies of the human clitoris. *Journal of Urology, 162,* 1015–1020.

Blackless, M., Charuvastra, A., Derryck A., Fasuto Sterling, A., Lauzanne, K., & Lee, E. (2000). How sexually dimorphic are we? Review and synthesis. *American Journal of Human Biology, 12,* 151–166.

Blizzard, R. M. (2002). Intersex issues: A series of continuing conundrums. *Pediatrics, 1103,* 616–621.

Brain, C., Creighton, S., Mushtaq, I., Carmichael, P., Barnicoat, A., Honour, J., . . . Achermann, J. (2010). Holistic management of DSD. *Best Practices Research in Clinical Endocrinological Metabolism, 242*(2), 335–354.

Bullough, V. (2003). The contributions of John Money: A personal view. *Journal of Sex Research, 40,* 230–236.

Chase, C. (1997). *Hermaphrodites speak!* [Videotape]. Rohnert Park: Intersex Society of North America.

Chase, C. (1998). Hermaphrodites with attitude: Mapping the emergence of intersex political activism. *GLQ: A Journal of Gay and Lesbian Studies, 4*(2), 189–211.

Cohen-Kettenis, P. T. (2005). Gender change in 46,XY persons with 5alpha-reductase-2 deficiency and 17beta-hydroxysteroid dehydrogenase-3 deficiency. *Archives of Sexual Behavior, 34*(4), 399–410.

Colapinto, J. (2001). *As nature made him: The boy who was raised as a girl.* New York: HarperCollins.

Creighton, S., & Minto, C. (2001). Managing intersex: Most vaginal surgery in childhood should be deferred. *BMJ, 323,* 1264–1265.

Daston, L., & Park, K. (2001). *Wonders and the orders of nature, 1150–1750.* New York: Zone Books.

Davidson, R. J. (2009). DSD debates: Social movement organizations' framing disputes surrounding the term "disorders of sex development." www.liminalis.de/2009_03/Artikel_Essay/Liminalis-2009-Davidson.pdf

Dessens, A. B., Froujke, M. E., & Slijper L. S. D. (2005). Gender dysphoria and gender change in chromosomal females with congenital adrenal hyperplasia. *Archives of Sexual Behavior, 34*(4), 389–397.

Dreger, A. (2003). Shifting the paradigm of intersex treatment. In E. Koyama (Ed.), *Teaching intersex issues* (2nd ed.). Portland, OR: Intersex Initiative Portland.

Dreger, A. D. (1998). *Hermaphrodites and the medical invention of sex.* Cambridge, MA: Harvard University Press.

Dreger, A. D. (2004). "Ambiguous sex"—or ambivalent medicine? Ethical problems in the treatment of intersexuality. In A. L. Caplan, J. J. McCartney, D. A. Sisti, & E. D. Pellegrino (Eds.), *Health, disease, and illness: Concepts in medicine* (pp. 25–35). Washington, DC: Georgetown University Press.

Elder, G., Johnson, M. K., & Crosnoe, R. (2003). The emergence and development of the life course. In J. T. Mortimer & M. J. Shanahan (Eds.), H. Kaplan (Series Ed.), *Handbook of the life course* (pp. 3–19). New York: Plenum Press.

Eugenides, J. (2002). *Middlesex.* New York: Farrar, Straus and Giroux.

Fausto-Sterling, A. (2000). *Sexing the body: Gender, politics, and the construction of human sexuality.* New York: Basic Books.

Frader, J., Alderson, P., Asch, A., Aspinall, C., Davis, D., Dreger, A., . . . Parens, E. (2004). Health care professionals and intersex conditions. *Archives of Pediatric and Adolescent Medicine, 158,* 424–428.

Gedro, J. (2009). LGBT career development. *Advances in Developing Human Resources, 11,* 54–66.

Harrison, J. (2005). Pink, lavender, and grey: Gay, lesbian, bisexual, transgender, and intersex ageing in Australian gerontology. *Gay and Lesbian Issues and Psychology Review, 1,* 11–16.

Hausman, B. (2000). Review of *Lessons from the intersexed,* by Suzanne Kessler. *American Journal of Sociology, 105,* 1471–1472.

Hughes, I. A. (2007). Early management and gender assignment in disorders of sexual differentiation. *Endocrinological Development, 11,* 47–57.

Karkazis, K. (2008). *Fixing sex: Intersex, medical authority, and lived experience.* Durham, NC: Duke University Press.

Karkazis, K., & Rossi, W. C. (2010). Ethics for the pediatrician. Disorders of sex development: Optimizing care. *Pediatrics in Review, 31,* e82–e85.

Karkazis, K., Tamar-Mattis, A., & Kon, A. A. (2010). Genital surgery for disorders of sex development: Implementing a shared decision-making approach. *Journal of Pediatric Endocrinology and Metabolism, 23,* 789–806.

Kessler, S. (1998). *Lessons from the intersexed.* New Brunswick, NJ: Rutgers University Press.

Lee, P., & Gruppuso, P. (1999). Should cosmetic surgery be performed on the genitals of children born with ambiguous genitals? *Physician's Weekly, 16.*

Lee, P., Houk C., Ahmed S., & Hughes I. (2006). Consensus statement on management of intersex disorders. *Pediatrics, 118,* e488–e500.

Lorber, J. (1993). Believing is seeing: Biology as ideology. *Gender and Society, 7,* 568–581.

Mazur, T. (2005). Gender dysphoria and gender change in androgen insensitivity or micropenis. *Archives of Sexual Behavior, 34*(4), 411–421.

Meyer-Bahlburg, H. F. (2005). Gender identity outcome in female-raised 46,XY persons with penile agenesis, cloacal exstrophy of the bladder, or penile ablation. *Archives of Sexual Behavior, 34*(4), 423–438.

Money, J. (1968). *Sex errors of the body.* Baltimore: Johns Hopkins Press.

Money, J., & Ehrhardt, A. A. (1972). *Man and woman, boy and girl: Differentiation and dimorphism of gender identity from conception to maturity.* Baltimore: Johns Hopkins University Press.

Navarro, M. (2004, November 28). The most private of makeovers. *New York Times.*

Preves, S. E. (2002). Sexing the intersexed: An analysis of sociocultural responses to intersexuality. *Signs, 27,* 523–558.

Preves, S. E. (2003). *Intersex and identity: The contested self.* New Brunswick, NJ: Rutgers University Press.

Sax, L. (2002). How common is intersex? A response to Anne Fausto-Sterling. *Journal of Sex Research, 39,* 174–179.

Schober, J. M. (1999). Long-term outcomes and changing attitudes towards intersexuality. *British Journal of Urology, 83,* 39–50.

Terry, J. (1999). *An American obsession: Science, medicine, and homosexuality in modern society.* Chicago: University of Chicago Press.

Thomson, R. G. (1996). *Freakery: Cultural spectacles of the extraordinary body.* New York: New York University Press.

Ward, Phyllis, & Associates; ISNA. (2000, March 6). *Is it a boy or a girl?* [Broadcast]. A Discovery Channel documentary on medical management of children with ambiguous sex anatomy [Cable broadcast]. Great Falls, VA: Discovery Channel.

Zucker, K. J. (2005). Measurement of psychosexual differentiation. *Archives of Sexual Behavior, 34*(4), 375–388.

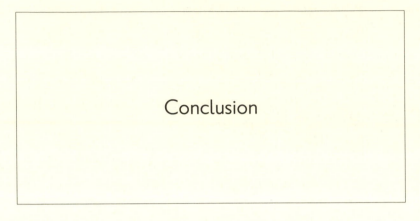

CHAPTER EIGHT

Conclusion

A. EVAN EYLER, M.D., M.P.H.

Older adults will be the largest demographic group in North America for approximately the next two decades, as the cohort of persons born in the 20 years following World War II enters the elder years. This weighty population cohort will continue to expand the ranks of each subgroup of older adults, including, ultimately, the oldest old, until approximately 2030.

Health and human service professionals who work with older adults are well advised to study both the common history shared by people of this age and the specific beliefs and customs of the cultural subgroups within this age cohort. Many stages of development shaped the shared history, perspectives, and expectations of persons who are now entering older adulthood and the elder years. These include *childhood*, during the postwar manufacturing and economic boom; *adolescence*, or *young adulthood*, during the Vietnam War and the years of struggle for civil rights for women and members of racial minorities; and *middle adulthood*, during decades of growth in information technology.

Within this larger cohort of older persons, particular experiential histories have influenced the beliefs and customs of members of specific population subgroups. Life as a member of a particular gender, racial, or ethnic group, living in defined economic circumstances and within the influence of religion and regional culture, shapes the experience of aging and the hopes and skills with which individuals enter the elder years.

Members of sexual* and gender minorities, including gay, lesbian, bisexual, and transgender persons, have always been present in the elderly population but only recently have become identifiable. Although variation in sex development, gender identity, sexual orientation, and partner choice is inherent in human biological and social evolution, Western cultures have usually regarded sex, gender, and sexual orientation as existing within a binary system and have attempted to eliminate evidence of variations in sex development and gender identity through medical treatment, mental health interventions, and sometimes social harassment. Homosexual and bisexual orientation and behavior also have been suppressed, through legal sanctions, psychological and medical "treatments," and social victimization.

During the last four decades of the twentieth century, sexual and gender minorities emerged as visible cultural groups. As a result of vigorous activism by members of these communities, their families, and supporters, substantial progress has been made in eroding stigma, harassment, and legal discrimination, although much remains to be gained.

The expanding population of older adults and the greater visibility of sexual and gender minority persons—of all ages—within North American culture mean that helping professionals will interact with clients, patients, and service consumers who self-identify as gay, lesbian, bisexual, intersex,† gender atypical, or transgender with increasing frequency. Demographic estimates regarding sexual and gender minority populations in the United States and worldwide are discussed by Tarynn M. Witten in chapter 1.

Most educational and training programs in medicine, nursing, psychology, social work, health administration, and related fields include instruction in the beliefs and practices of a variety of religious, ethnic, and cultural groups, with the goal of improving their graduates' *cultural competency*. Sexual and gender

---

* The terms *sexual minority* and *sexuality minority* are used interchangeably. Both appear in the current LGBT literature with generally equivalent meaning, most often referring to persons who are lesbian, gay, bisexual, or queer identified.

† The professional terminology and political culture regarding intersex/DSD/variation in sex development is currently evolving and, in some respects, being contested. The term *intersex* is employed in this discussion because it refers to an aspect of personal identity rather than medical biology and is employed by many adults who consider this a crucial aspect of their personhood. DSD is also used because this has come into greater usage in recent years. Please refer to chapter 6 for additional discussion regarding terminology and its implications in this regard.

minorities are now sometimes included in these curricula. However, the specific concerns of older sexual and gender minority persons have rarely been addressed. This book is a beginning effort in that regard.

Minority status and particular community culture influence the experience of aging in a variety of ways. However, some common themes characterize the experience of the elder years. The chapter authors have discussed the perspectives and specific needs of sexual and gender minority groups represented in this volume within the context of Western culture and certain general principles of gerontology.

Aging involves the progressive diminution of physical and, eventually, mental abilities. Older persons often require increased assistance and support to remain functional and independent. Caregiving, defined by Karen Fredriksen-Goldsen in chapter 2 as "unpaid assistance, provided by family members, friends, and neighbors, to help ill and disabled individuals remain in the community," is therefore a frequent necessity in the lives of elderly people. Although caregiving is nearly universal in the lives of the oldest old, caregiving and resources available for assistance are influenced by cultural, legal, and economic aspects of sexual and gender minority group community membership.

As in majority culture, family members provide the most caregiving in sexual and gender minority communities. Fredriksen's groundbreaking (1999) survey of gay men and lesbians found that 32% of respondents were caring for a friend, partner, or other family member; 23% were assisting an adult under 65 years of age; and 8% were caring for someone aged 65 years or older. These patterns persist despite negative stereotypes of gay men and lesbians as promiscuous single persons without family relationships. Caregivers were more likely to be older, partnered, and with less formal education, similarities shared with their heterosexually identified peers. More recent survey research (Fredriksen-Goldsen, Hyun-Jun, Muraco, & Mincer, 2009; MetLife, 2010) has also validated the frequent involvement of LGBT identified persons in caregiving responsibilities. See also Fredriksen-Goldsen and Muraco (2010).

Some differences in caregiving likely result from the patterns of kinship relations in gay and lesbian communities, the history of stigmatization by the helping professions, and the legal and economic consequences of lack of legal marriage rights. Lesbian and gay adults older than age 50 years are more likely to receive assistance from partners and friends and less likely to depend on adult children (deVries & Megathlin, 2009; MetLife, 2010; Muraco & Fredriksen-Goldsen, 2011). Also, men who identify as gay, bisexual, or transgender are significantly more likely to assume caregiving responsibilities than are their heterosexually identified peers (Fredriksen, 1999; MetLife, 2010). Bisexual women and men are more likely than gay men and lesbians to have been married and to have relationships with adult children and former spouses (Dworkin, 2006) and less likely to be out and well-connected to friends (MetLife, 2010), though further research regarding caregiving relationships is needed.

The current cohort of older sexual and gender minority persons grew up during an era of active and sometimes virulent hostility toward them, often including negative experiences with the helping professions. Some are therefore less likely to access assistance from formal service organizations. Lack of disclosure of same-gender-couple and other important relationships to service providers, because of fear of judgment and poor care, may reduce available support and hamper efforts to coordinate care.

Caregiving resources are also influenced by the economic status of the person in need of assistance, prior to the development of infirmity of functional loss. The legal right to marry, which allows couples access to a privileged taxation and inheritance status, enhances family economic health and is not available to many LGBT-identified couples in the United States. In addition, legal marriage bestows hundreds of other rights, many of which are the subject of federal law and are not influenced by state marriage and civil union statutes. Fredriksen-Goldsen notes in chapter 2 that "many federal and state laws and policies that provide family-based benefits use legal and structural forms inherently biased against LGBT caregivers and those that receive care." She continues:

> The range of institutional inequities includes allowing discrimination in employment, housing, and public accommodations, and denying same-sex partners health care benefits, family leave benefits, equivalent Medicaid spend-downs, Social Security benefits, and bereavement leave. Managed care and insurance policies are also often discriminatory (Garnets, Hancock, Cochran, Goodchilds, & Peplau, 1991; Kauth, Hartwig, & Kalichman, 2000; Phillips & Fischer, 1998; Winegarten, Cassie, Markowski, Kozlowski, & Yoder, 1994). If extensive legal planning is not completed in advance, LGBT caregivers and care recipients can be left highly vulnerable to the conflicting desires of members of the biological family, even if they have not been involved in the life of the LGBT individual for many years.

Discrimination in Medicaid spend-down limits and inheritance laws places partnered and widowed sexual and gender minority persons at risk for impoverishment and homelessness under circumstances that would be far less threatening to their heterosexual, legally married peers.

These contextual problems are shared by gay men and lesbians as well as by bisexual and transgender persons who are in coupled relationships excluded from legal marriage or who are identifiably outside the heteronormative ideal. In addition, differences in life experience between these population groups have implications for older adulthood and late life.

Older gay men have survived the AIDS crisis and are now entering a second wave of loss, during which their friends and partners who did not die during the early years of the epidemic are now approaching "the later years and a more normative expectation of mortality" (chapter 3). Brian de Vries and Gil Herdt discuss this "personal pool of grief" and its implications in chapter 3. In addition, the experience that family members—and society at large—often do not consider the death of a same-gender partner equal to the loss of a heterosexual husband or wife can resonate with the pattern of invalidation and homophobic harassment that has been an enduring theme in the lives of most older gay men.

Older gay men came of age during an era of overt harassment and often both legal and informal persecution, based on sexual behavior and lack of conformity to gender stereotypes in personal presentation. The frequent experience of harassment based on gender-atypical presentation in childhood has been associated with an increased risk of clinical depression during adulthood (Paul et al. 2002; Rawls, 2004), suggesting the need for medical and mental health professionals to remain alert for the potential for depression and substance abuse among their patients and clients. Nonetheless, despite the effects of homophobia, there is substantial evidence of resiliency among older gay men. As discussed by the authors, many gay men in late life are doing rather well.

Although sexual health and prevention and treatment of sexually transmissible infections (STI) remain important considerations in the health care of non-monogamous gay men, regardless of age, other chronic medical conditions, such as cardiovascular disease, diabetes, and cancer, are significant concerns during midlife and the elder years for both gay men and their heterosexually identified peers. Physicians, nurse practitioners, and physician assistants who care for older gay men should assess the risk of HIV/STI infection on an individual basis and apply standard health screening principles regarding the common chronic conditions of later life.

Older lesbians also are veterans of lifelong discrimination, both as women and as persons whose romantic, sexual, and committed relationships were judged as deviant and criminal by the larger society. As with their gay male peers, these experiences have had negative consequences and have also fostered resiliency that may serve them well in late life. Nancy M. Nystrom and Teresa C. Jones (chapter 4) note, "Aging and old lesbians, on the whole, are a highly self-sufficient group of women who have achieved personal and professional success despite numerous obstacles, including discrimination based on gender, sexual orientation, and age." Medical and mental health professionals should remain alert for the possibility of depression or substance abuse, and for a personal strength and resiliency that can be drawn on to enhance self-care and coping with the demands of old age.

Older lesbian women generally require the same medical treatments and preventive care as nonlesbian women, although relative risks of certain conditions probably differ in some respects on a population basis. For example, lesbian women are less likely than their heterosexual peers to be underweight and are more likely to be overweight or obese (Institute of Medicine, 2011). Women (and men) with higher body mass indices are at higher risk than their normal-weight peers to develop type 2 diabetes, hypertension, coronary artery disease, certain cancers, and arthritis and are less likely to develop osteoporosis. However, many lesbian women are average weight or slender, whereas the prevalence of obesity is increasing among all population groups. Therefore, medical treatment and screening practices must be individualized, based on the personal health history and physical characteristics. Lesbianism does not cause any health risks or diseases. In addition, most heterosexual sexual practices place women at higher risk for sexually transmissible infections than do most kinds of lesbian sex.

Social support for older lesbians exists in a variety of forms. Nystrom and Jones report that "although some women live in relatively small social circles, most old lesbians are actively involved in networks that include partners, family, friends, community groups, and religious affiliations. These women express their ardent desire to remain independent and healthy and to continue to maintain their own housing as they age. The possibility of living in lesbian communities appeals to many older lesbians."

Suggestions for actively including older lesbian women in existing health and social service programs, and for developing needed services, such as senior housing with a lesbian or a sexual and gender-minority focus, are also provided. (Readers tempted to consider such housing programs exclusivist are invited to consider the lifelong experience of discrimination that older lesbian and gay men have endured, as well as the large variety of specialized housing options available in majority culture.)

Older bisexual women and men share many similarities with their lesbian and gay peers and often have some significant differences in life experience and perspective. As Paula C. Rodríguez-Rust explains in chapter 5, "Bisexuality is a culturally marginalized concept, without a clear and universal definition. Bisexuality means different things to different people, and there are many ways to be bisexual." Many people with histories of sexual and romantic partnerships with both women and men do not self-identify as bisexual, and others without overt sexual experience with both genders do. Rodríguez Rust continues:

> The multiple dimensions of sexuality, including sexual identity, sexual behavior, sexual fantasies, sexual attractions, and romantic attractions, can be used to characterize the various forms of bisexuality . . . If a person can be regarded as bisexual on one or more of these dimensions (i.e., if she or he self-identifies as bisexual, has engaged in both same- and other-sex sexual activity, or has romantic, sexual, or fantasized attractions to both men and women), then his or her concerns during the aging process fall within the scope of this chapter.

The spectrum of bisexuality and the emergence of bisexuality as a recognized and enduring sexual identity rather than as a "transitional phase" or other invalidating characterization are discussed, along with the prevalent stereotypes regarding bisexual persons and their impact on bisexual older adults. For example, elderly people are caricatured as sexless, and bisexual people are caricatured as obsessed with sex. Further, bisexuality is often regarded as an unstable identity because women and men are stereotyped as opposites, whereas they are more alike than different, and considerable variation exists with regard to particular characteristics among individuals of each gender. Some bisexual persons are attracted to partners of either gender with particular attributes, others to members of both genders. Bisexual men and women who are now older adults have managed to live their lives despite the societal invalidation of their sense of sexual self, frequent disapproval by both heterosexually and homosexually identified peers, and persecution as homosexuals along with their gay and lesbian age-mates.

Social and biological science literatures are largely silent with regard to the experiences and concerns of bisexual older adults. The International Bisexual Identities, Communities, Ideologies, and Politics Study, conducted by Rodríguez Rust, is a beginning effort in that regard, and the first-person accounts from the study's respondents illuminate the realities of the lives of older bisexual women and men. Some materials and resources for professionals and service providers are available, as noted in this chapter. It is hoped that the concerns of bisexual elders will gain greater prominence within professional literatures and, indeed, within the larger society and its political discourse in the years ahead.

Middle-aged and older intersex-identified* persons remain a largely invisible minority. The intersex identity and DSD patients' rights/quality-of-life movement is still relatively young, and the inclusion of intersex concerns within the rubric of sexual and gender minority health care and civil rights is perhaps an even more recent development. In chapter 7, Heather Laine Talley and Monica J. Casper acknowledge that "it may seem strange to include DSD/intersex in this book alongside lesbian, gay, bisexual, transgender, and queer (LGBTQ) identities and issues. After all, intersex is not a sexual orientation or practice, nor is it a political identity for all but a handful of people." They continue:

> Yet there are some important reasons to talk about DSDs/intersex in relation to LGBTQ priorities and concerns. First, just as sexuality is profoundly shaped in our culture such that LGBTQ concerns are stigmatized, so too is intersex. Homophobia underlies some of the surgical treatment for intersex; what genitals look like matters tremendously in a culture rigidly organized around heterosexuality. Second, the bodies of people with intersex conditions have been pathologized and conceptualized as deviant, as are the bodies of gay, lesbian, and transgendered people (Terry, 1999). . . . the lives and experiences of people with DSDs, regardless of their sexuality, cannot help but be affected by social hierarchies of sexuality and power in which "LGBTQ" and its fictive kin are marginalized and stigmatized.

Despite this commonality, information regarding intersex and aging is currently more limited than the lesbian, gay, and bisexual aging literature. Until recently, medical and psychological professionals focused on treatment outcomes during childhood and adolescence, and intersex patients' rights advocates focused on stopping many infant genital surgeries and substituting treatment with family support and counseling. Casper and Laine Tally note that this has resulted in a "notable demographic myopia. Attention is focused on the beginning of the life cycle without much attention paid to the difficulties of aging and the later stages of life." As noted in the introduction to this chapter, this perspective is changing, but almost no information is currently available regarding the experiences and needs of intersex-identified older adults. Casper and Laine Talley therefore propose a research agenda for intersex and aging, including factors that may influence health and well-being across the life span, noting that "like all human beings, people who experience DSDs or identify as intersex are aging."

* See footnote on page 291.

It has been suggested that transgender and intersex/variations in sex development share similar biological determining factors. Indeed, the notion that psychological gender self-perception and physical signifiers of sex are closely related during development has intuitive appeal. However, the life experience of persons born with intersex/DSD conditions—many of whom wish that they had not been genitally surgerized as infants—and transgender persons—many of whom have actively sought surgical services for gender confirmation—is quite different. Nonetheless, sex development and gender identity are currently not well understood by most people, and both intersex-identified and transgender older adults often have histories of inappropriate or unhelpful interactions with health professionals, including mental health clinicians. In addition, members of both groups who transition gender, or who live as a third-gender person or with a gender identity other than female or male, may be regarded as homosexual by the larger society, with the attendant stigmatization and experiences of discrimination and harassment. Persons who do not conform to gender norms are often similarly victimized.

Similar to older adults who are intersex identified, elderly transgender women and men have participated in biological or social science research less commonly than their younger peers. Thus, many gaps remain with regard to understanding the lived experience of this group of people, as well as their current health and social service needs.

Older transgender persons are a heterogeneous group, composed of those who transitioned gender in adolescence or in young or middle adulthood and have matured into the elder years, and those who transitioned more recently, often after decades of confusion or frustration. Many older transgender persons in our clinical practices emphatically stated that they would have sought medical services for physical transition in their adolescence or early adulthood had these treatments been available, and would have lived as a gender-variant person (at least cross-dressing) had this been safe.

Transgender older adults have the same needs as their non-transgender peers for community support in maintaining independence, for legal recognition of important relationships regardless of the gender of the life partner, and for protection from discrimination. In addition, gender transition has implications for medical care during the later years and for end-of-life care and funerary practices.

The risks associated with using supplemental hormones increase during midlife and the elder years, and the need to use estrogens or androgens to maintain an appropriate gender presentation must be balanced with other health considerations. In addition, many transgender elders have not had genital surgery. The presence of genital anatomy that does not "match" the social gender presentation can result in the need for urgent education of nurses and caregiving personnel in the case of sudden, incapacitating illness or a new physical or cognitive disability. Postmortem care, such as autopsy and funereal practices, represents a last opportunity for outing as a transgender person due to breaches in confidentiality, as was the case for Billy Tipton, a transsexual man whose female genitalia were sensationalized in the tabloid press (Middlebrook, 1998).

Where do we stand, in 2012, regarding the well-being of sexual and gender minority persons during the elder years? Many older adults who identify as gay, lesbian, bisexual, intersex, or transgender have survived years—often lifetimes—of stigmatization, discrimination, and victimization. Nonetheless, they have survived to maturity, many developing a high degree of personal resilience despite the consequences of these experiences. The current civil rights movements, such as marriage equality, have been made possible by decades of earlier activism undertaken by persons who are now in late midlife or the elder years, as well as some who have died during recent years.

Older adults, regardless of minority status and life experience, are most likely to thrive in an environment of connectedness and social support. Sexual and gender minority persons also depend on relationships with family and chosen others. Communities of gay men and lesbians in many urban areas are moving beyond the youth focus of earlier decades and are beginning to offer more activities and services for their older members, as well as some intergenerational programming.

Unfortunately, the current political and legal environment in many parts of the United States (and many other nations) actively invalidates same-gender life-partner relationships and often impedes second-parent adoptions, thereby interfering with the most important supports in the lives of most elders—spouses and children. Discriminatory laws and policies regarding Medicaid spend-down, inheritance, and other important aspects of partnered life place sexual and gender minority persons at higher risk than their heterosexually married peers for impoverishment and homelessness.

Discrimination during the working years has also negatively impacted the earnings and savings—resources needed during old age—of the current cohort of older sexual and gender minority persons. Salient types of discrimination have included higher rates of taxation due to lack of legal marriage, lower earnings for women and racial minority men, and lack of protection from employment termination for gay, lesbian, bisexual, and transgender persons. Change in marriage and inheritance laws and achieving protection from discrimination in the workplace and other public spheres remain priorities for the current generation—building on the courage and perseverance of their elders.

Overall, older sexual and gender minority persons can experience increased vulnerability due to current and past discrimination and stigma but often have also gained strengths and connectedness that serve them well in later life. Much has been gained; however, much remains to be done.

Priorities for enhancing the well-being of older sexual and gender minority persons include improvements in health care, social support, legal status, and research. Specific recommendations are provided in the following sections.

HEALTH CARE

1. Creating a more welcoming environment for sexual and gender minority persons in existing health care settings. Examples include changing language on medical and mental health history forms from "married" to "married or partnered" and posting information regarding LGBT-specific services and resources on bulletin boards at health care facilities.

2. Including information about aging, and about sexual and gender minority concerns, in curricula for students of medicine, nursing, psychology, social work, health administration, and related fields.

3. Making resource lists, readings, and consultants available to professionals currently in practice.

4. Conducting outcomes research regarding the physical aspects of gender transition, including supplemental hormone use and surgical procedures, as they affect transgender persons across the life span.

5. Conducting research with, and on behalf of persons who are intersex identified, regarding physical and mental health in midlife and older age, in order to improve available health care services and enhance quality of life.

6. Developing and disseminating training for certified nursing assistants and other personal care attendants regarding the physical aspects of gender transition and intersex/DSD conditions, as well as the social aspects of sexual and gender minority living.

7. Improving the availability and use of living wills, advance directives, and durable power-of-attorney procedures for older adults in same-gender relationships.

8. Improving end-of-life and funerary practices on behalf of sexual and gender minority persons.

SOCIAL SUPPORT

1. Developing senior housing designed for, or at least welcoming of, older sexual and gender minority persons.
2. Developing senior social support and intergenerational programming, through both LGBT community centers and general service agencies (i.e., Area Agencies on Aging).
3. Publicizing the importance of estate planning, medical decision making, and related concerns, for same-gender couples; promoting affordable legal services to meet these needs.
4. Promoting documentation of decisions about end-of-life and funerary practices.

LEGAL

1. Gaining equal legal status for same-gender life-partner and second-parent relationships, including an end to discrimination in taxation, joint savings and assets, Medicaid spend-down, and related concerns.
2. Gaining full legal protection from discrimination in the workplace, public accommodation, and other spheres of public life.
3. Reversing recent erosions of civil rights and protections from discrimination based on gender and race.

RESEARCH

Each chapter describes pertinent agendas and priorities for research. As research progress is made, the heterogeneity of the LGBT communities with regard to race and ethnicity, specific gender identities, and other important characteristics will require consideration and respect.

Ultimately, the day may come when the purpose of writing about sexuality and gender minority–identified older adults will be to explore cultural, personal, and community contributions, rather than advocacy aimed at mitigating the harms wrought by decades of stigma and abuse. It is important both to celebrate the resilience of older gay, lesbian, bisexual, transgender, and intersex-identified persons and to work to eliminate the factors that have made "surviving in adversity" a way of life. It is hoped that efforts such as this one will contribute, at least in some beginning steps, to improving the lives of our elders now and in the future.

> Something there is that doesn't love a wall . . .
> That wants it down.
> —Robert Frost, "Mending Wall"

REFERENCES

DeVries, B., & Megathlin, D. (2009). The meaning of friendship for gay men and lesbians in the second half of life. *Journal of GLBT Family Studies, 5*(1/2), 82–98.

Dworkin, S. H. (2006). The aging bisexual: The invisible of the invisible minority. In D. C. Kimmel, T. Rose, & S. David (Eds.), *Lesbian, gay, bisexual, and transgender aging: Research and clinical perspectives* (pp. 36–52). New York: Columbia University Press.

Fredriksen, K. I. (1999). Family caregiving responsibilities among lesbians and gay men. *Social Work, 44*(2), 142–155.

Fredriksen-Goldsen, K. I., Hyun-Jun, K., Muraco, A., & Mincer, S. (2009). Chronically ill midlife and older lesbians, gay men, and bisexuals and their informal caregivers: The impact of social context. *Sexuality Research and Social Policy, 6*(4), 52–64.

Fredriksen-Goldsen, K. I., & Muraco, A. (2010). Aging and sexual orientation: A 25-year review of the literature. *Research on Aging, 32,* 372.

Institute of Medicine. (2011). *The health of lesbian, gay, bisexual, and transgender people: Building a foundation for better understanding* [Prepublication e-copy, uncorrected proofs]. Washington, DC: National Academies Press. Retrieved from www.nap.edu/catalog/13128.html

MetLife. (2010). *Still out, still aging: The MetLife Study of Lesbian, Gay, Bisexual, and Transgender Baby Boomers.* Westport, CT: MetLife Mature Market Institute.

Middlebrook, D. W. (1998). *Suits me: The double life of Billy Tipton.* New York: Houghton Mifflin.

Muraco, A., & Fredriksen-Goldsen, K. I. (2011). "That's what friends do": Informal caregiving for chronically ill midlife and older lesbian, gay and bisexual adults. *Journal of Social and Personal Relationships.* doi:10.1177/0265407511402419.

Paul, J. P., Catania, J., Pollack, L., Moskowitz, J., Canchola, J., Mills, T., . . . Stall, R. (2002). Suicide attempts among gay and bisexual men: Lifetime prevalence and antecedents. *American Journal of Public Health, 92,* 1338–1345.

Rawls, T. (2004). Disclosure and depression among older gay and homosexual men: Findings from the Urban Men's Health Study. In G. Herdt & B. de Vries (Eds.), *Gay and lesbian aging: Research and future directions* (pp. 117–141). New York: Sage.

Suggested Further Reading

This section contains literature references relevant to various chapter discussions in this text. We have endeavored to make it as up to date as possible before going to press. In order not to overwhelm the chapters with reference citations, these supplemental references are provided.

Highwire+Pubmed, Ovid, Silver Platter, and Google Scholar search engines were searched using the following keyword phrases "aging and ——" where "——" was either "gay," "homosexual," "lesbian," "queer," "bisexual," "transgender," "transsexual," or "cross-dressing," "cross-dresser." These searches included all references available through April 30, 2011. We have avoided Google web searches, as there are numerous web-related citations that could also be included. The interested reader is encouraged to perform additional web-related searches.

Acierno, R., Hernandez, M. A., Amstadter, A. B., Resnick, H. S., Steve, K., Muzzy, W., & Kilpatrick, D. G. (2010). Prevalence and correlates of emotional, physical, sexual, and financial abuse and potential neglect in the United States: The National Elder Mistreatment Study. *American Journal of Public Health, 100,* 292–297.

Adams, J. M., & White, M. (2004). Biological ageing: A fundamental, biological link between socio-economic status and health? *European Journal Public Health, 14,* 331–334.

Allen, J. D. (2003). *Gay, lesbian, bisexual and transgender people with developmental disabilities and mental retardation: Stories of the Rainbow Support Group.* Binghamton, NY: Haworth Press.

Alliance for Health Reform. (2006). *Covering health issues.* Retrieved from www .allhealth.org/sourcebook2006/pdfs/sourcebook2006.pdf

Almack, K. (2010). Review: Conceptualising social exclusion and lesbian, gay, bisexual and transgender people: The implications for promoting equity in nursing policy and practice. *Journal of Research in Nursing, 15,* 313–314.

Alwin, D. F., & Wray, L. A. (2005). Life-span developmental perspective on social status and health [Special issue 2]. *Journal of Gerontology, Series B, Psychological Sciences and Social Sciences, 60B,* 7–14.

Anderson, R. M., & Davidson, P. L. (1997). Ethnicity, aging and oral health outcomes: A conceptual framework. *Advances in Dentistry Research, 11*(2), 203–209.

Andrews, J. G., & Muzumdar, T. (2009). Rethinking the applied: Public gerontology, global responsibility. *Journal of Applied Gerontology*, 29, 143–154.

Angus, J., & Reeve, P. (2006). Ageism: A threat to "aging well" in the 21st century. *Journal of Applied Gerontology*, 25, 137–152.

Ariel, J. (2008). Women aging together in community. *Journal of Lesbian Studies*, 12(2–3), 283–292.

Arndt, S., Gunter, T. D., & Acion, L. (2005). Older admissions to substance abuse treatment in (2001). *American Journal of Geriatric Psychiatry*, 13(5), 385–392.

Ash, M. A., & Lee Badgett, M. V. (2006). Separate and unequal: The effect of unequal access to employment-based health insurance on same-sex and unmarried different-sex couples. *Contemporary Economic Policy*, 24(4), 582–599.

Atkins, D. (Ed.). (1998). *Looking queer: Body image and identity in the lesbian, bisexual, gay and transgender communities*. Binghamton, NY: Haworth Press.

Ayala, J., & Coleman, H. (2000). Predictors of depression among Lesbian women. *Journal of Lesbian Studies*, 4(3), 71–86.

Balsam, K. F., Lehavot, K., & Beadnell, B. (2011). Sexual revictimization and mental health: A comparison of lesbians, gay men and heterosexual women. *Journal of Interpersonal Violence*, 26, 1798–1814.

Barrett, A. E. (1999). Social support and life satisfaction among the never married. *Research on Aging*, 6, 46–72.

Barrett, A. E., & Robbins, C. (2008). The multiple sources of women's aging anxiety and their relationship with psychological distress. *Journal of Aging in Health*, 20, 32–65.

Bear, M. (1989). Network variables on determinants of the elderly entering adult residential care facilities. *Aging and Society*, 9, 149–163.

Becker, J. T., Kingsley, L., Mullen, J., Cohen, B., Martin, E., Miller, E. N., . . . Visscher, B. R. (2009). Vascular risk factors, HIV serostatus, and cognitive dysfunction in gay and bisexual men. *Neurology*, 73, 1292–1299.

Biggs, S. (2005). Beyond appearances: Perspectives on identity in late life and some implications for method. *Journal of Gerontology, Series B, Psychological Sciences and Social Sciences*, 60B(3), S118–S128.

Boehmer, U. (2002). Twenty years of public health research: Inclusion of lesbian, gay, bisexual and transgender populations. *American Journal of Public Health*, 92, 1125–1130.

Bradley, L. J., Whiting, P. P., Hendricks, B., & Wheat, L. S. (2010). Ethical imperatives for intervention with elder families. *Family Journal*, 18, 215–221.

Braithwaite, D. O., Wackernagael Bach, B., Baxter, L. A., DiVerniero, R., Hammonds, J. R., Hozek, A. M., . . . Wolf, B. M. (2010). Constructing family: A typology of voluntary kin. *Journal of Social and Personal Relationships*, 27, 388–407.

Brandl, B., Dyer, C. B., Heisler, C. J., Otto, J. M., Stiegel, L. A., & Thomas, R. W. (2006). *Elder abuse detection and intervention: A collaborative approach*. New York: Springer.

Brandt, M. J., & Reyna, C. (2010). The role of prejudice and the need for closure in religious fundamentalism. *Personal Social Psychology Journal*, 36, 715–725.

Braun, K. L., Mokuau, N., Hun, G. H., Kaanoi, M., & Gotay, C. C. (2002). Supports and obstacles to cancer survival for Hawaii's native people. *Cancer Practice*, 10(4), 192–200.

Brecher, E. (1984). *Love, sex, and aging*. Boston: Little, Brown.

Brodowsky, G., Granitz, N., & Anderson, B. (2008). The best of times is now: A study of the gay subculture's attitudes. *Time and Society*, 17, 233–260.

Brown, D. R., & Sankar, A. (1998). HIV/AIDS and aging minority populations. *Research on Aging*, 20, 865–884.

Brown, S. (2002). "Con discriminación y represión no hay democracia": The lesbian and gay movement in Argentina. *Latin American Perspectives*, 29, 119–138.

Brownlee, K., Graham, J. R., Doucette, E., Hotson, N., & Halverson, G. (2010). Have communication technologies influenced social work practice? *British Journal of Social Work*, 40, 622–637.

Burbank, P. (2006). *Vulnerable older adults*. New York: Springer.

Burdge, B. J. (2007). Blending gender, ending gender: Theoretical foundations for social work practice with the transgender community. *Social Work*, 52(3), 243–250.

Butler, R. N. (2002). The study of productive aging. *Journal of Gerontology, Series B, Psychological Sciences and Social Sciences*, 57B(6), S363.

Butler, S. S., & Hope, B. (1999). Health and well-being for late middle-aged and old lesbians in a rural area. *Journal of Gay and Lesbian Social Services*, 9(4), 27–46.

Byrd, L., Fletcher, A., & Menifield, C. (2007). Disparities in health care: Minority elders at risk. *ABNF Journal*, 18(2), 51–55.

Cahill, S., & Jones, K. T. (2001). *Leaving our children behind: Welfare reform and the LGBT community*. Washington, DC: National Gay and Lesbian Task Force. Retrieved from www.ngltf.org

Carlson, H. M., & Steuer, J. (1985). Age, sex-role categorization and psychological health in American homosexual and heterosexual men and women. *Journal of Social Psychology*, 125(2), 203–211.

Cartwright, C. (2011). Advance care planning for GLBTI people: Results from a state-wide survey. *British Medical Journal of Supportive & Palliative Care*, 1, 79.

Casas-Zamora, J. A., & Ibrahim, S. A. (2004). Confronting health inequity: The global dimension. *American Journal of Public Health*, 94(12), 2055–2058.

Cavenagh, S. L. (2003). Teacher transsexuality: The illusion of sexual difference and the idea of adolescent trauma in the Dana Rivers case. *Sexualities*, 6(3–4), 361–383.

Centers for Disease Control and Prevention. (2003). Public health and aging: Trends in aging, United States and worldwide. *JAMA*, 289, 1371.

Chae, D. H., & Walters, K. L. (2009). Racial discrimination and racial identity attitudes in relation to self-rated health and physical pain and impairment among Two-Spirit American Indians/Alaska Natives. *American Journal of Public Health*, 99, S144–S151.

Chartier, M., Araneta, A., Duca, L., McGlynn, L. M., Gore-Felton, C., Goldblum, P., & Koopman, C. (2009). Personal values and meaning in the use of methamphetamine among HIV-positive men who have sex with men. *Qualitative Health Research*, 19, 504–518.

Cheng, S.-T., & Chan, A. C. M. (2006). Relationship with others and life satisfaction in later life: Do gender and widowhood make a difference? *Journal of Gerontology, Series B, Psychological Sciences and Social Sciences, 61B*(1), P46–P53.

Choudhury, S., & Leonescio, M. V. (1997). Life-cycle aspects of poverty among older women. *Social Security Bulletin, 60*(2), 17–36.

Cigolle, C. T., Langa, K. M., Kabeto, M. U., Tian, Z., & Blaum, C. S. (2007). Geriatric conditions and disability: The Health and Retirement Study. *Annals of Internal Medicine, 147,* 156–164.

Clark, F., Carlson, M., Zemke, R., Frank, G., Patterson, K., Ennevor, B. L., . . . Lipson, L. (1996). Life domains and adaptive strategies of a group of low-income, well older adults. *American Journal of Occupational Therapy, 50*(2), 99–108.

Clark, M. E., Landers, S., Linde, R., & Sperber, J. (2001). The GLBT Health Access Project: A state-funded effort to improve access to care. *American Journal of Public Health, 91,* 895–896.

Clover, D. (2006). Overcoming barriers for older gay men in the use of health services: A qualitative study of growing older, sexuality and health. *Health Education Journal, 65,* 41–52.

Cochran, B. N., & Cauce, A. M. (2006). Characteristics of lesbian, gay, bisexual and transgender individuals entering substance abuse treatment. *Journal of Substance Abuse Treatment, 30*(2), 135–146.

Cochran, B. N., Peavy, K. M., & Robohm, J. S. (2007). Do specialized services exist for LGBT individuals seeking treatment for substance misuse? A study of available treatment programs. *Substance Use and Misuse, 42*(1), 161–176.

Cochran, B. N., Stewart, A. J., Ginzler, J. A., & Cauce, A. M. (2002). Challenges faced by homeless sexual minorities: Comparison of gay, lesbian, bisexual and transgender homeless adolescents with their heterosexual counterparts. *American Journal of Public Health, 92,* 773–777.

Cohen, C. I. (1999). Aging and homelessness. *Gerontologist, 39,* 5.

Colton, H. (1983). *The gift of touch.* New York: Seaview and Putman.

Comerford, S. A., Henson-Stroud, M. M., Sionainn, C., & Wheeler, E. (2004). Crone songs: Voices of lesbian elders on aging in a rural environment. *Affilia, 19,* 418–436.

Committee on Population (CPOP). (2004). *Understanding racial and ethnic differences in health in late life: A research agenda.* Washington, DC: National Academies Press.

Comstock, G. (1989). Victims of anti-gay/lesbian violence. *Journal of Interpersonal Violence, 4*(1), 101–106.

Concannon, L. (2009). Developing inclusive health and social care policies for older LGBT citizens. *British Journal of Social Work, 39,* 403–417.

Connor, R. P., & Sparks, D. H. (2004). *Queering Creole spiritual traditions: Lesbian, gay, bisexual and transgender participation in African-inspired traditions in the Americas.* Binghamton, NY: Haworth Press.

Conron, K. J., Mimiaga, M. J., & Landers, S. J. (2010). A population-based study of sexual orientation identity and gender differences in adult health. *American Journal of Public Health, 100,* 1953–1960.

Cooper, C., Selwood, A., & Livingston, G. (2008). The prevalence of elder abuse and neglect: A systematic review. *Age and Ageing*, 37, 151–160.

Coppin, A. K., Ferrucci, L., Lauretani, F., Phillips, C., Chang, M., Bandinelli, S., & Guralnik. (2006). Low socioeconomic status and disability in old age: Evidence from the In Chianti study for the mediating role of physiological impairments. *Journal of Gerontology Medical Science*, 61A (1), 86–91.

Corbett, K. (2007). Lesbian women and gay men found that nurses often assumed they were heterosexual, which led to feelings of discomfort and insecurity. *Evidenced Based Nursing*, 10, 94. doi:10.1136/ebn.10.3.94.

Corliss, H. L., Grella, C. E., Mays, V. M., & Cochran, S. D. (2006). Drug use, drug severity and help-seeking behaviors of lesbian and bisexual women. *Journal of Women's Health (Larchmt)*, 15(5), 556–568.

Corliss, H. L., Shankle, M. D., & Moyer, M. B. (2007). Research, curricula and resources related to lesbian, gay, bisexual and transgender health in US schools of public health. *American Journal of Public Health*, 97, 1023–1027.

Coustasse, A., Singh, K. P., & Trevino, F. M. (2007). Disparities in access to healthcare: The case of a drug and alcohol abuse detoxification treatment program among minority groups in a Texas hospital. *Hospital Topics*, 85(1), 27–34.

Cox, R. L. (2004). Global health disparities: Crisis in the diaspora. *Journal of the National Medical Association*, 96(4), 546–49.

Craft, E. M., & Mulvey, K. P. (2001). Addressing lesbian, gay, bisexual and transgender issues from the inside: One federal agency's approach. *American Journal of Public Health*, 91, 889–891.

Cramer, R. J., Chandler, J. F., & Wakeman, E. E. (2010). Blame attribution as a moderator of perceptions of sexual orientation-based hate crimes. *Journal of Interpersonal Violence*, 25, 848–862.

Creighton, S. (2001). Surgery for intersex. *Journal of the Royal Society of Medicine*, 94, 218–220.

Crimmins, E. M. (2004). Trends in the health of the elderly. *Annual Reviews of Public Health*, 25, 79–98.

Cronin, A., Ward, R., Pugh, S., King, A., & Price, E. (2011). Categories and their consequences: Understanding and supporting the caring relationships of older lesbian, gay and bisexual people. *International Social Work*, 5, 421–435.

Crystal, S., Johnson, R. W., Harman, J., Sambamoorthi, U., & Kumar, R. (2000). Out-of-pocket healthcare costs among older Americans. *Journal of Gerontology Social Science*, 55B(1), S51–S62.

Curry, L., & Jackson, J. (Eds.). (2003). *The science of inclusions: Recruiting and retaining racial and ethnic elders in health research*. Washington, DC: Gerontological Society of America.

Daaleman, T. P., & VandeCreek, L. (2000). Placing religion and spirituality in end-of-life care. *JAMA*, 284(19), 2514–2517.

Daiski, I. (2005). The health bus: Healthcare for marginalized populations. *Policy Politics Nursing Practice*, 6, 30–38.

Dang, A., & Vianney, C. (2007). Living in the margins: A national survey of lesbian, gay, bisexual and transgender Asian and Pacific Islander Americans. New York: National Gay and Lesbian Task Force Policy Institute.

Darkwa, K., Mazibuko, F. N., & Candidate, P. H. (2002). Population aging and its impact on elderly welfare in Africa. *International Journal of Aging and Human Development, 54*(2), 107–123.

Das, J., & Gertler, P. J. (2007). Variations in practice quality in five low-income countries: A conceptual overview. *Health Affairs, 26*(3), w296–w309.

D'Augelli, A. R. (2002). Mental health problems among lesbian, gay and bisexual youths ages 14 to 21. *Clinical Child Psychology and Psychiatry, 7,* 433–456.

David, S., & Knight, B. G. (2008). Stress and coping among Gay men: Age and ethnic differences. *Psychology and Aging, 23*(1), 62–69.

Davies, M., Harries, P., Cairns, D., Stanley, D., Gilhooly, M., Hilhooly, K., . . . Hennessy, C. (2011). Factors used in the detection of elder financial abuse: A judgement and decision-making study of social workers and their managers. *International Journal of Social Work, 54,* 404–420.

Deanow, C. G. (2011). Relational development through the life cycle: Capacities, opportunities, challenges, and obstacles. *Affilia, 26,* 125–138.

Dempsey, C. L. (1994). Health and social issues of gay, lesbian, and bisexual adolescents. *Families in Society, 75*(3), 160–167.

Devor, H. (1994). Transsexualism, dissociation and child abuse: An initial discussion based on non-clinical data. *Journal of Psychology and Human Sexuality, 6*(3), 49–72.

Dibble, S., Eliason, M. J., Dejoseph, J. F., & Chinn, P. (2008). Sexual issues in special populations: Lesbian and gay individuals. *Seminars in Oncological Nursing, 24,* 127–130.

DiPietro, L. (2001). Physical activity in aging: Changes in patterns and their relationships to health and function. *Journal of Gerontology, Series B, Psychological Sciences and Social Sciences, 56*(2), 13–22.

DiStefano, A. S., & Cayetano, R. T. (2011). Health care and social service providers' observations on the intersection of HIV/AIDS and violence among their clients and patients. *Qualitative Health Research, 21,* 884–899.

Dobson, R. (2007). Report calls for urgent action on ageism in treating stroke patients. *BMJ, 334,* 607.

Doyal, L. (2001). Sex, gender, and health: The need for a new approach. *BMJ, 323,* 1061–1063.

Dressler, W. W., & Bindon, J. R. (1997). Social status, social context, and arterial blood pressure. *American Journal of Physical Anthropology, 102*(1), 55–66.

Dunlop, D. D., Manheim, L. M., Song, J., & Chang, R. W. (2002). Gender and ethnic/racial disparities in health care utilization among older adults. *Journal of Gerontology, Series B, Psychological Sciences and Social Sciences, 57B,* 221.

Dyer, C. B., Goodwin, J. S., Pickens-Pace, S., Burnett, J., & Kelly, P. A. (2007). Self-neglect among the elderly: A model based on more than 500 patients seen by a geriatric medicine team. *American Journal of Public Health, 97*(9), 1–6.

Ebinger, M., Sievers, C., Ivan, D., Schneider, H. J., & Stalla, G. K. (2009). Is there a neuroendocrinological rationale for testosterone as a therapeutic option in depression. *Journal of Psychopharmacology, 23,* 841–853.

Elford, J., Ibrahim, F., Bukutu, C., & Anderson, J. (2008). Over fifty and living with HIV in London. *Sexually Transmitted Infections, 84,* 468–472.

Eliason, M. J., & Hughes, T. (2004). Treatment counselor's attitudes about lesbian, gay, bisexual, and transgender clients: Urban vs. rural settings. *Substance Use and Misuse, 39,* 625–644.

Emlet, C. A. (2006). "You're awfully old to have *this* disease": Experiences of stigma and ageism in adults 50 years and older living with HIV/AIDS. *Gerontologist, 46,* 781–790.

Emlet, C. A., Tozay, S., & Ravels, V. H. (2010). "I'm not going to die from the AIDS": Resilience in aging with HIV disease. *Gerontologist.* doi:10.1093/geront/gnq060.

Ettrich, K. U., & Fischer-Cyrulies, A. (2005). Substance abuse in middle and old age: Everyday drug alcohol and nicotine. Use and abuse. *Zeitschrift für Gerontologie und Geriatrie, 38*(1), 47–59.

Fagan, K. (2006). *S.F.'s homeless aging on the street: Chronic health problems on the rise as median age nears 50.* Retrieved from http://sfgate.com/cgi-bin/article.cgi ?file=/c/a/2006/08/04/MNGILKB9KV1.DTL

Feder, E. K. (2009). Imperatives of normality: From "intersex" to "disorders of sex development." *GLQ: A Journal of Lesbian and Gay Studies, 15,* 225–247.

Federal Interagency Forum on Aging-Related Statistics. (2000). *Older Americans 2000: Key indicators of well-being.* Washington, DC: Government Printing Office.

Feinberg, L. (1996). *Transgender warriors.* Boston: Beacon Press.

Feinglass, J., Lin, S., Thompson, J., Sudano, J., Dunloop, D., Song, J., & Baker, D. W. (2007). Baseline health, socioeconomic status, and 10-year mortality among older middle-aged Americans: Findings from the Health and Retirement Study, 1992–2002. *Journal of Gerontology, Series B, Psychological Sciences and Social Sciences, 62B*(4), S209–S217.

Fenge, L.-A. (2008). Striving towards inclusive research: An example of participatory action research with older lesbians and gay men. *British Journal of Social Work.* doi:10.1093/bjsw/bcn144.

Fenge, L.-A., Fannin, A., Armstrong, A., Hicks, C., & Taylor, V. (2009). Lifting the lid on sexuality and aging: The experiences of volunteer researchers. *Qualitative Social Work, 8,* 509–524.

Fenge, L.-A., & Jones, K. (2011, May). Gay and pleasant land? Exploring sexuality, ageing and rurality in a multi-method, performative project. *British Journal of Social Work.* doi:10.1093/bjsw/bcr058.

Ferron, P., Young, S., Boulanger, C., Rodriguez, A., & Moreno, J. (2010). Integrated care of an aging HIV-infected male-to-female transgender patient. *Journal of the Association of Nurses AIDS Care, 2*(3), 278–282.

Fetner, T. (2005). Ex-gay rhetoric and the politics of sexuality: The Christian antigay/pro-family movement's "truth in love" ad campaign. *Journal of Homosexuality, 50*(1), 71–75.

Fikree, F. F., & Pasha, O. (2004). Role of gender in health disparity: The South Asian context. *BMJ, 328,* 823–826.

Fingerhood, M. (1991). Substance abuse in older people. *Journal of the American Geriatrics Society, 48,* 985–995.

Fiori, K. L., Antonucci, T. C., & Cortina, K. S. (2006). Social network typologies and mental health among older adults. *Journal of Gerontology, Series B, Psychological Sciences and Social Sciences, 61B*(1), P25–P32.

Fiscella, K., Franks, P., Gold, M. R., & Clancy, C. M. (2000). Inequality in quality: Addressing socioeconomic, racial and ethnic disparities in health care. *JAMA, 283,* 2579–2584.

Fish, J. (2010). Conceptualizing social exclusion and lesbian, gay, bisexual and transgender people: The implications for promoting equity in nursing policy and practice. *Journal of Research in Nursing, 15,* 303–312.

Fisher, B. J., & Specht, D. K. (1999). Successful aging and creativity in later life. *Journal of Aging Studies, 13*(4), 457–472.

Flaherty, M. P. (2010). Constructing a world beyond intimate partner abuse. *Affilia, 25,* 224–235.

Flint, A. (2005). Generalized anxiety disorder in elderly patients: Epidemiology, diagnosis, and treatment options. *Drugs and Aging, 22*(2), 101–114.

Flores, G., Olsen, L., & Tomany-Korman, S. C. (2005). Racial and ethnic disparities in early childhood health and health care. *Pediatrics, 115,* e183–e193.

Flowers, P. (2009). How does an emergent LGBTQ health psychology reconstruct its subject? *Feminism Psychology, 19,* 555–560.

Fredriksen-Goldsen, K. I. (2005). Multigenerational health, development and equality. *Gerontologist, 45,* 125–130.

Fredriksen-Goldsen, K. I., & Muraco, A. (2010). Aging and sexual orientation: A 25-year review of the literature. *Research on Aging, 32,* 371–413.

Fried, L. P. (2000). Epidemiology of aging. *Epidemiologic Review, 22*(1), 95–106.

Friend, R. A. (1987). The individual and social psychology of aging: Clinical implications for lesbians and gay men. *Journal of Homosexuality, 14*(1–2), 307–331.

Fullmer, E. M. (1995). Challenging biases against families of older gays and lesbians. In G. C. Smith, S. S. Tobin, E. A. Robertson-Tchabo, & P. W. Power (Eds.), *Strengthening aging families: Diversity in practice and policy.* Thousand Oaks, CA: Sage.

Fullmer, E. M., Shenk, D., & Eastland, L. J. (1999). Negating identity: A feminist analysis of the social invisibility of older lesbians. *Journal of Women and Aging, 11*(2–3), 131–148.

Galea, J. T., Kinsler, J. J., Salazar, X., Lee, S.-J., Giron, M., Sayles, J. N., . . . Cunningham, W. E. (2011). Acceptability of pre-exposure prophylaxis as an HIV prevention strategy: Barriers and facilitators to pre-exposure prophylaxis uptake among at-risk Peruvian populations. *International Journal of STD AIDS, 22,* 256–262.

Galobardes, B., Lynch, J. W., & Davey Smith, G. (2004). Childhood socioeconomic circumstances and cause-specific mortality in adulthood: Systematic review and interpretation. *Epidemiologic Review, 26,* 7–21.

Gelber, R. P., McCarthy, E. P., Davis, J. W. & Seto, T. B. (2006). Ethnic disparities in breast cancer management among Asian Americans and Pacific Islanders. *Annals of Surgical Oncology, 13*, 977–984.

Getov, S. V., Lee, R. W., Dockery, F., & Rajkumar, C. (2008). Androgens, ageing and vascular function. *Age Ageing, 37*, 361–363.

Giles, H., & Reid, S. A. (2005). Ageism across the lifespan: Towards a self-categorization model of ageing. *Journal of Social Issues, 61*(2), 389–404.

Gluffre, P. (2010). Doing gender diversity: Readings in theory and real-world experience [Book review]. *Teaching Sociology, 38*, 269–271.

Goh, V. H.-H., & Tong, T. Y.-Y. (2010). Sleep, sex steroid hormones, sexual activities and aging in Asian men. *Journal of Andrology, 31*, 131–137.

Goltz, D. (2009). Investigating queer future meetings: Destructive perceptions of "The harder path." *Qualitative Inquiry, 15*, 561–586.

Goodson, P. O. (2010). Sexual activity in middle to later life. *BMJ, 340*, c850.

Gooren, L. J., Giltay, E. J., & Bunck, M. C. (2008). Long-term treatment of transsexuals with cross-sex hormones: Extensive personal experience. *Journal of Clinical and Endocrinological Metabolism, 93*, 19–25.

Gornick, M. E. (2003). A decade of research on disparities in Medicare utilization: Lessons from the health and healthcare of vulnerable men. *American Journal of Public Health, 93*, 753–759.

Graham, C. L., Ivey, S. L., & Neuhauser, L. (2009). From hospital to home: Assessing the transitional care needs of vulnerable seniors. *Gerontologist, 49*, 23–33.

Graham-Garcia, J., Raines, T. L., Andrews, J. O., & Mensah, G. A. (2001). Race, ethnicity and geography: Disparities in heart disease in women of color. *Journal of Transcultural Nursing, 12*, 56–67.

Grant, A. M. (2001). Health of socially excluded groups: Lessons must be applied. *BMJ, 323*, 1071.

Grant, J. M. (2009). *Outing Age 2010: Public policy issues affecting lesbian, gay, bisexual and transgender elders.* Washington, DC: National Gay and Lesbian Task Force.

Green, A. I. (2008). Health and sexual status in an urban Gay enclave: An application of the stress process model. *Journal of Health and Social Behavior, 49*, 436–451.

Green, L., & Grant, V. (2008). "Gagged grief and beleaguered bereavements?" An analysis of multidisciplinary theory and research relating to same sex partnership bereavement. *Sexualities, 11*, 275–300.

Grossman, A. H., D'Augelli, A. R., & Hershberger, S. L. (2000). Social support networks of lesbian, gay, and bisexual adults 60 years of age and older. *Journal of Gerontology, Series B, Psychological Sciences and Social Sciences, 55B*(3), P171–P179.

Haber, D. (2009). Gay aging. *Gerontology & Geriatrics Education, 30*(3), 267–280.

Hartley, D. (2004). Rural health disparities, population health and rural culture. *American Journal of Public Health, 94*, 1675–1678.

Hatzenbuehler, M. L., Keyes, K. M., & Hasin, D. S. (2009). State-level policies and psychiatric morbidity in lesbian, gay and bisexual populations. *American Journal of Public Health, 99*, 2275–2281.

Hatzenbuehler, M. L., McLaughlin, K. A., Keyes, K. M., & Hasin, D. S. (2010). The impact of institutional discrimination in psychiatric disorders in lesbian, gay and bisexual populations: A prospective study. *American Journal of Public Health, 100*, 452–459.

Haviland, M. G., Morales, L. S., Dial, T. H., & Pincus, H. A. (2005). Race/ethnicity, socioeconomic status, and satisfaction with health care. *American Journal of Medical Quality, 20*, 195–203.

Haynes, M. O. (1996). Geriatric gynecologic care of minorities. *Clinical Obstetrics and Gynecology, 39*, 946–958.

Heaphy, B. (2007). Sexualities, gender, and ageing: Resources and social change. *Current Sociology, 55*, 193–210.

Heintz, A. J., & Melendez, R. M. (2006). Intimate partner violence and HIV/STD risk among lesbian, gay, bisexual, and transgender individuals. *Journal of Interpersonal Violence, 21*, 193–208.

Hellman, R. E., & Drescher, J. (2004). *Handbook of LGBT issues in community mental health*. Binghamton, NY: Haworth Press.

Hembree, W. C., Cohen-Kettenis, P., Delemarre-van de Waal, H. A., Gooren, L. J., Meyer, W. J., III, Spack, N. P., . . . Montori, V. M. (2009). Endocrine treatment of transsexual persons: An Endocrine Society clinical practice guideline. *Journal of Clinical and Endocrinological Medicine, 94*, 3132–3154.

Herek, G. M. (1989). Hate crimes against lesbians and gay men. *American Psychologist, 44*(6), 948–955.

Herek, G. M., & Garnets, L. D. (2007). Sexual orientation and mental health. *Annual Reviews of Clinical Psychology, 3*, 353–375.

Hernandez, L., Robson, P., & Sampson, A. (2010). Towards integrated participation: Involving seldom heard users of social care services. *British Journal of Social Work, 40*(3), 714–736.

Hinchliff, S. (2009). Ageing and sexual health in the UK: How should health psychology respond to the challenges? *Journal of Health Psychology, 14*, 355–360.

Hinton, L., Zweifach, M., Oishi, S., Tang, L., & Unützer, J. (2006). Gender disparities in the treatment of late-life depression: Qualitative and quantitative findings from the IMPACT trial. *American Journal of Geriatric Psychiatry, 14*, 884–892.

Holkup, P. A., Salois, E. M., Tripp-Reimer, T., & Weinert, C. (2007). Drawing on wisdom from the past: An elder abuse intervention with tribal communities. *Gerontologist, 47*(2), 248–254.

Holt, M. (2009). "Just take Viagra": Erectile insurance, prophylactic certainty and deficit correction in gay men's accounts of sexuopharmaceutical use. *Sexualities, 12*, 746–764.

Horberg, M. A. (2008). Fenway guide to lesbian, gay, bisexual and transgender health. *Annals of Internal Medicine, 149*, 368.

House, A., Van Horn, E., Coppeans, C., & Stepelman, L. (2011). Interpersonal trauma and discriminatory events as predictors of suicidal and nonsuicidal self-injury in gay, lesbian, bisexual and transgender persons. *Traumatology.* doi:10.1177/1534765610395621.

Hu, M. (2005). *Selling us short: How the Social Security privatization will affect lesbian, gay, bisexual and transgender Americans.* New York: National Gay and Lesbian Task Force Policy Institute.

Huang, F. Y., Chung, H., Kroenke, K., & Spitzer, R. L. (2006). Racial and ethnic differences in the relationship between depression severity and functional status. *Psychiatric Service, 57,* 498–503.

Huang, H.-H., & Coker, A. D. (2010). Examining issues affecting African-American participation in research studies. *Journal of Black Studies, 40,* 619–636.

Hughes, M., & Kentlyn, S. (2011). Older LGBT people's care networks and communities of practice: A brief note. *International Social Work, 54,* 436–444.

Hurley, R. E., Pham, H. H., & Claxton, G. (2005). A widening rift in access and quality: Growing evidence of economic disparities. *Health Affairs.* doi:10.1377/hlthaff .w5.566.

Hutchins, C. K. (2001). Holy ferment: Queer philosophical destabilizations and the discourse on lesbian, gay, bisexual and transgender lives in Christian institutions. *Theology Sexuality, 8,* 9–22.

Hyde, J., Perez, R., & Forester, B. (2007). Dementia and assisted living. *Gerontologist, 47,* 51–67.

Iasenza, S. (2008). Queering the new view. *Feminism Psychology, 18,* 537–548.

Irwin, A., Valentine, N., Brown, C., Loewenson, R., Solar, O., Brown, H., . . . Vega, J. (2006). The Commission on Social Determinants of Health: Tackling the roots of health inequities. *PLoS Medicine, 3*(6), 749–751.

Ivery, J. M. (2008). Balancing priorities in gerontological social work. *Gerontologist, 48,* 844–847.

Jackson, N. C., Johnson, M. J., & Roberts, R. (2008). The potential impact of discrimination fears of older gays, lesbians, bisexuals and transgender individuals living in small-to moderate-sized cities on long-term health care. *Journal of Homosexuality, 54*(3), 325–339.

Jackson, P. B. (2005). Health inequalities among minority populations [Special issue 2]. *Journal of Gerontology, Series B, Psychological Sciences and Social Sciences, 60B,* 63–67.

Jacobs, S.-E., Thomas, W., & Lang, S. (Eds.). (1997). *Two-Spirit people: Native American gender identity, sexuality and spirituality.* Urbana: University of Illinois Press.

Jacobzone, S. (2000). Coping with aging: International challenges. *Health Affairs, 19,* 213–225.

Jatoi, I., Becher, H., & Leake, C. R. (2003). Widening disparity in survival between white and African-American patients with breast carcinoma treated in the U.S. Department of Defense healthcare system. *Cancer, 98*(5), 894–899.

John, R., Kerby, D. S., & Hennessy, C. H. (2003). Patterns and impact of comorbidity and multimorbidity among community-resident American Indians. *Gerontologist, 43,* 649–60.

Johnson, C. J., & McGee, M. (2004). Expressions of manhood: Reconciling sexualities and masculinities of aging. *Gerontologist, 44*(5), 714–722.

Johnson, M. K. (2005). Gay and lesbian perceptions of discrimination in retirement care facilities. *Journal of Homosexuality, 49*(2), 83–102.

Johnson, M. K., Rowatt, W. C., & LaBouff, J. (2010). Priming Christian religious concepts increases racial prejudice. *Social Psychological and Personality Science, 1*, 119–126.

Jones, J. W. (1996). *In the middle of this road we call our life: The courage to search for something more.* San Francisco: HarperSanFrancisco.

Jowett, A., & Peel, E. (2009). Chronic illness in non-heterosexual contexts: An on-line survey of experiences. *Feminism Psychology, 19*, 454–474.

Kahn, J. R., & Fazio, E. M. (2005). Economic status over the life course and racial disparities in health. *Journal of Gerontology, Psychological Sciences and Social Sciences, 60*, S76–S84.

Kahn, J. R., & Pearlin, L. I. (2006). Financial strain over the life course and health among older adults. *Journal of Health and Social Behavior, 47*(1), 17–31.

Kales, H. C., Neighbors, H. W., Blow, F. C., Taylor, K. K. K., Gillon, L., Welsh, D. E., . . . Mellow, A. M. (2005). Race, gender and psychiatrists' diagnosis and treatment of major depression among elderly patients. *Psychiatric Services, 56*, 721–728.

Kaminski, E. (2000). Lesbian health: Social context, sexual identity, and well-being. *Journal of Lesbian Studies, 4*(3), 87–101.

Kausch, O. (2002). Cocaine abuse in the elderly: A series of three case reports. *Journal Nervous and Mental Disease, 190*(8), 562–565.

Kearney, F., Moore, A. R., Donegan, C. F., & Lambert, J. (2010). The aging of HIV: Implications for geriatric medicine. *Age Ageing, 39*, 536–541.

Kehoe, M. (1986). A portrait of an older lesbian. *Journal of Homosexuality, 12*(3–4), 157–161.

Kehoe, M. (1989). *Lesbians over sixty speak for themselves.* Binghamton, NY: Haworth Press.

Kelly, R. J., & Robinson, G. C. (2011). Disclosure of membership in the lesbian, gay, bisexual and transgender community by individuals with communication impairments: A preliminary web-based survey. *American Journal of Speech & Language Pathology, 20*, 86–94.

Kennedy, J., & Erb, C. (2002). Prescription noncompliance due to cost among adults with disabilities in the United States. *American Journal of Public Health, 92*, 1120–1124.

Kerbs, J. J., & Jolley, J. M. (2009). A commentary on age segregation for older prisoners: Philosophical and pragmatic considerations for correctional systems. *Criminal Justice Review, 34*, 119–139.

Kindle, P. A. (2010). *Social work practice with men at risk.* New York: Columbia University Press.

Kite, S. (2006). Palliative care for older people. *Age and Aging, 35*, 459–469.

Kitts, R. L. (2011). Barriers to optimal care between physicians and lesbian, gay, bisexual transgender, and questioning adolescent patients. *Journal of Homosexuality, 57*(6), 730–747.

Kleinschmidt, K. C. (1997). Elder abuse: A review. *Annals of Emergency Medicine*, 30, 463–472.

Knochel, K. A., Quam, J. K., & Croghan, C. F. (2011). Are old lesbian and gay people well served? Understanding the perceptions, preparation and experiences of aging services providers. *Journal of Applied Gerontology*, 30, 370–389.

Knudsen, H. K., Ducharme, L. J., & Roman, P. M. (2007). Racial and ethnic disparities in SSRI availability in substance abuse treatment. *Psychiatric Services*, 58, 55–62.

Kolsky, K. (2008). *End of life: Helping with comfort and care*. Publication No. 08-0636. Bethesda, MD: US Department of Health and Human Services, National Institutes of Health, National Institute on Aging.

Kuh, D. (2007). A life course approach to healthy aging, frailty, and capability. *Journal of Gerontology, Series A, Biological Sciences and Medical Sciences*, 62, 717–721.

Kuhns, L. M., Vazquez, R., & Ramirez-Valles, J. (2008). Researching special populations: Retention of Latino gay and bisexual men and transgender persons in longitudinal health research. *Health Education Research*, 23, 814–825.

Kuschner, W. G. (2011). Racial disparities in end-of-life care. *Archives of Internal Medicine*, 171, 949–950.

Kushel, M. B., Evans, J. L., Perry, S., Robertson, M. J., & Moss, A. R. (2003). No door to lock. Victimization among homeless and marginally housed persons. *Archives of Internal Medicine*, 163, 2492–2499.

Kuyper, L., & Fokkema, T. (2009). Loneliness among older lesbian, gay and bisexual adults in the Netherlands. *Archives of Sexual Behavior*, 38(2), 264–275.

Kuyper, L., & Fokkema, T. (2010). Loneliness among older lesbian, gay and bisexual adults: The role of minority stress. *Archives of Sexual Behavior*, 39(4), 1171–1180.

Lacks, M. S., Williams, C. S., O'Brien, S., Charlson, M. E., & Pillemer, K. A. (2002). Adult protective service use and nursing home placement. *Gerontologist*, 42(6), 734–739.

Lacks, M. S., Williams, C. S., O'Brien, S., Pillemer, K. A., & Charlson, M. E. (1998). The mortality of elder mistreatment. *JAMA*, 280(5), 428–432.

Lamster, I. B. (2004). Oral health care services for older adults: A looming crisis. *American Journal of Public Health*, 94(5), 700–702.

Landers, S., Mimiaga, M. J., & Krinsky, L. (2010). The Open Door Project Task Force: A qualitative study on LGBT aging. *Journal of Gay and Lesbian Social Services*, 22, 316–336.

Lawton, M. P. (1991). Functional status and aging well. *Generations*, 15, 31–35.

Lee, J. A. (1987). What can homosexual aging studies contribute to theories of aging? *Journal of Homosexuality*, 13(4), 43–71.

Leichtentritt, R. D., & Rettig, K. D. (2001). The construction of a good death: A dramaturgy approach. *Journal of Aging Studies*, 15, 85–103.

Leon, D. A., Walt, G., & Gilson, L. (2001). International perspectives on health inequalities and policy. *BMJ*, 322, 591–594.

Letizia, M., & Reinbolz, M. (2005). Identifying and managing acute alcohol withdrawal in the elderly. *Geriatric Nursing, 26*(3), 176–183.

Levin, A. (2009). Legal barriers, bias complicate aging for gays, lesbians. *Psychiatric News, 44,* 24–26.

Levin, J. S. (Ed.). (2001). *Religion in aging and health.* Thousand Oaks, CA: Sage.

Li, R. M., McCardle, P., Clark, R. L., Kinsella, K., & Berch, D. (Eds.). (2001). *Diverse voices. Inclusion of language-minority populations in national studies: Challenges and opportunities.* Bethesda, MD: NIA and NICHD.

Liebig, P. S. (1996). Area agencies on aging and the National Affordable Housing Act: Opportunities and challenges. *Journal of Applied Gerontology, 15*(4), 486–500.

Lindau, S. T., & Gavrilova, N. (2009). Sex, health and years of sexually active life gained due to good health: Evidence from two US population based cross-sectional surveys of ageing. *BMJ, 340,* c810.

Linder, J. F., Enders, S. R., Craig, E., Richardson, J., & Meyers, F. J. (2002). Hospice care for the incarcerated in the United States: An introduction. *Journal of Palliative Medicine, 5,* 4549–4552.

Lipworth, W. L., Hooker, C., & Carter, S. M. (2011). Balance, balancing and health. *Qualitative Health Research, 21,* 714–725.

Litwin, H. (2001). Social network type and morale in old age. *Gerontologist, 41*(4), 516–524.

Litwin, H., & Landow, R. (2000). Social network type and social support among the old-old. *Journal of Aging Studies, 14,* 213–28.

Loeb, S. J., & Steffensmeier, D. (2006). Older male prisoners: Health status, self-efficacy beliefs and health-promoting behaviors. *Journal of Correctional Health Care, 12,* 269–278.

Loewy, M. (2004). Aging in the Americas. *Perspectives in Health—Magazine of the Pan American Health Organization, 9*(1). Retrieved from www.paho.org/English /DD/PIN/Number19_article02.htm

Lothian, K., & Phillip, I. (2001). Care of older people: Maintaining the dignity and autonomy of older people in the healthcare setting. *BMJ, 322,* 668–670.

Lothstein, L. M. (1979). The aging gender dysphoria (transsexual) patient. *Archives of Sexual Behavior, 8*(5), 431–444.

Lunney, J. R., Foley, K. M., Smith, T. J., Gelband, H. (Eds.). (2003). *Describing death in America: What we need to know.* Washington, DC: National Academy Press.

Luo, Y., & Waite, L. J. (2010). Mistreatment and psychological well-being among older adults: Exploring the role of psychological resources and deficits. *Journal of Gerontology, Series B, Psychological Sciences and Social Sciences, 66B*(2), 217–229.

Lyons, A., Pitts, M., Grierson, J., Thorpe, R., & Power, J. (2010). Aging with HIV: Health and psychosocial well-being of older gay men. *AIDS Care, 22*(10), 1236–1244.

Mackie, V. (2001). The trans-sexual citizen: Queering sameness and difference. *Australian Feminist Studies, 16*(35), 185–192.

Magee, J. C., Bigelow, L., DeHaan, S., & Mustanski, B. S. (2011). Sexual health information seeking behavior online: A mixed-methods study among lesbian, gay, bisexual and transgender young people. *Health and Education Behavior*. doi:10.1177 /1090198111401384.

Malebranche, D. J., Peterson, J. L., Fullilove, R. E., & Stackhouse, R. W. (2004). Race and sexual identity: Perceptions about medical culture and healthcare among Black men who have sex with men. *Journal of the National Medical Association*, 96(1), 97–107.

Mangin, D., Sweeney, K., & Heath, I. (2007). Preventative health care in elderly people needs rethinking. *BMJ*, 335(7614), 285–287.

Manton, K. G., Singer, B. H., & Suzman, B. M. (Eds.). (1993). *Forecasting the health of elderly populations*. New York: Springer-Verlag.

Marmot, M. (1999). Epidemiology of socioeconomic status and health: Are determinants within countries the same as between countries? *Annals of the New York Academy of Sciences*, 896, 16–29.

Martin, A. D., & Hetrick, E. S. (1988). The stigmatization of the gay and lesbian adolescent. *Journal of Homosexuality*, 15(1–2), 163–183.

Martin, L. J. (2010). Anticipating infertility: Egg freezing, genetic preservation and risk. *Gender Society*, 24, 526–545.

Masiongale, T. (2009). Ethical service delivery to culturally and linguistically diverse populations: A specific focus on gay, lesbian, bisexual and transgender populations. *Communication Disorders and Sciences in Culturally and Linguistically Diverse Populations*, 16, 20–30.

Mathieson, K. M., Kronenfeld, J. J., & Keith, V. M. (2002). Maintaining functional independence in elderly adults: The roles of health status and financial resources in predicting home modifications and use of mobility equipment. *Gerontologist*, 42(1), 24–31.

May, V. (2011). Self, belonging and social change. *Sociology*, 45, 363–378.

Mays, V. M., Yancey, A. K., Cochran, S. D., Weber, M., & Fielding, J. E. (2002). Heterogeneity of health disparities among African American, Hispanic, and Asian American women: Unrecognized influences of sexual orientation. *American Journal of Public Health*, 92, 632–639.

McAuley, E., & Blissmer, B. (2000). Self-efficacy determinants and consequences of physical activity. *Exercise and Sport Sciences Reviews*, 28(2), 85–88.

McAuley, E., Courneya, K. S., Rudolph, D. L., & Lox, C. L. (1994). Enhancing exercise adherence in middle-aged males and females. *Preventative Medicine*, 23, 498–506.

McAuley, E., Jerome, G. J., Elavsky, S., Marquez, D. X., & Ramsey, S. N. (2003). Predicting long-term maintenance of physical activity in older adults. *Preventative Medicine*, 37, 110–118.

McDaniel, S. A. (2008). Families caring across borders: Migration, ageing and transnational caregiving. *Contemporary Sociology: A Journal of Reviews*, 37, 32–33.

McIntyre, L., Szewchuk, A., & Munro, J. (2010). Inclusion and exclusion in mid-life lesbians' experiences of the Pap test. *Culture, Health and Sexuality*, 1.

McLean, A. J., & Le Couteur, D. G. (2004). Aging biology and geriatric clinical pharmacology. *Pharmacological Reviews*, 56, 163–184.

McMahon, E. (2003). The older homosexual: Current concepts of lesbian, gay, bisexual and transgender older Americans. *Clinical Geriatric* Medicine, 19(3), 587–593.

Meckler, G. D., Elliot, M. N., Kanouse, D. E., Beals, K. P., & Schuster, M. A. (2006). Nondisclosure of sexual orientation to a physician among a sample of gay, lesbian and bisexual youth. *Archives of Pediatric Medicine, 160,* 1248–1254.

Menec, V. H. (2003). The relation between everyday activities and successful aging: A 6-year longitudinal study. *Journal of Gerontology, Series B, Psychological Sciences and Social Sciences, 58B*(2), S74–S82.

Meyer, I. H. (2001). Why gay, lesbian, bisexual and transgender public health? *American Journal of Public Health,* 91(6), 856–559.

Meyer, I. H., & Northridge, M. E. (Eds.). (2007). *The health of sexual minorities: Public health perspectives on lesbian, gay, bisexual and transgender populations.* New York: Springer.

Mezuk, B., Rafferty, J. A., Kershaw, K. N., Hudson, D., Abdou, C. M., Lee, H., . . . Jackson, J. S. (2010). Reconsidering the role of social disadvantage in physical and mental health: Stressful life events, health behaviors, race, and depression. *American Journal of Epidemiology, 172,* 1238–1249.

Miksad, R. A., Bubley, G., Church, P., Sanda, M., Rofsky, N., Kaplan, I., & Cooper, A. (2006). Prostate cancer in a transgender woman 41 years after initiation of feminization. *JAMA, 296L,* 2316–2317.

Millet, X., Raoux, N., Le Carret, N., Bouisson, J., Dartigues, J.-F., & Amieva, H. (2009). Gender-related differences in visuospatial memory persist in Alzheimer's disease. *Archives of Clinical Neuropsychology, 24,* 783–789.

Miner-Rubino, K., Winter, D. G., & Stewart, A. J. (2004). Gender, social class and the subjective experience of aging: Self-perceived personality change from early adulthood to late midlife. *Personality and Social Psychology Bulletin, 30,* 1599–1610.

Miville, M. I.., Duan, C., Nutt, R. L., Waehler, C. A., Suzuki, L., Pistole, M. C., . . . Corpus, M. (2009). Integrating practice guidelines into professional training: Implications for diversity competence. *Counseling Psychologist, 37,* 519–563.

Moody, H. (1988). Generational equity and social insurance. *Journal of Medical Philosophy,* 13(1), 31–56.

Moore, S. E. H. (2010). Is the healthy body gendered? Toward a feminist critique of the new paradigm of health. *Body Society, 16,* 95–118.

Morrow, D. F., & Messinger, L. (2006). *Sexual orientation and gender expression in social work practice: Working with LGBT people.* New York: Columbia University Press.

Moskowitz, D. A., & Roloff, M. E. (2010). Moderators of sexual behavior in gay men. *Archives of Sexual Behavior, 39*(4), 950–958.

Mueller, A., & Gooren, L. (2008). Hormone-related tumors in transsexuals receiving treatment with cross-sex hormones. *European Journal of Endocrinology, 159,* 197–202.

Mueller, A., Gooren, L. J., Naton-Schötz, S., Cupisti, S., Beckmann, M. W., & Dittrich, R. (2008). Prevalence of polycystic ovary syndrome and hyperandrogenemia in female-to-male transsexuals. *Journal of Clinical Endocrinology & Metabolism*, 93, 1408–1411.

Munford, R., Oka, T., & Desai, M. (2009). Qualitative social work research in the Asia-Pacific region. *Qualitative Social Work*, 8, 419–426.

Mustanski, B. S., Garofalo, R., & Emerson, E. M. (2010). Mental health disorders, psychological distress, and suicidality in a diverse sample of lesbian, gay, bisexual and transgender youths. *American Journal of Public Health*, 100, 2426–2432.

Nadien, M. B. (2006). Factors that influence abusive interactions between aging women and their caregivers. *Annals of the New York Academy of Sciences*, 1087, 158–169.

National Center on Elder Abuse. (2005). *Fact sheet on elder abuse prevalence and incidence*. Washington, DC: Author.

National Gay and Lesbian Task Force (NGLTF). (2005). *Make room for all: Diversity, cultural competency and discrimination in an aging America*. Retrieved from www .thetaskforce.org/reslibrary/list.cfm?pubTypeID=2#pub304

National Institute on Aging (NIA). (2007a). *Why population aging matters: A global perspective*. (NIA/NIH Publication No. 07-6134). Bethesda, MD: Author

National Institute on Aging (NIA). (2007b). *Review of minority aging research at the NIA*. Retrieved from www.nia.nih.gov/AboutNIA/MinorityAgingResearch.htm

National Research Council. (2004). *Eliminating health disparities: Measurement and data needs*. Washington, DC: National Academies Press.

Newman, C., Kippax, S., Mao, L., Saltman, D., & Kidd, M. (2008). GP's understanding of how depression affects gay and HIV positive men. *Australian Family Physician*, 37(8), 678–680.

Nichols, S. (2010). The body in bioethics. *Medical Law Review*, 18, 120–125.

Norton, C. K., Hobson, G., & Kulm, E. (2011). Palliative and end of life care in the emergency department: Guidelines for nurses. *Journal of Emergency Nursing*, 37(3), 240–245.

O'Connell, J. J. (2004). Dying in the shadows: The challenge of providing healthcare for homeless people. *Canadian Medical Association Journal*, 170, 1251–1252.

Odubanjo, E., Bennett, K., & Feely, J. (2004). Influence of socioeconomic status on the quality of prescribing in the elderly: A population based study. *British Journal of Clinical Pharmacology*, 58(5), 496–502.

Oggins, J., & Eichenbaum, J. (2002). Engaging transgender substance users in substance use treatment. *International Journal of Transgenderism*, 6(2). Retrieved from www.symposion.com/ijt/ijtvoo6noo2_03.htm

Orel, N., Stelle, C., Watson, W. K., & Bunner, B. L. (2010). No one is immune: A community education partnership addressing HIV/AIDS and older adults. *Journal of Applied Gerontology*, 29, 352–370.

Osterwell, A. (2010). A body is not a metaphor: Barbara Hammer's x-ray vision. *Journal of Lesbian Studies*, 14(2), 185–200.

Otis, M. D. (2007). Perceptions of victimization risk and fear of crime among lesbians and gay men. *Journal of Interpersonal Violence*, 22, 198–217.

Ott, B. R., Lapane, K. L., & Gambassi, G. (2000). Gender differences in the treatment of behavior problems in Alzheimer's disease. *Neurology*, 54, 427.

Ozdemir, V., Fourie, J., Busto, U., & Naranjo, C. A. (1996). Pharmacokinetic changes in the elderly: Do they contribute to drug abuse and dependence. *Clinical Pharmacokinetics*, 31(5), 372–385.

Pampel, F. C., Krueger, P. M., & Denney, J. T. (2010). Socioeconomic disparities in health behaviors. *Annual Reviews of Sociology*, 36, 349–370.

Parry, D. C., & Glover, T. D. (2011). Living with cancer? Come as you are. *Qualitative Inquiry*, 17, 395–403.

Patton, C. (2006). *Anti-lesbian, gay, bisexual and transgender violence in 2005: A report of the National Coalition of Anti-Violence Programs.* Retrieved from www.ncavp.org

Pattussi, M. P., Hardy, R., & Sheiham, A. (2006). Neighborhood social capital and dental injuries in Brazilian adolescents. *American Journal of Public Health*, 96(8), 1462–1468.

Paul, J. P., Catania, J., Pollack, L., Moskowitz, J., Canchola, J., Mills, T., . . . Stall, R. (2002). Suicide attempts among gay and bisexual men: Lifetime prevalence and antecedents. *American Journal of Public Health*, 92, 1338–1345.

Penny, L. (2005). Functioning and health service use among elderly nursing home residents with alcohol use disorders: Findings from the National Nursing Home Survey. *American Journal of Geriatric Psychiatry*, 13(6), 475–483.

Persson, D. I. (2009). Unique challenges of transgender aging: Implications from the literature. *Journal of Gerontological Social Work*, 52(6), 633–646.

Pesquera, A. (1999, September 3). Court to decide what's changed in sex operations. *San Antonio Express News*.

Petersen, P. E., & Yamamoto, T. (2005). Improving the oral health of older people: The approach of the WHO Global Oral Health Programme. *Community Dentistry and Oral Epidemiology*, 33, 81–92.

Phillips, L. L., Allen, R. S., Harris, G. M., Presnell, A. H., DeCoster, J., & Cavanaugh, R. (2011). Aging prisoner treatment selection: Does prospect theory enhance understanding of end-of-life medical decisions? *Gerontologist*. doi:10.1093/geront/gnr039.

Phillips, L. R., & Guo, G. (2011). Mistreatment in assisted living facilities: Complaints, substantiations and risk factors. *Gerontologist*, 51(3), 343–353.

Phillips-Angeles, E., Wolfe, P., Meyers, R., Dawson, P., Marrazzo, J., Soltner, S., & Dzieweczynski, M. (2004). Lesbian health matters: A Pap test education campaign nearly thwarted by discrimination. *Health Promotion Practice*, 5, 314–325.

Pinquart, M., & Sorenson, S. (2000). Influences of socio-economic status, social network, and competence on subjective well-being in later life: A meta-analysis. *Psychology and Aging*, 14(2), 187–224.

Pinquart, M., & Sorenson, S. (2006). Gender differences in caregiver stressors, social resources, and health: An updated meta-analysis. *Journal of Gerontology, Series B, Psychological Sciences and Social Sciences*, 61B(1), P33–P45.

Pisani, E., Girault, P., Gultom, M., Sukartini, N., Kumalawati, J., Jazan, S., & Donegan, E. (2004). HIV, syphillus infection, and sexual practices among transgenders, male sex workers, and other men who have sex with men in Jakarta, Indonesia. *Sexually Transmitted Infections*, 80, 536–540.

Pittman, P. M. (1999). Gendered experiences of health care. *International Journal of Qualitative Health Care*, 11(5), 397–405.

Pitts, M. K., Couch, M., Mulcare, H., Croy, S., & Mitchell, A. (2009). Transgender people in Australia and New Zealand: Health, well-being and access to health services. *Feminism & Psychology, 19*, 475–496.

Pitzer, L. M., & Fingerman, K. L. (2010). Psychosocial resources and associations between childhood physical abuse and adult well-being. *Journal of Gerontology, Series B, Psychological Sciences and Social Sciences, 65B*, 425–433.

Porter, K., Oala, C. R., & Witten, T. M. (2011). *Spirituality and aging in the transsexual and transgendered community.* Manuscript in preparation.

Post, L., Page, C., Conner, T., Prokhorov, A., Fang, Y., & Biroscak, B. J. (2010). Elder abuse in longterm-care: Types, patterns and risk factors. *Research on Aging, 32*, 323–348.

Poteat, V. P., & Espelage, D. L. (2007). Predicting psychosocial consequences of homophobic victimization in middle school students. *Journal of Early Adolescence, 27*, 175–191.

Prather, J. E. (2008). Brave new stepfamilies: Diverse paths toward stepfamily living. *Contemporary Sociology: A Journal of Reviews, 37*, 33–34.

Price, E. (2008). Pride or prejudice? Gay men, lesbians and dementia. *British Journal of Social Work, 38*, 1337–1352.

Pringle, K. E., Ahern, F. M., Heller, D. A., Gold, C. H., & Brown, T. V. (2005). Potential for alcohol and prescription drug interactions in older people. *Journal of the American Geriatrics Society, 53*(11), 1930–1936.

Quam, J. K., & Whitford, G. S. (1992). Adaptation and age-related expectations of older gay and lesbian adults. *Gerontologist, 32*, 367–374.

Read, J. G., & Gorman, B. K. (2010). Gender and health equality. *Annual Reviews of Sociology, 36*, 371–386.

Rejeski, W. J., & Mihalko, S. L. (2001). Physical activity and quality of life in older adults. *Journal of Gerontology, Series A, Biological Sciences and Medical Sciences, 56A*(Suppl 2), 23–35.

Reker, G. T., & Chamberlain, K. (Eds.). (2000). *Exploring existential meaning: Optimizing human development across the lifespan.* Thousand Oaks, CA: Sage.

Rhoades, D. A. (2005). Racial misclassification and disparities in cardiovascular disease among American Indians and Alaska Natives. *Circulation, 111*, 1250–1256.

Riorden, D. C. (2004). Interaction strategies of lesbian, gay, and bisexual healthcare practitioners in the clinical examination of patients: Qualitative study. *BMJ, 328.* doi:10.1136/bmj.38071.774525.EB.

Ritchie, C. S., & Wieland, G. D. (2007). Improving end-of-life care for older adults: An international challenge [Editorial]. *Journal of Gerontology, Series A, Biological Sciences and Medical Sciences, 62A*(4), 393–394.

Robertson, M. J., Clark, R. A., Charlebois, E. D., Tulsky, J., Long, H. L., Bangsberg, D. R., & Moss, A. R. (2004). HIV seroprevalence among homeless and marginally housed adults in San Francisco. *American Journal of Public Health, 94*, 1207–1217.

Robinson, K. (2000). *Older Americans 2000: Key indicators of well-being.* Hyattsville, MD: Federal Interagency Forum on Aging-Related Statistics. Retrieved from www.agingstats.gov

Rodriguez, M. A., Ward, L. M., & Perez-Stable, E. J. (2005). Breast and cervical cancer screening: Impact of health insurance status, ethnicity and nativity of Latinas. *Annals of Family Medicine, 3*, 235–241.

Rondahl, G., Innala, S., & Carlsson, M. (2006). Heterosexual assumptions in verbal and non-verbal communication in nursing. *Journal of Advanced Nursing, 56*(4), 373–381.

Rose, S. M., & Mechanic, M. B. (2002). Psychological distress, crime features, and help-seeking behaviors related to homophobic bias incidents. *American Behavioral Scientist, 46*(1), 14–26.

Rosenfeld, D. (2009). Heteronormativity and homonormativity as practical and moral resources: The case of lesbian and gay elders. *Gender Society, 23*, 617–638.

Rowe, J. R., & Kahn, R. L. (1997). Successful aging. *Gerontologist, 37*(4), 433–440.

Rowe, J. R., & Kahn, R. L. (1998). *Successful aging.* New York: Pantheon Books.

Russell, A. (2009). Lesbians surviving culture: Relational-culture theory applied to lesbian connection. *Affilia, 24*, 406–416.

Ryan, C., Huebner, D., Diaz, R. M., & Sanchez, J. (2009). Family rejection as a predictor of negative health outcomes in White and Latino lesbian, gay and bisexual young adults. *Pediatrics, 123*, 346–352.

Ryan, C., Russell, S. T., Huebner, D., Diaz, R., & Sanchez, J. (2010). Family acceptance in adolescence and the health of LGBT young adults. *Journal of Child & Adolescent Psychiatric Nursing, 23*(4), 205–213.

Saewyc, E. M., Skay, C. L., Pettingell, S. L., Reis, E. A., Bearinger, L., Resnick, M., . . . Combs, L. (2006). Hazards of stigma: The sexual and physical abuse of gay, lesbian and bisexual adolescents in the United States and Canada. *Child Welfare, 85*(2), 195–213.

Salari, S. (2002). Invisible in aging research: Arab Americans, Middle Eastern immigrants, and Muslims in the United States. *Gerontologist, 42*, 580.

Sanchez, D. T., Crocker, J., & Boike, K. R. (2005). Doing gender in the bedroom: Investing gender norms and the sexual experience. *Personality & Social Psychology Bulletin, 31*, 1445–1455.

Sarkisian, C. A., Hays, R. D., & Magione, C. M. (2002). Do older adults expect to age successfully? The association between expectations regarding aging and beliefs regarding healthcare seeking among older adults. *Journal of the American Geriatrics Society, 50*(11), 1837–1843.

Satariano, W. A., & McAuley, E. (2003). Promoting physical activity among older adults: From ecology to individual. *American Journal of Preventive Medicine, 25*(Suppl 2), 184–192.

Schaie, K. W., & Carstensen, L. L. (2006). *Social structures, aging, and self-regulation in the elderly.* New York: Springer.

Schechtman, K. B., & Ory, M. G. (2001). The effects of exercise on the quality of life of frail older adults: A preplanned meta-analysis of the FICSIT trials. *Annals of Behavioral Medicine, 23*(3), 186–197.

Schlit, K. (2006). Just one of the guys? How transmen make gender visible at work. *Gender and Society, 20,* 465–490.

Schoeni, R. F., Martin, L. G., Andreski, P. M., & Freedman, V. A. (2005). Persistent and growing socioeconomic disparities in disability among the elderly, 1982–2002. *American Journal of Public Health, 95,* 2065–2070.

Schulz, R., & Heckhausen, J. (1996). A lifespan model of successful aging. *American Psychologist, 51*(7), 702–714.

Scott, S. (2010). How to look good (nearly) naked: The performative regulation of the swimmer's body. *Body & Society, 16,* 143–168.

Scout, J. B., & Fields, C. (2001). Removing the barriers: Improving practitioners' skills in providing health care to lesbians and women who partner with women. *American Journal of Public Health, 91,* 892–894.

Servaty-Seib, H. L., & Taub, D. J. (2010). Bereavement and college students: The role of counseling psychology. *Counseling Psychologist, 38,* 947–975.

Shankle, M. D. (Ed.). (2006). *The handbook of lesbian, gay, bisexual, and transgender public health: A practitioner's guide to service.* New York: Harrington Park Press.

Shapiro, A. (2010). The modern family and aging: New insights and directions. *Gerontologist, 50,* 714–716.

Sherr, L., Harding, R., Lampe, F., Johnson, M., Anderson, J., Zetler, S., . . . Edwards, S. (2009). Clinical and behavioral aspects of aging with HIV infection. *Psychology Health Medicine, 14*(3), 273–279.

Shippy, R. A., & Karpiak, S. E. (2005). The aging HIV/AIDS population: Fragile social networks. *Aging and Mental Health, 9*(3), 246–254.

Shuey, K. M., & Willson, A. E. (2008). Cumulative disadvantage and Black-White disparities in life-course health trajectories. *Research on Aging, 30,* 200–225.

Singh, G. K., & Siahpush, M. (2006). Widening socioeconomic inequalities in US life expectancy, 1980–2000. *International Journal of Epidemiology, 35,* 969–979.

Sleven, K. F., & Linneman, T. J. (2009). Old gay men's bodies and masculinities. *Men & Masculinities.* doi:10.1177/1097184X08325225.

Smedley, B. D., Stith, A. Y., & Nelson, A. R. (Eds.). (2003). *Unequal treatment: Confronting racial and ethnic disparities in healthcare.* Washington, DC: National Academies Press.

Smith, M. D. (2002). Culture and quality: Joining the levers. In *Advancing effective health care through systems development, data, and measurement.* Paper presented at the Third National Conference on Quality Health Care for Culturally Diverse Populations, October 2, Chicago. Retrieved from www.diversityrx.org/CCCONF /02/CultureandQuality

Smyer, T., & Clark, M. C. (2011). A cultural paradox: Elder abuse in the Native American community. *Home Health Care Management Practice, 23,* 201–206.

Sobsey, D. (1994). *Violence and abuse in the lives of people with disabilities: The end of silent acceptance?* Baltimore: Paul H. Brookes.

Solimeo, S. (2008). Sex and gender in older adult's experience of Parkinson's disease. *Journal of Gerontology, Series B, Psychological Sciences and Social Sciences, 63B,* S42–S48.

Soumerai, S. B., Pierre-Jacques, M., Shang, F., Ross-Degnan, D., Adams, A. S., Gurwitz, J., . . . Safran, D. G. (2006). Cost-related medication nonadherence among elderly and disabled Medicare beneficiaries: A national survey 1 year before the Medicare drug benefit. *Archives of Internal Medicine, 166,* 1829–1835.

States, R. A., Susman, W. M., Riquelme, L. F., Godwin, E. M., & Greer, E. (2006). Community health education: Reaching ethnically diverse elders. *Journal of Allied Health,* 35(4), 215–222.

Steckley, R. G. (2009). Gay, lesbian, bisexual and transgender people: An introduction and discussion of terminology and demographics. *Communication Disorders and Sciences in Culturally and Linguistically Diverse Populations, 16,* 4–10.

Steele, L. S., Tinmouth, J. M., & Lu, A. (2006). Regular health care use by lesbians: A path analysis of predictive factors. *Family Practice, 23,* 631–636.

Steinberg, A., Brooks, J., & Remtulla, T. (2003). Youth hate crimes: Identification, prevention, and intervention. *American Journal of Psychiatry, 160,* 979–989.

Stevens, P., Carlson, L. M., & Hinman, J. M. (2004). An analysis of tobacco industry marketing to lesbian, gay, bisexual and transgender (GLBT) populations: Strategies for mainstream tobacco control and prevention. *Health Promotion and Practice, 5,* 129S–134S.

Strawbridge, W. J., Cohen, R. D., Shema, S. J., & Kaplan, G. A. (1996). Successful aging: Predictors and associated activities. *American Journal of Epidemiology,* 144(2), 135–141.

Substance Abuse and Mental Health Services Administration (SAMSA). (2003). *A provider's introduction to substance abuse treatment for lesbian, gay, bisexual, and transgender individuals.* Center for Substance Abuse Treatments, DHHS Publication No. [SMA] 03-3819. NCADI Publication No. BKD392. Rockville, MD: U.S. Government Printing Office.

Sussman, S. (1997). Marijuana use in the elderly. *Clinical Geriatrics, 5,* 109–119.

Suto, I., & Arnaut, G. L. Y. (2010). Suicide in prison: A qualitative study. *Prison Journal, 90,* 288–312.

Svartberg, J., Brækkan, S. K., Laughlin, G. A., & Hanson, J.-B. (2009). Endogenous sex hormone levels in men are not associated with risk of venous thromboembolism: The Tromsø Study. *European Journal of Endocrinology, 160,* 833–838.

Teaster, P. B., & Roberto, K. A. (2004). Sexual abuse of older adults: APS cases and outcomes. *Gerontologist,* 44(6), 788–796.

Ten Kulve, J. S., de Jong, F. H., & de Ronde, W. (2010). The effect of circulating estradiol concentrations on gonadotropin secretion in young and old castrated male-to-female transsexuals. *Aging Male,* 14(3), 155–161.

Timiras, P. S., Quay, W. B., & Vernadakis, A. (Eds.). (1995). *Hormones and aging.* Boca Raton, FL: CRC Press.

Tornstam, L. (2005). *Gerotranscendence: A developmental theory of positive aging.* New York: Springer.

TranScience Longitudinal Aging Research Study (TLARS). (2007). Retrieved from www.people.vcu.edu/~tmwitten

TranScience Research Institute. (2006). Retrieved from www.transcience.org

Trivedi, A. N., Zaslavsky, A. M., Schneider, E. C., & Ayanian, J. Z. (2005). Trends in the quality of care and racial disparities in Medicare managed care. *New England Journal of Medicine, 353*, 692–700.

Tsoi, W. F. (1992). Male and female transsexuals: A comparison. *Singapore Medical Journal, 33*(2), 182–185.

Turra, C. M., & Goldman, N. (2007). Socioeconomic differences in mortality among U.S. adults: Insights into the Hispanic paradox. *Journal of Gerontology, Series B, Psychological Sciences and Social Sciences, 62B*(3), S184–S192.

Turrell, G., Lynch, J. W., Kaplan, G. A., Everson, S. A., Helkala, E.-L., Kauhanen, J., & Salonen, J. T. (2002). Socioeconomic position across the lifecourse and cognitive function in late middle age. *Journal of Gerontology, Series B, Psychological Sciences and Social Sciences, 57*, 43.

Turrell, S. C. (2000). A descriptive analysis of same-sex relationship violence for a diverse sample. *Journal of Family Violence, 15*(3), 281–93.

Umberson, D., Brosnoe, R., & Reczek, C. (2010). Social relationships and health behavior across the life course. *Annual Reviews of Sociology, 36*, 139–157.

U.S. Department of Health and Human Services (USDHHS). (2000). *Healthy people 2010* (2nd ed.). *With understanding and improving health and objectives for improving health.* 2 vols. Washington, DC: U.S. Government Printing Office, Healthy People 2010 Online Documents. Retrieved from www.healthypeople.gov/document

U.S. House of Representatives, Select Committee on Aging, Subcommittee on Health and Long-term Care. (1990). *Elder abuse: A decade of shame and inaction.* Washington, DC: U.S. Government Printing Office.

Velkoff, V. A., & Kinsella, K. (1998). Gender stereotypes: Data needs for ageing research. *Aging International, 24*(4), 18–38.

Vellas, B. J., Albarede, J. L., & Garry, P. J. (1992). Diseases and aging. Patterns of morbidity with age: Relationship between aging and age-associated diseases. *American Journal of Clinical Nutrition, 55*, 1225S–1230S.

Victoria, C. G. (2006). The challenge of reducing health inequalities. *American Journal of Public Health, 96*(1), 10–11.

Von Faber, M., Bootsma-van der Weil, A., van Exell, E., Gussekloo, J., Lagaay, A. M., van Dongen, E., . . . Westendorp, R. G. J. (2001). Successful aging in the oldest old. Who can be characterized as successfully aged? *Archives of Internal Medicine, 161*, 2695–2700.

Walker, A. (2002). Ageing in Europe: Policies in harmony or discord? *International Journal of Epidemiology, 31*, 758–761.

Wallace, P. M. (2010). Finding self: A qualitative study of transgender, transitioning and adulterated silicone. *Health Education Journal, 69*, 439–446.

Walsh, C. A., Ploeg, J., Lohfeld, L., Horne, J., MacMillan, H., & Lai, D. (2007). Violence across the lifespan: Interconnections among forms of abuse as described by marginalized Canadian elders and their care-givers. *British Journal of Social Work, 37*, 491–514.

Wang, J., Noel, J. M., Zuckerman, I. H., Miller, N. A., Shaya, F. T., & Mullins, C. D. (2006). Disparities in access to essential new prescription drugs between non-Hispanic whites, non-Hispanic blacks, and Hispanic whites. *Medical Care Research and Review, 63,* 742–763.

Ward, R., Vass, A. A., Aggarwal, N., Garfield, C., & Cybyk, B. (2005). A kiss is still a kiss? The construction of sexuality in dementia care. *Dementia, 4,* 49–72.

Wassersug, R., Gray, R. E., Barbara, A., Trosztmer, C., Raj, R., & Sinding, C. (2007). Experiences of transwomen with hormone therapy. *Sexualities, 10,* 101–122.

Watt, G. (2001). Policies to tackle social exclusion. *BMJ, 323,* 175–176.

Waxman, B. F. (1991). Hatred: The unacknowledged dimension in violence against disabled people. *Sexuality and Disability, 9*(3), 185–199.

Waysdorf, S. L. (2002). The aging of the AIDS epidemic: Emerging legal and public health issues for elderly persons living with HIV/AIDS. *Elder Law Journal, 10*(1), 47–89.

Webster, J. D., Bohlmeijer, E. T., & Westerhof, G. J. (2010). Mapping the future of reminiscence: A conceptual guide for research and practice. *Research on Aging, 32,* 527–564.

Wei, W., Akincigil, A., Crystal, S., & Sambamoorthi, U. (2006). Gender differences in out-of-pocket prescription drug expenditures among the elderly. *Research on Aging, 28,* 427–453.

Weinick, R. M. (2003). Researching disparities: Strategies for primary data collection. *Academic Emergency Medicine, 10,* 1161–1168.

Wells, K., Klap, R., Koike, A., & Sherbourne, C. (2001). Ethnic disparities in unmet need for alcoholism, drug abuse, and mental health care. *American Journal of Psychiatry, 158,* 2027–2032.

Wen, X. (2004). Trends in the prevalence of disability and chronic conditions among the older population: Implications for survey design and measurement of disability. *Australasian Journal of Ageing, 23*(1), 3–6.

Whipple, V. (2006). *Lesbian widows: Invisible grief.* Binghamton, NY: Harrington Park Press.

Wiking, E., Johansson, S.-E., & Sundquist, J. (2003). Ethnicity, acculturation, and self-reported health: A population based study among immigrants from Poland, Turkey, and Iran in Sweden. *Journal of Epidemiology & Community Health, 58,* 574–582.

Willging, C. E., Salvador, M., & Kano, M. (2006a). Pragmatic help-seeking: How sexual and gender minority groups access mental health care in a rural state. *Psychiatric Services, 57,* 871–874.

Willging, C. E., Salvador, M., & Kano, M. (2006b). Unequal treatment: Mental health care for sexual and gender minority groups in a rural state. *Psychiatric Services, 57,* 867–870.

Williams, D. (2005). The health of U.S. racial and ethnic populations [Special issue 2]. *Journal of Gerontology, Series B, Psychological Sciences and Social Sciences, 60B,* 53–62.

Witten, T. M. (2002). *The Tao of gender.* Atlanta, GA: Humanics Press.

Witten, T. M. (2006). End of life concerns for transgender elders and their caregivers: Graceful exits. *Outward*.

Witten, T. M. (2010). Graceful exits: III. Intersections of aging, transgender identities and the family/community. In C. A. Fruhauf & D. Mahoney (Eds.), *Older GLBT family and community life*. London: Routledge.

Witten, T. M., & Eyler, A. E. (1997). *HIV, AIDS and the elderly transgendered/transsexual: Risk and invisibility*. Presented at the Gerontological Society of America, Cincinnati, Ohio.

Wolf, D. A., Hunt, K., & Knickman, J. (2005). Perspectives on the recent decline in disability at older ages. *Milbank Quarterly, 83*, 365–395.

Wolinsky, F. D., Coe, R. M., Miller, D. K., & Prendergast, J. M. (1985). Correlates of change in subjective well-being among the elderly. *Journal of Community Health, 10*, 93–107.

Wong, M. D., Shapiro, M. F., Boscardin, W. J., & Ettner, S. L. (2002). Contribution of major diseases to disparities in mortality. *New England Journal of Medicine, 347*, 1585–1592.

World Health Organization. (2000). *Health systems: Improving performance*. Geneva, Switzerland: World Health Organization.

Wright, N. M. J., Tompkins, C. N. E., Oldham, N. S., & Kay, D. J. (2004). Homelessness and health: What can be done in general practice? *Journal of the Royal Society of Medicine, 97*, 170–173.

Wrubel, J., Stumbo, S., & Johnson, M. O. (2010). Male same-sex couple dynamics and received social support for HIV medication adherence. *Journal of Social and Personal Relationships, 27*, 553–572.

Wykle, M. L., Whitehouse, P. J., & Morris, D. L. (Eds.). (2005). *Successful aging through the lifespan: Intergenerational issues in health*. New York: Springer.

Xu, K. T. (2003). Financial disparities in prescription drug use between elderly and nonelderly Americans. *Health Affairs, 22*, 210–221.

Yeo, G., & Gallagher-Thompson, D. (2006). *Ethnicity and the dementias*. New York: Routledge.

Yoakam, J. R. (2005). Three videos on gay and lesbian elders. *Gerontologist, 45*(2), 284–286.

Zablotska, I., Frankland, A., Crim, M., Imrie, J., Adam, P., Westacott, R., . . . Prestage, G. (2009). Current issues in care and support for HIV-positive gay men in Sydney. *International Journal of STD AIDS, 20*, 628–633.

Zack, M. M., Moriarty, D. G., Stroup, D. F., Ford, E. S., & Mokdad, A. H. (2004). Worsening trends in adult health-rated quality of life and self-rated health, United States, 1993–2001. *Public Health Reports, 119*(5), 493–505.

Zarit, S. H., & Pearlin, L. I. (Eds.). (2005). Health inequities across the life course [Special issue 2]. *Journal of Gerontology, Series B, Psychological Sciences and Social Sciences, 60B*, 5–139.

Index